Shoulder Instability

Guest Editor

WILLIAM N. LEVINE, MD

ORTHOPEDIC CLINICS OF NORTH AMERICA

www.orthopedic.theclinics.com

July 2010 • Volume 41 • Number 3

SAUNDERS an imprint of ELSEVIER, Inc.

W.B. SAUNDERS COMPANY
A Division of Elsevier Inc.

1600 John F. Kennedy Blvd. • Suite 1800 • Philadelphia, PA 19103-2899.

http://www.orthopedic.theclinics.com

ORTHOPEDIC CLINICS OF NORTH AMERICA Volume 41, Number 3
July 2010 ISSN 0030-5898, ISBN-13: 978-1-4377-2474-5

Editor: Debora Dellapena

Orthopedic Clinics of North America (ISSN 0030-5898) is published quarterly by Elsevier Inc., 360 Park Avenue South, New York, NY 10010-1710. Months of issue are January, April, July, and October. Business and Editorial Offices: 1600 John F. Kennedy Blvd., Suite 1800, Philadelphia, PA 19103-2899. Customer Service Office: 3251 Riverport Lane, Maryland Heights, MO 63043. Periodicals postage paid at New York, NY and additional mailing offices. Subscription prices are $251.00 per year for (US individuals), $458.00 per year for (US institutions), $297.00 per year (Canadian individuals), $549.00 per year (Canadian institutions), $366.00 per year (international individuals), $549.00 per year (international institutions), $126.00 per year (US students), $182.00 per year (Canadian and international students). Foreign air speed delivery is included in all *Clinics* subscription prices. All prices are subject to change without notice. **POSTMASTER:** Send change of address to *Orthopedic Clinics of North America*, **Elsevier Health Sciences Division, Subscription Customer Service, 3251 Riverport Lane, Maryland Heights, MO 63043. Customer Service (orders, claims, online, change of address): Elsevier Health Sciences Division, Subscription Customer Service, 3251 Riverport Lane, Maryland Heights, MO 63043. Tel: 1-800-654-2452 (U.S. and Canada); 314-447-8871 (outside U.S. and Canada). Fax: 314-447-8029. E-mail: journalscustomerservice-usa@elsevier. com (for print support); journalsonlinesupport-usa@elsevier.com (for online support).**

Reprints. For copies of 100 or more, of articles in this publication, please contact the Commercial Reprints Department, Elsevier Inc., 360 Park Avenue South, New York, NY 10010-1710. Tel.: 212-633-3812; Fax: 212-462-1935; E-mail: reprints@elsevier. com.

Orthopedic Clinics of North America is covered in *MEDLINE/PubMed (Index Medicus), Cinahl, Excerpta Medica, and Cumulative Index to Nursing and Allied Health Literature.*

Printed and bound in the United Kingdom
Transferred to Digital Print 2011

Contributors

GUEST EDITOR

WILLIAM N. LEVINE, MD
Vice Chairman and Professor, Department of
Orthopaedic Surgery, Columbia University
Medical Center, New York, New York

AUTHORS

CHRISTOPHER S. AHMAD, MD
Associate Professor, Department of
Orthopaedic Surgery, Center for Shoulder,
Elbow, and Sports Medicine, Columbia-
Presbyterian Hospital, Columbia University,
New York, New York

ROBERT A. ARCIERO, MD
Professor, Orthopaedic Surgery; Director,
Sports Medicine Fellowship, Department of
Orthopaedic Surgery, University of
Connecticut Health Center, Farmington,
Connecticut

MARSHAL S. ARMITAGE, MD, FRCSC
Fellow, Department of Orthopedic Surgery,
St Joseph's Health Care, The Hand and
Upper Limb Centre, University of Western
Ontario, London, Ontario, Canada

GEORGE S. ATHWAL, MD, FRCSC
Assistant Professor, Department of
Orthopedic Surgery, St Joseph's Health Care,
The Hand and Upper Limb Centre, University
of Western Ontario, London, Ontario, Canada

JOHN-ERIK BELL, MD
Assistant Professor of Orthopaedic Surgery,
Shoulder, Elbow, and Sports Medicine,
Dartmouth-Hitchcock Medical Center,
Lebanon, New Hampshire

LOUIS U. BIGLIANI, MD
Director, Chief, Center for Shoulder, Elbow and
Sports Medicine; Frank E. Stinchfield Professor
and Chairman, Department of Orthopaedic
Surgery, Columbia University Medical Center,
New York, New York

PASCAL BOILEAU, MD
Professor and Chairman, Department of
Orthopaedic Surgery and Sports
Traumatology, Hôpital de L'Archet 2, University
of Nice-Sophia-Antipolis, Nice, France

JULIENNE L. BOONE, MD
Department of Orthopedic Surgery,
Washington University School of Medicine,
St Louis, Missouri

KAREN J. BOSELLI, MD
Fellow, Center for Shoulder, Elbow and Sports
Medicine, Department of Orthopaedic Surgery,
Columbia University Medical Center,
New York, New York

SIMON BOYLE, MSc, FRCS(Tr & Orth)
Alps Surgery Institute, Clinique Generale,
Annecy, France

JAMES P. BRADLEY, MD
Head Team Physician, Pittsburgh Steelers;
Clinical Professor, Department of Orthopaedic
Surgery, University of Pittsburgh Medical
Center; Burke and Bradley Orthopaedics,
Pittsburgh, Pennsylvania

EDWIN R. CADET, MD
Assistant Professor, Clinical Orthopaedic
Surgery, Columbia University; Assistant
Attending Surgeon of Orthopaedic Surgery,
Columbia–Presbyterian Medical Center,
New York, New York

ELIZABETH A. CODY, BA
Columbia University College of Physicians and
Surgeons, New York, New York

JOE F. DE BEER, MBChB, MMed(Orth)
Cape Shoulder Institute, Cape Town,
South Africa

DARREN S. DROSDOWECH, MD, FRCSC
Assistant Professor, Department of
Orthopedic Surgery, St Joseph's Health Care,
The Hand and Upper Limb Centre, University
of Western Ontario, London, Ontario, Canada

KENNETH J. FABER, MD, MHPE, FRCSC
Associate Professor, Department of
Orthopedic Surgery, St Joseph's Health Care,
The Hand and Upper Limb Centre, University
of Western Ontario, London, Ontario, Canada

NEIL GHODADRA, MD
Department of Orthopaedic Surgery, Rush
University, Chicago, Illinois

R. MICHAEL GREIWE, MD
Fellow, Department of Orthopaedic Surgery,
Center for Shoulder, Elbow, and Sports
Medicine, Columbia-Presbyterian Hospital,
Columbia University, New York, New York

MIKEL GUTIERREZ-ARAMBERRI, MD
Alps Surgery Institute, Clinique Generale,
Annecy, France

LAURENT LAFOSSE, MD
Alps Surgery Institute, Clinique Generale,
Annecy, France

WILLIAM N. LEVINE, MD
Vice Chairman and Professor,
Department of Orthopaedic Surgery,
Columbia University Medical Center,
New York, New York

ROBERT B. LITCHFIELD, MD, FRCSC
Professor, Department of Orthopedic Surgery,
Fowler-Kennedy Sports Medicine Clinic,
University of Western Ontario, London,
Ontario, Canada

RUPERT MELLER, MD
Alps Surgery Institute, Clinique Generale,
Annecy, France

NUMA MERCIER, MD
Orthopaedic Surgeon, Department of
Orthopaedic Surgery and Sports
Traumatology, Hôpital de L'Archet 2, University
of Nice-Sophia-Antipolis, Nice, France

JASON OLD, MD, FRCSC
Assistant Professor, Section of Orthopaedic
Surgery, University of Manitoba; Pan Am Clinic,
Winnipeg, Manitoba, Canada

**CDR MATTHEW T. PROVENCHER,
MD, MC, USN**
Director, Section of Shoulder and Elbow,
Division of Sports Medicine, Department of
Orthopaedic Surgery, Naval Medical Center
San Diego; Associate Professor of Surgery,
Department of Surgery, Orthopaedics,
Uniformed Services University of Health
Sciences, San Diego, California

CHRISTOPHER ROBERTS, FRCS(Tr & Orth)
Ipswich Hospital NHS Trust, Ipswich, Suffolk,
United Kingdom

ANTHONY A. ROMEO, MD
Director, Section of Shoulder and Elbow,
Division of Sports Medicine; Professor,
Department of Orthopaedics; Section Head
Shoulder and Elbow Surgery; Team Physician,
Chicago White Sox, Division of Sports
Medicine, Department of Orthopaedic Surgery,
Rush University Medical Center, Chicago,
Illinois

ANUP SHAH, MD
Alps Surgery Institute, Clinique Generale,
Annecy, France

SAM G. TEJWANI, MD
Department of Orthopaedic Surgery, Division
of Sports Medicine, Southern California
Permanente Medical Group, Kaiser
Permanente Hospital, Fontana, California

JESSE VELLA
Department of Orthopedic Surgery, Columbia
University Medical Center, New York,
New York

BOB YIN, MD
Postdoctoral Resident, Department of
Orthopedic Surgery, Columbia University
Medical Center, New York, New York

Contents

Preface   xi

William N. Levine

Evaluation of Glenohumeral Instability   287

Edwin R. Cadet

> Glenohumeral instability is a common cause of shoulder disability. A wide spectrum of causes and presentations can make diagnosing subtle instability very difficult. This article describes clinical evaluation of the glenohumeral joint using pertinent components of the patient history, physical examination, and selective imaging to arrive at the diagnosis of glenohumeral instability in the symptomatic patient.

Arthroscopic Alphabet Soup: Recognition of Normal, Normal Variants, and Pathology   297

Bob Yin, Jesse Vella, and William N. Levine

> The capsule, labrum, glenohumeral ligaments, and rotator cuff represent the static and dynamic stabilizers of the glenohumeral joint. Various injuries can occur to one or more of these structures during traumatic shoulder dislocation, predisposing the patient to recurrent instability. Improved understanding of shoulder anatomy and biomechanics, and advancements in arthroscopic technique led to the recognition of various pathologic lesions that may contribute to instability. The ability to identify and address these lesions during arthroscopy will allow the surgeon to more fully tailor operative treatments for each individual patient suffering from shoulder instability. Furthermore, the ability to differentiate pathologic lesions from normal anatomic variants is critical to avoid inadvertent repair that will lead to loss of normal function and worsening symptoms.

Management of the Throwing Shoulder: Cuff, Labrum and Internal Impingement   309

R. Michael Greiwe and Christopher S. Ahmad

> Repetitive throwing or other overhead activity places great stress on the shoulder. As a result, the shoulder is a common site of injury in athletes. Addressing throwing-related injuries requires an understanding of throwing biomechanics and pathology. Nonoperative treatment is directed at restoring strength, flexibility, and neuromuscular control to the entire kinetic chain. Surgery is indicated when nonoperative treatment fails, and is directed at correcting labral, capsular, and rotator cuff pathology.

Arthroscopic Management of Anterior Instability: Pearls, Pitfalls, and Lessons Learned   325

Matthew T. Provencher, Neil Ghodadra, and Anthony A. Romeo

> Despite advances in the understanding of anterior shoulder instability, failure rates after open and arthroscopic surgery have been reported to be as high as 30%. In general, a successful operative outcome for patients with shoulder instability requires the surgeon to perform a complete preoperative evaluation, a thorough diagnostic arthroscopy to evaluate for concomitant co-pathology, and implement an effective postoperative therapy program tailored to the repair strategy. In addition to the Bankart lesion, the treating surgeon must be aware of other co-pathologies,

such as the HAGL lesion, ALPSA lesion, and SLAP tears, that can occur in concert with capsular pathology and present as potential barriers to a successful outcome. This article focuses specifically on the pearls and pitfalls that are important to recognize in the preoperative workup, intraoperative evaluation, and arthroscopic surgery to optimize surgical outcomes for anterior instability.

Arthroscopic Management of Posterior Instability

339

James P. Bradley and Sam G. Tejwani

In comparison with anterior shoulder instability, posterior instability is uncommon, occurring in 2% to 10% of cases, and covering a wide clinical spectrum ranging from locked posterior dislocation to the often subclinical recurrent posterior subluxation (RPS). With increased clinical awareness, imaging advances such as magnetic resonance arthrography, and the development of specific provocative physical examination tests, the identification of RPS in the athletic population is improving. This article describes the anatomic-based arthroscopic approach to treatment of RPS, which allows for enhanced identification and repair of intra-articular pathology including posterior capsular laxity, complete or incomplete detachment of the posterior capsulolabral complex, and inferior capsular tears. While postoperative results are generally good to excellent after stabilization for RPS, there is room for improvement.

Arthroscopic Management of Multidirectional Instability

357

John-Erik Bell

The most critical step in successful treatment of shoulder instability does not lie in surgical technique, but in accurate assessment of factors contributing to instability. Multidirectional instability (MDI) is initially treated with rehabilitation. The primary goal of rehabilitation is strengthening of the dynamic stabilizers, including the rotator cuff and scapular stabilizers. There are several surgical techniques described to manage MDI, ranging from the classic Neer inferior capsular shift to a variety of arthroscopic procedures. This article focuses on the arthroscopic management of MDI.

Management of Failed Instability Surgery: How to Get It Right the Next Time

367

Julienne L. Boone and Robert A. Arciero

Traumatic anterior shoulder dislocations are the most frequent type of joint dislocation and affect approximately 1.7% of the general population. The literature supports the consideration of primary stabilization in high-risk patients because of reported recurrences as high as 80% to 90% with nonoperative treatment regimens. Successful stabilization of anterior glenohumeral instability relies on not only good surgical techniques but also careful patient selection. Failure rates after open and arthroscopic stabilization have been reported to range from 2% to 8% and 4% to 13%, respectively. Recurrent shoulder instability leads to increased morbidity to the patient, increased pain, decreased activity level, prolonged time away from work and sports, and a general decrease in quality of life. This article reviews the potential pitfalls in anterior shoulder stabilization and discusses appropriate methods of addressing them in revision surgery.

Arthroscopic Bankart-Bristow-Latarjet (2B3) Procedure: How to Do It and Tricks To Make it Easier and Safe

381

Pascal Boileau, Numa Mercier, and Jason Old

The all-arthroscopic technique that the authors propose combines a Bristow-Latarjet procedure with a Bankart repair. This combined procedure provides a triple blocking of the shoulder (the so-called 2B3 procedure): (1) the labral repair recreates the anterior bumper and protects the humeral head from direct contact with the coracoid bone graft (Bumper effect); (2) the transferred coracoid bone block compensates for anterior glenoid bone loss (Bony effect); and (3) the transferred conjoined tendon creates a dynamic sling that reinforces the weak anteroinferior capsule by lowering the inferior part of the subscapularis when the arm is abducted and externally rotated (Belt or sling effect). The procedure combines the theoretic advantages of the Bristow-Latarjet procedure and the arthroscopic Bankart repair, eliminating the potential disadvantages of each. The extra-articular positioning of the bone block together with the labral repair and capsule retensioning allows the surgeon to perform a nearly anatomic shoulder repair. This novel procedure allows the surgeon to extend the indications of arthroscopic shoulder reconstruction to the subset of patients with recurrent anteroinferior shoulder instability with glenoid bone loss and capsular deficiency. It is an attractive surgical option to treat patients with a previous failed capsulolabral repair for which the surgical solutions are limited.

Arthroscopic Latarjet Procedure

393

Laurent Lafosse, Simon Boyle, Mikel Gutierrez-Aramberri, Anup Shah, and Rupert Meller

Although soft tissue stabilization procedures in the shoulder yield good results, arthroscopy and radiological investigations have identified more complex soft tissue and bony lesions that can be successfully treated using a Latarjet procedure. The authors have advanced this technique to make it possible arthroscopically, thereby conferring all the benefits that arthroscopic surgery offers. This article describes how and why the arthroscopic Latarjet procedure is a valuable tool in the treatment of complex shoulder instability and how the procedure can be introduced into practice. This technique has shown excellent results at short- to mid-term follow-up, with minimal complications. As such, this procedure is recommended to surgeons with good anatomic knowledge, advanced arthroscopic skills, and familiarity with the instrumentation.

Glenoid Bone Defects—Open Latarjet with Congruent Arc Modification

407

Joe F. de Beer and Christopher Roberts

Recurrent anterior shoulder instability is commonly associated with glenoid bone defects. When the defect is significant, bony reconstruction is typically necessary. The congruent arc modification of the Latarjet procedure uses the concavity of the undersurface of the coracoid to optimally reconstruct the glenoid. Outcomes are maximized and complications minimized.

Humeral Head Bone Defects: Remplissage, Allograft, and Arthroplasty

417

Marshal S. Armitage, Kenneth J. Faber, Darren S. Drosdowech, Robert B. Litchfield, and George S. Athwal

The Hill-Sachs lesion is a well-known entity that threatens recurrent instability, but the treatment options are multiple and the surgical indications remain undefined. The evidence for each operative technique is limited to retrospective reviews and small case series without controls. The decision of which technique to use resides with the surgeon. Older, osteopenic patients, especially those with underlying arthritis and large defects, should be managed with complete humeral resurfacing. Humeralplasty is best used in younger patients with good quality bone in an acute setting with small- to moderate-sized bone defects. Partial resurfacing and remplissage are best used with small to moderate lesions, and both require further study.

Allograft humeral reconstruction is an established technique for patients with moderate to large defects, and is best applied to nonosteopenic bone. Surgeons must be able to recognize the presence of humeral bone loss via specialized radiographs or cross-sectional imaging and understand its implications. The techniques to manage humeral bone loss are evolving and further biomechanical and clinical studies are required to define the indications and treatment algorithms.

Open Capsular Shift: There Still Is A Role!   **427**

Karen J. Boselli, Elizabeth A. Cody, and Louis U. Bigliani

As our understanding of the pathoanatomy of glenohumeral instability has improved, surgical techniques for the treatment of anterior instability have progressed. Many stabilization procedures are now successfully performed arthroscopically; open capsular shift, however, continues to play an important role in the management of instability in certain patients, providing an accurate and selective means of capsular plication. When performed with proper surgical technique, shoulder range of motion can be preserved with low recurrence rates and high subjective satisfaction, making the open capsular shift a durable and effective option in the modern management of shoulder instability.

Index   **437**

Orthopedic Clinics of North America

FORTHCOMING ISSUES

October 2010

Orthopedic Management of Cerebral Palsy
Hank Chambers, MD, *Guest Editor*

January 2011

Obesity in Orthopaedics
George V. Russell, MD, *Guest Editor*

RECENT ISSUES

April 2010

Evidence Based Medicine in Orthopedic Surgery
Safdar N. Khan, MD, Mark A. Lee, MD, and
Munish C. Gupta, MD, *Guest Editors*

January 2010

**Autologous Techniques to Fill Bone Defects
for Acute Fractures and Nonunions**
Hans C. Pape, MD, FACS,
and Timothy G. Weber, MD,
Guest Editors

October 2009

**Minimally Invasive Surgery in Orthopedic
Surgery**
Nicola Maffulli, MD, MS, PhD, FRCS (ORTH),
Guest Editor

THE CLINICS ARE NOW AVAILABLE ONLINE!

Access your subscription at:
www.theclinics.com

Preface

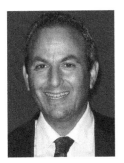

William N. Levine, MD
Guest Editor

Treatment for the unstable shoulder has evolved from Hippocrates' "hot poker" treatment to the open repairs popularized by Bankart, Rowe, and Neer to arthroscopic labral and capsular repairs. This special issue of *Orthopedic Clinics of North America* focuses on the arthroscopic and open management of shoulder instability, and we have enlisted experts from around the world to share their pearls, pitfalls, and insights in managing these challenging problems. Specific emphasis is placed on the proper management of the unstable shoulder in association with bone defects, as this variable has been associated with significantly higher failure rates. Although the open Latarjet and Bristow have just recently enjoyed a renaissance in North America and are highlighted in the excellent contribution from de Beer and colleagues, exciting break through techniques are presented by Lafosse and Boileau, who have paved the way for transition to all-arthroscopic Latarjet and Bristow procedures.

I would like to thank Ms Debora Dellapena from Elsevier and Ms Michele Roberts from the Columbia University Center for Shoulder, Elbow and Sports Medicine for their assistance. Of course, as always, I would like to thank my wife, Jill, and our daughters, Sonya and Clare, for their support and love. Finally, I would like to thank Dr Louis Bigliani, my mentor, partner, and friend, for teaching me shoulder surgery and affording me this incredible opportunity to do what I love on a daily basis.

William N. Levine, MD
Department of Orthopaedic Surgery
Columbia University Medical Center
622 West 168th Street, PH-1117
New York, NY 10032, USA

E-mail address:
wnl1@columbia.edu

Evaluation of Glenohumeral Instability

Edwin R. Cadet, MD

KEYWORDS

- Glenohumeral instability • Glenohumeral laxity
- Physical examination • Imaging

The glenohumeral joint is a ball-and-socket joint that achieves the greatest mobility when compared with any other joint in the human body. The overall glenohumeral to scapulothoracic motion ration is 2:1. Because of the great extremes of motion achievable by the shoulder joint, in addition to its complex anatomy that relies on a combination of bone and soft tissue structures for stability, it is not surprising that the shoulder is the most commonly dislocated joint. Although many patients who sustain an initial glenohumeral joint dislocation never experience an additional instability episode, subjective and objective recurrent instability can persist in others and may result in increased morbidity depending on the demands placed on the affected shoulder.

Despite numerous studies dedicated toward the topic, no consensus exists on what is defined as normal glenohumeral laxity. There have been many efforts to quantify glenohumeral laxity based on the amount of humeral head translation relative to the glenoid when the scapula has been stabilized. Reis and colleagues[1] sought to quantify normal humeral head translation in cadaveric models. Mean anterior and posterior glenohumeral translation measured between 9 and 11 mm. Harryman and colleagues[2] quantified anterior and posterior humeral head translation as 7.8 mm ± 4.0 and 7.9 mm ± 5.6, respectively, in asymptomatic volunteers using electromagnetic sensors to track humeral translation relative to the scapula. However, the difficulty in providing accurate and reproducible measuring reference points on cadaveric specimens or patients, and the great variability in humeral translation found in other studies, have raised questions regarding the validity of any of these measurements.

Historically, glenohumeral instability has been classified based on either cause or direction of instability. In general, causes of glenohumeral instability can be classified as either traumatic or atraumatic. Traumatic instability is defined as the result of an inciting event that causes subjective or objective glenohumeral subluxation or frank dislocation that is either spontaneously reduced or requires reduction by a practitioner. Atraumatic glenohumeral instability can result as the sequelae of generalized ligamentous laxity or secondary to repetitive motion; eg, activities in the overhead-throwing athlete. Glenohumeral instability can also be classified based on direction: anterior, posterior, inferior, or multidirectional. The concept of inferior and multidirectional instability was first proposed by Neer and Foster[3] in 1980. In their report, the presence of a sulcus sign, or inferior subluxation of the humeral head relative to the glenoid with applied downward traction of the arm, with the presence of symptoms (eg, discomfort, pain, persistent episodes of dislocation, or subluxation) confirmed the presence of multidirectional instability. They identified redundancy of the glenohumeral capsule and laxity in the inferior glenohumeral ligaments as the cause for multidirectional instability.

The distinction between normal glenohumeral laxity and pathologic instability is often difficult to ascertain from history alone. The clinician must rely on the physical examination and interpretation

Center for Shoulder, Elbow and Sports Medicine, Clinical Orthopaedic Surgery, Columbia University, 622 West 168th Street, PH-11, New York, NY 10032, USA
E-mail address: ec2195@columbia.edu

Orthop Clin N Am 41 (2010) 287–295
doi:10.1016/j.ocl.2010.02.005

of selective imaging to make the diagnosis of glenohumeral instability. This article describes the evaluation of glenohumeral instability, including pertinent parts of the patient history, clinical examination, and selective imaging used to arrive at the diagnosis of glenohumeral instability in the symptomatic patient.

PATIENT HISTORY

The examiner must obtain a thorough history from the patient regarding symptoms. Determining whether trauma to the involved extremity (eg, car accident, collision during athletic competition) preceded an initial instability event may help to determine the cause of disability to the patient. The patient may recall sustaining a frank dislocation that required manual reduction by a practitioner or a subjective feeling of instability of the shoulder "popping out," which may represent a subluxation event. The position of the arm at the time of the instability event is a critical clue in determining the direction of instability. Patients with traumatic anterior glenohumeral instability will generally describe the instability event occurring with the arm in the abducted, externally rotated, and extended position. Patients with posterior instability, conversely, describe the arm being held in forward flexion, internal rotation, and adduction.

Many patients cannot attribute a discrete event to their symptoms. This is generally seen in patients with generalized ligamentous laxity causing pathologic instability or overhead-throwing athletes (eg, volleyball, swimming, baseball). For example, the overhead-throwing athlete may present with complaints of pain during specific phases in the throwing cycle. Pain due to anterior instability is generally experienced during the late phase of cocking. This has been suggested to be the result of repetitive stresses and attenuation of the anteroinferior, capsule-ligament complex. Posterior instability can elicit pain during the follow-through phase. Furthermore, impingement of the posterosuperior rotator cuff with the labrum can also result in pain in these patients.

Rowe and Zarins[4] first described the "dead arm syndrome" where patients with transient anterior instability have debilitating or "paralyzing" pain or subluxation that results in brief loss of control of the affected extremity when the arm is in maximum external rotation, abduction, and extension.[5] Jobe and colleagues[6] further popularized this concept of instability as a source of pain in the overhead-throwing athlete. These patients may also complain of vague neurologic complaints

with inferior or multidirectional instability. When neurologic symptoms exist, a history of neck pain followed by a thorough cervical spine examination must follow.

The degree of disability and the number of discrete instability events must be obtained from the history. Recurrent instability may impair the patient's ability to perform activities of daily living (eg, carrying heavy loads, reaching for overhead objects) or may only be experienced during athletic activities (eg, pitching, striking). The ability to voluntarily dislocate the glenohumeral joint must be carefully drawn from the history, as surgical management of instability in this patient population may result in high rates of recurrence. Psychological factors may contribute to the patient voluntarily dislocating the glenohumeral joint and may necessitate psychological evaluation. However, not all voluntary glenohumeral instability patients have an underlying psychological cause. Selective activation of muscle groups can elicit instability.[7] Patients with voluntary instability can be addressed with physical therapy focusing on biofeedback techniques.[5]

IMAGING

Selective imaging of the shoulder can provide critical information when assessing the patient with glenohumeral instability. Radiographic imaging of the shoulder should include; a true anteroposterior (AP) view of the glenohumeral joint in neutral, external, and internal rotation; a lateral or Y view in the scapular plane; and an axillary view (**Fig. 1**). In the case of significant trauma, a trauma series of the affected shoulder should include a true AP view, Y view in the scapular plane, and an axillary, or a Velpeau axillary view. Hill-Sachs

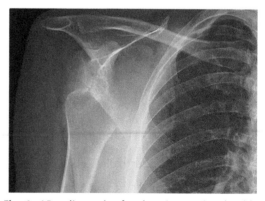

Fig. 1. AP radiograph of a chronic anterior shoulder dislocation in a 45 year-old, right-hand dominant male who presented for medical attention 5.5 months after a traumatic episode. (*Courtesy of* Center for Shoulder, Elbow and Sports Medicine, Columbia University.)

lesions (posterolateral impression fractures) following anterior glenohumeral dislocation can be best appreciated on the AP view in internal rotation or a notch view. The notch view, as initially described by Hall and colleagues,[8] is performed with the patient lying supine with the cassette placed posterior to the shoulder. The hand of the affected extremity is placed on top of the head with the elbow pointing straight upward. The radiograph beam is directed 10° superior toward the head and centered over the coracoid process. Avulsion fractures and deficiency of the inferior glenoid (bony Bankart lesions) can occasionally be detected on the AP shoulder views, but are best visualized with a standard, Velpeau, or West Point axillary view. The West Point axillary view, as described by Rokous and colleagues[9] is performed with the patient lying prone with the affected shoulder resting on a pad. The radiograph beam is aimed 25° from the horizontal plane (angled toward the table surface) and 25° toward the patient's midline.

CT scan is a useful adjuvant test when assessing bone defects on either the humeral or the glenoid side. CT scan is particularly useful in the setting of failed shoulder stabilization surgery to determine whether bone deficiencies contribute to recurrent instability that were not adequately addressed at the index procedure. Although CT arthrography was widely used in the past,[10–12] MRI and MR arthrography has become the gold standard for evaluating glenohumeral instability. Chandnani and colleagues[13] prospectively studied the sensitivity of CT arthrography, MRI, and MR arthrography for their ability to detect glenoid labral lesions for shoulder instability. They found that MR arthrography was the most sensitive of the three techniques for detecting a detached, labral fragment and labral degeneration (**Figs. 2** and **3**). Furthermore, MR arthrography afforded the best visualization of the inferior part of the labrum and the inferior glenohumeral ligament. Other studies have demonstrated high accuracy when using noncontrast, enhanced MR imaging for the detection of labral tears.[14] In addition, recent studies have demonstrated the improved techniques of assessing capsular laxity in patients with recurrent anterior shoulder instability with MR imaging.[15]

PHYSICAL EXAMINATION

Physical examination must always begin with both shoulders exposed for visual inspection. Visual inspection of the back during active shoulder forward flexion with the examiner positioned behind the patient can detect subtle scapulothoracic dyskinesia or scapular winging. Active and passive range of motion should be assessed and compared with the unaffected extremity. Deficits with internal rotation can suggest posterior capsule contractures that are common in the throwing athlete with internal impingement. Extreme deficits with internal and external rotation can be seen in the setting of unrecognized anterior and posterior dislocations, respectively. An assessment of generalized laxity (eg, hypermobile patella, hyperextension of elbows, metacarpophalangeal joints, and the ability to reach the ipsilateral forearm with the abducted thumb) must be performed.

The physical examination for shoulder instability can be divided into two main groups: (1) tests for the assessment of glenohumeral laxity and (2) provocative, or instability, tests. The following sections will describe these tests in detail.

LAXITY TESTING
Anterior Drawer Test

The anterior drawer test was first described by Gerber and Ganz[16] in 1984. This test attempts to quantify anterior translation of the humeral head

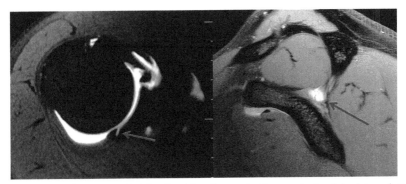

Fig. 2. (*Right panel*) MR arthrogram of right shoulder demonstrating posterior labral tear (*arrow*) with (*left panel*) associated paralabral cyst in spinoglenoid notch (*arrow*). (*Courtesy of* Center for Shoulder, Elbow and Sports Medicine, Columbia University.)

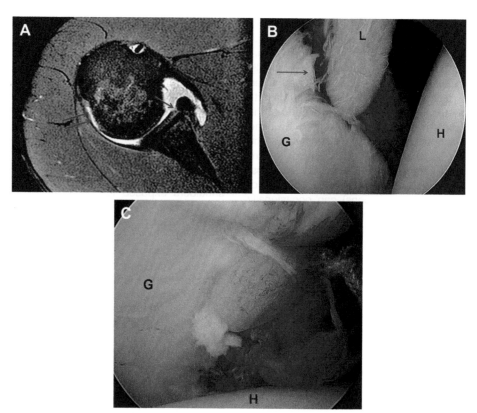

Fig. 3. (A) Noncontrast, enhanced MRI of right shoulder demonstrating subtle detachment of anteroinferior labrum from adjacent glenoid cartilage (*arrow*) and small posterolateral impaction fracture or Hill-Sachs lesion (*double arrow*). This patient sustained a traumatic anterior shoulder dislocation that was manually reduced. (B) Arthroscopic image from posterior viewing portal of the labral tear. The arrow depicts detachment of the anteroinferior labrum from glenoid surface. (C) Labro-ligamentous repair. G, glenoid; H, humerus; L, labrum. (*Courtesy of* Center for Shoulder, Elbow and Sports Medicine, Columbia University.)

on the face of the glenoid (**Fig. 4**). The test should be performed with the patient lying supine. The examiner stands at the ipsilateral side of the affected extremity. The patient's hand is positioned in the examiner's axilla. The shoulder is in 80° to 120° of abduction, 0° to 20° of forward flexion, and 0° to 30° of external rotation. One of the examiner's hands is used to stabilize the scapula by placing the fingers on the scapular spine and the thumb on the coracoid. The other hand grasps the proximal humeral shaft. An anterior force is applied to the proximal humerus and the amount of translation is quantified. To elicit maximum translation, the patient must be relaxed.

McFarland and colleagues[17] and Bahk and colleagues[18] have described techniques for performing the anterior drawer test. When examining a left shoulder, the examiner uses his or her left hand to support the left wrist and his or her right hand to support the patient's upper arm. The affected shoulder is abducted to 60° to 70° with slight internal rotation with an axial load applied perpendicular to the glenoid. The examiner applies an anterior force to "translate the humeral head onto the chest in one motion." The investigators contend that their technique may provide

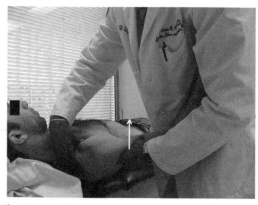

Fig. 4. Anterior shoulder drawer test. The arrow demonstrates anterior force applied to the arm. Examiner's right hand is stabilizing the scapula. (*Courtesy of* Center for Shoulder, Elbow and Sports Medicine, Columbia University.)

increased stability to scapular rotation when performing the test.

Posterior Drawer

Gerber and Ganz[16] also described this test to determine posterior humeral head translation. The patient is in the supine position (**Fig. 5**). If the left shoulder is being examined, the examiner holds the patient's left wrist and forearm with the elbow flexed to 120°. The left shoulder is in 80° to 120° of abduction and 20° to 30° of forward flexion. The examiner stabilizes the patient's scapula by placing his or her right second and third fingers on the scapula spine and the thumb just lateral to the coracoid process, so that "its ulnar aspect remains in contact with the coracoid while performing the test."[16] The examiner slightly rotates the affected extremity medially and flexes the shoulder to between 60° to 80°. During the maneuver, the examiner's thumb attempts to subluxate the humeral head posteriorly. The examiner can appreciate the amount of posterior translation in two ways: (1) the examiner's thumb can detect the position of the humeral head where it lies relative to the anterior glenoid rim and (2) depending on the amount of posterior translation, the humeral head may be increasingly palpable by the examiner's fingers positioned on the scapular spine. "The maneuver is pain-free but often associated with a slight to moderate degree of apprehension, enabling the patient to identify the position of instability with certainty."[16,19]

Bahk and colleagues[18] have described a modified technique of the posterior shoulder drawer test. The affected shoulder is abducted to 50° to 60° in neutral rotation. They state that this position unloads the posterior capsule to enhance maximum laxity. Assuming the left shoulder is being examined, the examiner holds the left wrist and forearm with his or her left hand. The examiners right thumb is placed on the anterior humeral head and the fingers are positioned on the posterior humeral head. "As the thumb pushes the humeral head posteriorly, the arm is flexed forward toward the examiner. The fingers placed posteriorly can be used to feel the humeral head subluxate over the posterior glenoid rim."[18]

Anterior and Posterior Load and Shift Test

The load and shift test was initially described by Silliman and Hawkins[20] in 1993. The patient can be in either a supine or seated position. In the supine position, the arm is placed in 20° of abduction, 20° of forward flexion, and neutral rotation. If in the upright position, the examiner stands behind

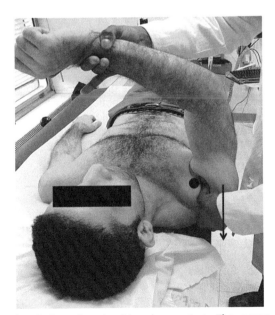

Fig. 5. Posterior shoulder drawer test. The arrow demonstrates a posterior-applied force exerted on the humeral head. Black circle; coracoid. (*Courtesy of* Center for Shoulder, Elbow and Sports Medicine, Columbia University.)

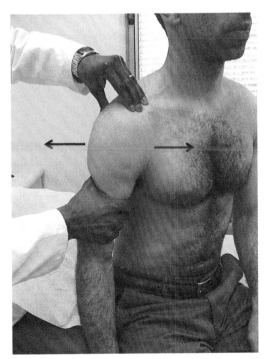

Fig. 6. Anterior and posterior load and shift test in the upright position. Arrows demonstrate anterior (*right arrow*) or posterior (*left arrow*) force applied to the arm. (*Courtesy of* Center for Shoulder, Elbow and Sports Medicine, Columbia University.)

the patient on the ipsilateral side of the examined extremity (**Fig. 6**). Assuming the right shoulder is being examined, the examiner places his or her left hand on the scapula to stabilize scapular motion. The examiner grasps the humeral head with his or her right hand and applies an axial load perpendicular to the articular surface of the glenoid. Anterior or posterior-directed forces are then applied the humeral head and translation relative to the glenoid is measured.

Tzannes and colleagues[21] described a modification to the load and shift tests. In this variation, the examiner sits on a stool adjacent to the patient lying in the supine position (**Fig. 7**). The scapula is stabilized on the examining table and the humeral head hangs over the edge of the table. The patient's elbow is gently flexed with one of the examiner's hand. The humeral head is stabilized with the other hand. The examiner translates the humeral head in the anterior, posterior, and inferior directions with the shoulder in 90° of abduction. The amount of humeral translation is then graded. Grade 0 is defined as little-to-no movement of the humeral head; grade 1, the humeral head is translated onto the glenoid labrum; grade 2, the humeral head is translated over the glenoid but spontaneously reduced; and grade 3, the humeral head is translated over the glenoid and remains dislocated once the applied force is removed.

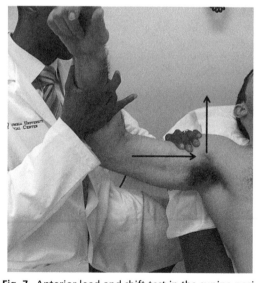

Fig. 7. Anterior load and shift test in the supine position. Axial and anterior forces (*arrows*) are exerted onto the humeral head to load the glenoid. The scapula is stabilized posteriorly by the examining table. (*Courtesy of* Center for Shoulder, Elbow and Sports Medicine, Columbia University.)

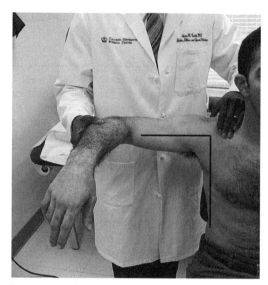

Fig. 8. Gagey hyperabduction test. Lines demonstrate the measurement of the passive motion of the shoulder in abduction (RPA). In this patient, the RPA measures approximately 90°. (*Courtesy of* Center for Shoulder, Elbow and Sports Medicine, Columbia University.)

Gagey Hyperabduction Test

Gagey and Gagey[22] initially described this test as a measure of laxity of the inferior glenohumeral ligament complex. The test is performed with the patient sitting and the examiner standing behind (**Fig. 8**). The examiner uses one hand to stabilize the scapula. The other hand is used to abduct the affected shoulder. The amount of abduction measured before the initiation of scapula motion is then recorded. The investigators termed the amount of abduction where glenohumeral motion ends and scapulothoracic motion begins as the passive motion of the shoulder in abduction (RPA). An RPA greater than 105° was suggestive of inferior glenohumeral ligament laxity.

Sulcus Sign

The sulcus sign was initially described by Neer and Foster[3] in 1980. They observed increased inferior translation of the humeral head relative to the glenoid with applied downward traction in patients with inferior and multidirectional instability (**Fig. 9**). Although the authors did not formally coin the term "sulcus sign," their report demonstrates photos of patients with an increased acromiohumeral interval and inferior translation of the humeral head relative to the glenoid with stressed radiographs. Silliman and Hawkins[20] described a similar approach with the patient lying in the supine position. With the patient in the supine

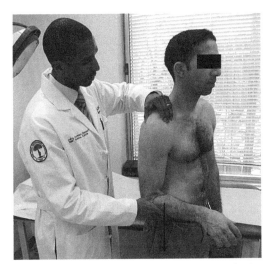

Fig. 9. Sulcus sign. Downward traction is applied to the arm (*arrow*). The examiner then grades the amount of inferior translation of the humeral head relative to the inferior acromion in centimeters. (*Courtesy of* Center for Shoulder, Elbow and Sports Medicine, Columbia University.)

position, the shoulder is held in 20° of abduction and forward flexion in neutral rotation. An inferior stress is applied and inferior translation of the humeral head is observed and quantified. The sulcus sign has been graded in many studies.[20,23,24] In general, grade 0 translation is defined as minimal inferior translation, grade I is less than 1 cm translation, grade II is 1 to 2 cm of translation, and grade 3 is greater than 2.0 cm of translation. The patient should be asked if inferior translation reproduces symptoms. The presence of symptoms can help the examiner differentiate whether the sulcus is a measurement of normal glenohumeral laxity in that specific individual or pathologic instability. In addition, the sulcus should be measured at both neutral and 30° of external rotation. Elimination of the sulcus sign with external rotation suggests competency of the rotator interval; persistence of the sulcus sign at 30° of external rotation suggests a lax rotator interval.

Grading of Humeral Translation

Although many systems for grading humeral head translation exist, no consensus has been reached regarding the efficacy of one grading system over the other. One method describes grading humeral head translation by estimating distance in millimeters. For example, four grades of anterior and posterior translation has been previously described[18,24]: grade 0 is defined as no or minimal translation; grade 1, 0 to 1 cm of translation; grade II, 1 to 2 cm of translation or humeral head translation to the glenoid rim; and grade III, greater than 2 cm of translation or translation over the glenoid rim. Altchek and colleagues[23] quantified laxity of the glenohumeral joint (anterior, posterior, inferior) in patients under anesthesia undergoing shoulder stabilization for instability. Translation of the glenohumeral joint was graded from 1+ to 3+. A grade of 1+ was defined as increased glenohumeral translation relative to the contralateral shoulder without subluxation. A translation of 2+ indicated that the humeral head could be translated over the glenoid, but would spontaneously reduce once the applied force was removed. A translation of 3+ was defined as translation of the humeral head over the glenoid that remained dislocated after the applied force was removed. Others have graded humeral translation based on the percentage of humeral head translation relative to the center of the glenoid[18,25]: grade 0, 0% to 25%; grade 1, 25% to 50%; grade II, greater than 50%; and grade III, 100%, or complete translation of the humeral head over the glenoid rim.

INSTABILITY TESTS
Apprehension Test

The apprehension test was first described by Rowe and Zarins[4] in 1981 (**Fig. 10**). The test can

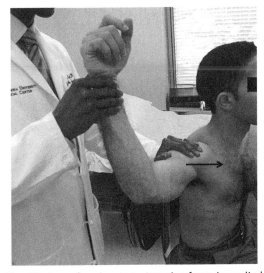

Fig. 10. Apprehension test. Anterior force is applied to the posterior humeral head (*arrow*) in the position of shoulder abduction and external rotation. A positive test will reproduce symptoms of apprehension and pain. (*Courtesy of* Center for Shoulder, Elbow and Sports Medicine, Columbia University.)

be performed with the patient in the supine or upright position. The affected shoulder is passively moved to abduction and maximum external rotation. At the same time, a gentle anterior force is placed on the posterior humeral head. A test is positive when the patient becomes "apprehensive" (eg, subjective feeling as the shoulder is "coming out") and experiences pain. Posterior apprehension can also be appreciated when performing the posterior drawer or posterior load and shift (as previously described).

Apprehension-Relocation Test

Jobe and colleagues[6] described this test in 1989. The first part of the examination incorporates the apprehension test. The patient is supine and the affected arm is placed in abduction and external rotation. An anterior-directed force is placed on the posterior humeral head. This position will produce apprehension and pain in patients who have sustained recurrent dislocations. Patients who have sustained anterior subluxation will complain of pain but not apprehension with this maneuver. The relocation test is performed by applying a posterior-directed force to the anterior humeral head. According to the investigators, "patients with primary impingement will have no change in their pain, whereas patients with instability (subluxation) and impingement will have pain relief and will tolerate maximal external rotation with the humeral head maintained in the reduced position."[6] The relief of apprehension with application of the posteriorly directed force on the humeral head is also known as "Fowler's sign" (**Fig. 11**).[20] When apprehension is used as

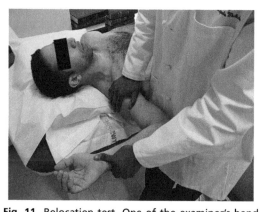

Fig. 11. Relocation test. One of the examiner's hand places a posterior force to the anterior humeral head while maintaining the shoulder in abduction and maximum external rotation. A positive test alleviates apprehension and pain. (*Courtesy of* Center for Shoulder, Elbow and Sports Medicine, Columbia University.)

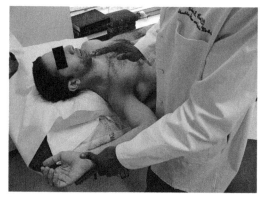

Fig. 12. Release test. The posterior directed force in the relocation test is removed. A positive test will reproduce symptoms of apprehension and pain. (*Courtesy of* Center for Shoulder, Elbow and Sports Medicine, Columbia University.)

the diagnostic criteria compared with pain, sensitivity of the test was 68%, specificity 100%, positive predictive value 100%, and negative predictive value 78%.

Anterior Release and Surprise Test

The anterior release test was first described in 1997.[26] The test is performed with the patient in the supine position. The affected shoulder is held over the edge of the examiner's table. The arm is positioned in 90° of abduction. A posterior-directed force is applied to the anterior humeral head while simultaneously moving the shoulder to maximum external rotation. The posterior force is then released. A positive test is defined as when the patient experiences pain and apprehension. The sensitivity of the test was cited as 92%, specificity 89%, positive predictive value 87%, and negative predictive value 93%.[19,26] Furthermore, if the posterior force is suddenly removed and symptoms (eg, pain and apprehension) are elicited, this is termed a "surprise" test[27] (**Fig. 12**).

SUMMARY

Glenohumeral instability is a common cause of shoulder disability, particularly in the young athlete. A wide spectrum of causes and presentation can make diagnosing subtle instability very difficult. Evaluation of the glenohumeral joint begins with obtaining a thorough patient history, supplemented by a comprehensive physical examination and selective imaging. Only with the combination of all these components can an accurate treatment plan be established for the patient with symptomatic glenohumeral instability.

REFERENCES

1. Reis MT, Tibone JE, McMahon PJ, et al. Cadaveric study of glenohumeral translation using electromagnetic sensors. Clin Orthop Relat Res 2002; 400:88–92.

2. Harryman DT 2nd, Sidles JA, Harris SL, et al. Laxity of the normal glenohumeral joint: a quantitative in vivo assessment. J Shoulder Elbow Surg 1992;1: 66–76.

3. Neer CS 2nd, Foster CR. Inferior capsular shift for involuntary inferior and multidirectional instability of the shoulder. A preliminary report. J Bone Joint Surg Am 1980;62:897–908.

4. Rowe CR, Zarins B. Recurrent transient subluxation of the shoulder. J Bone Joint Surg Am 1981;63:863–72.

5. Pollock RG, Bigliani LU. Glenohumeral instability: evaluation and treatment. J Am Acad Orthop Surg 1993;1:24–32.

6. Jobe FW, Kvitne RS, Giangarra CE. Shoulder pain in the overhand or throwing athlete. The relationship of anterior instability and rotator cuff impingement. Orthop Rev 1989;18:963–75.

7. Fronek J, Warren RF, Bowen M. Posterior subluxation of the glenohumeral joint. J Bone Joint Surg Am 1989;71:205–16.

8. Hall RH, Isaac F, Booth CR. Dislocations of the shoulder with special reference to accompanying small fractures. J Bone Joint Surg Am 1959;41-A: 489–94.

9. Rokous JR, Feagin JA, Abbott HG. Modified axillary roentgenogram. A useful adjunct in the diagnosis of recurrent instability of the shoulder. Clin Orthop Relat Res 1972;82:84–6.

10. Rafii M, Firooznia H, Golimbu C, et al. CT arthrography of capsular structures of the shoulder. AJR Am J Roentgenol 1986;146:361–7.

11. Shuman WP, Kilcoyne RF, Matsen FA, et al. Double-contrast computed tomography of the glenoid labrum. AJR Am J Roentgenol 1983;141: 581–4.

12. Sanders TG, Morrison WB, Miller MD. Imaging techniques for the evaluation of glenohumeral instability. Am J Sports Med 2000;28:414–34.

13. Chandnani VP, Yeager TD, DeBerardino T, et al. Glenoid labral tears: prospective evaluation with MRI imaging, MR arthrography, and CT arthrography. AJR Am J Roentgenol 1993;161:1229–35.

14. Gusmer PB, Potter HG, Schatz JA, et al. Labral injuries: accuracy of detection with unenhanced MR imaging of the shoulder. Radiology 1996;200: 519–24.

15. Ng AW, Chu CM, Lo WN, et al. Assessment of capsular laxity in patients with recurrent anterior shoulder dislocation using MRI. AJR Am J Roentgenol 2009;192:1690–5.

16. Gerber C, Ganz R. Clinical assessment of instability of the shoulder. With special reference to anterior and posterior drawer tests. J Bone Joint Surg Br 1984;66:551–6.

17. McFarland EG, Torpey BM, Curl LA. Evaluation of shoulder laxity. Sports Med 1996;22:264–72.

18. Bahk M, Keyurapan E, Tasaki A, et al. Laxity testing of the shoulder: a review. Am J Sports Med 2007;35: 131–44.

19. Tennent TD, Beach WR, Meyers JF. A review of the special tests associated with shoulder examination. Part II: laxity, instability, and superior labral anterior and posterior (SLAP) lesions. Am J Sports Med 2003;31:301–7.

20. Silliman JF, Hawkins RJ. Classification and physical diagnosis of instability of the shoulder. Clin Orthop Relat Res 1993;7–19.

21. Tzannes A, Paxinos A, Callanan M, et al. An assessment of the interexaminer reliability of tests for shoulder instability. J Shoulder Elbow Surg 2004; 13:18–23.

22. Gagey OJ, Gagey N. The hyperabduction test. J Bone Joint Surg Br 2001;83:69–74.

23. Altchek DW, Warren RF, Skyhar MJ, et al. T-plasty modification of the Bankart procedure for multidirectional instability of the anterior and inferior types. J Bone Joint Surg Am 1991;73:105–12.

24. Hawkins RJ, Schutte JP, Janda DH, et al. Translation of the glenohumeral joint with the patient under anesthesia. J Shoulder Elbow Surg 1996;5:286–92.

25. Cooper RA, Brems JJ. The inferior capsular-shift procedure for multidirectional instability of the shoulder. J Bone Joint Surg Am 1992;74:1516–21.

26. Gross ML, Distefano MC. Anterior release test. A new test for occult shoulder instability. Clin Orthop Relat Res 1997;339:105–8.

27. Lo IK, Nonweiler B, Woolfrey M, et al. An evaluation of the apprehension, relocation, and surprise tests for anterior shoulder instability. Am J Sports Med 2004;32:301–7.

Arthroscopic Alphabet Soup: Recognition of Normal, Normal Variants, and Pathology

Bob Yin, MD, Jesse Vella, William N. Levine, MD*

KEYWORDS

- Arthroscopy • Instability • Shoulder • Bankart
- Humeral avulsion of the glenohumeral ligaments
- Anterior labroligamentous periosteal sleeve avulsion

The importance of diagnostic arthroscopy in the management of patients with acute and recurrent shoulder instability is well recognized.[1–4] Prior to the use of arthroscopy to diagnose and repair pathologic causes of shoulder instability, the patient's age at time of initial dislocation and to a lesser degree the period of immobilization were the main risk factors determining recurrent dislocation.[5,6] Recent level I evidence showed that primary arthroscopic repair in patients with first-time shoulder dislocation reduces the risk of recurrent dislocation and improves the patient's functional outcome.[7] Improved understanding of shoulder anatomy and biomechanics led to the recognition of various pathologic lesions that may contribute to instability. The ability to identify and address these lesions during arthroscopy will allow the surgeon to more fully tailor operative treatments for each individual patient suffering from shoulder instability.

Although the Bankart lesion is still the most common lesion associated with shoulder instability, various other lesions have been identified and must be addressed during shoulder arthroscopy to prevent significant disability associated with recurrent dislocations. In 1993 Norlin[3] reviewed 24 patients with first-time anterior shoulder dislocation who were evaluated with examination under anesthesia and arthroscopy. He found that all shoulders sustaining anterior dislocations had

Bankart and Hill-Sachs lesions, and concluded that these uniform arthroscopic findings did not allow them to be used as predictors for recurrent instability.

NORMAL ANATOMY

The shoulder joint has few restraints to motion, thus providing it with 6° of freedom to allow for a wide array of actions ranging from the activities of daily living to high-intensity athletics. To strike a balance between broad functionality and frank instability, the shoulder is equipped with many important anatomic structures that act in concert to maintain stability while facilitating function.

Labrum

The glenohumeral joint has been analogized to a golf ball sitting on a tee, to highlight the glenoid's relative lack of depth and surface area when compared with the larger spherical humeral articular surface.[8] The fibrocartilagenous labrum compensates for this relative deficiency by acting to maintain glenohumeral congruency via several mechanisms.

First it acts as an attachment for the capsule and ligamentous structures, anchoring these stabilizers to the glenoid rim. The labrum itself is firmly attached to the glenoid in its inferior hemisphere

Department of Orthopedic Surgery, Columbia University Medical Center, 622 West 168th Street, PH-11 Center, New York, NY 10032, USA
* Corresponding author.
E-mail address: wnl1@columbia.edu

Orthop Clin N Am 41 (2010) 297–308
doi:10.1016/j.ocl.2010.02.003

through a narrow rim of fibrocartilagenous tissue that directly transitions into the glenoid articular cartilage.[9] The inferior glenohumeral ligament (IGHL) blends in directly with the inferior labrum (**Fig. 1**). In its superior half above the glenoid equator, the labrum is more loosely and variably inserted, leading to anatomic variants that may be confused as pathologic when identified during arthroscopy. The superior labrum receives fibers directly from the long head of the biceps tendon (LHBT) that inserts onto the supraglenoid tubercle in close proximity to the superior edge of the glenoid (**Fig. 2**). Cooper and colleagues[9] demonstrated that the labrum is vascularized only in its periphery, and is more perfused in the posterosuperior and inferior portions.

Furthermore, the labrum significantly enhances the concavity of the glenoid socket. Howell and Galinat[10] showed that the labrum deepens the glenoid by 9 mm in the superoinferior plane and 5 mm in the anteroposterior plane, and that loss of the labrum would reduce glenoid depth by more than 50% in both directions. The labrum also increases the surface area of contact for the humeral head, and may function as a load-bearing structure loosely analogous to the meniscus in the knee.[11]

Superior Glenohumeral Ligament, Coracohumeral Ligament, and Rotator Interval

The rotator interval (RI) is a medially based triangular space within the glenohumeral joint capsule. The RI contains 3 structures in close association

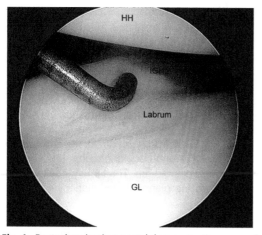

Fig. 1. Posterior viewing portal demonstrating normal labrum and inferior glenohumeral ligament attachment (RIGHT shoulder lateral decubitus position: HH, humeral head; GL, glenoid; IGHL, inferior glenohumeral ligament). (*Courtesy of* Center for Shoulder, Elbow and Sports Medicine, Columbia University.)

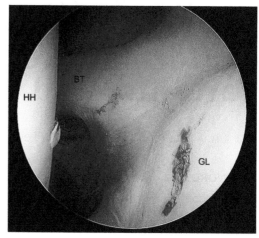

Fig. 2. Posterior viewing portal demonstrating normal biceps attachment to the superior labrum (LEFT shoulder Beach chair position: HH, humeral head; GL, glenoid; BT, biceps tendon). (*Courtesy of* Center for Shoulder, Elbow and Sports Medicine, Columbia University.)

(coracohumeral ligament [CHL], superior glenohumeral ligament [SGHL], and long head of the biceps tendon), and is considered important to shoulder stability because sectioning of the interval leads to increased anterior, posterior, and inferior humeral head translation.[12] The borders of the interval are as follows: the medial base is formed by the lateral aspect of the coracoid, the superior border is formed by the anterior margin of the supraspinatus tendon, and the inferior border is formed by the superior margin of the subscapularis tendon (**Fig. 3**). The CHL is a broad (1–2 cm), thin structure that originates on the lateral aspect of the coracoid and courses through the RI to insert onto the greater and lesser tuberosities on either side of the bicipital groove. Deep to the CHL in the RI lies the SGHL, which is variable in size and is present in more than 90% of cases.[13] The SGHL is usually small and variably originates from the supraglenoid tubercle and anterosuperior labrum, running just anterior to the long biceps tendon and parallel to the CHL as it inserts onto the humerus just superior to the lesser tuberosity. The intra-articular portion of the long biceps tendon pierces the interval at its apex during the tendon's course out of the joint, after which it immediately enters the bicipital groove.

The biomechanical role of the CHL and SGHL has been extensively studied and there exists various opinions regarding their relative importance in maintaining stability.[13] These 2 structures have similar roles because they share a parallel course, and act to limit inferior translation and

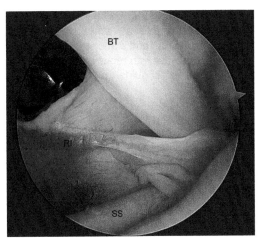

Fig. 3. Posterior viewing portal demonstrating normal rotator interval (RIGHT shoulder Beach Chair position: BT, biceps tendon; RI, rotator interval; SS, subscapularis). (*Courtesy of* Center for Shoulder, Elbow and Sports Medicine, Columbia University.)

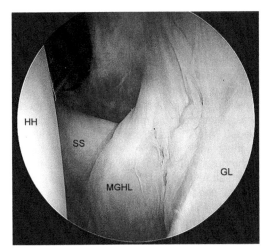

Fig. 4. Posterior viewing portal demonstrating normal middle glenohumeral ligament (MGHL) (LEFT shoulder Beach chair position: HH, humeral head; GL, glenoid; SS, subscapularis; MGHL, middle glenohumeral ligament). (*Courtesy of* Center for Shoulder, Elbow and Sports Medicine, Columbia University.)

external rotation when the arm is adducted.[14,15] There is also evidence that they limit posterior translation when the shoulder is in forward flexion, adduction, and internal rotation.[16]

Middle Glenohumeral Ligament

The middle glenohumeral ligament (MGHL) is the most variable in size and appearance of all the glenohumeral ligaments. Typically, the MGHL originates from the supraglenoid tubercle and anterosuperior labrum in close relation to the SGHL and inserts just anterior to the lesser tuberosity, blending with the fibers of the subscapularis tendon (**Fig. 4**). The MGHL acts to limit anterior and posterior humeral head translation when the arm is abducted between 60° and 90° and limits inferior translation when the arm is adducted.[17,18]

Inferior Glenohumeral Ligament Complex

The IGHL originates from the inferior half of the labrum and adjacent glenoid neck and inserts just inferior to the MGHL on the humerus (see **Fig. 1**). Arthroscopic, gross, and histologic studies by O'Brien and colleagues[19] delineated the IGHL as a complex of 3 components: the anterior band, the axillary pouch, and the posterior band. Later studies by Ticker and colleagues[20] indicated that the posterior band was less discrete and showed greater variation than the anterior band and axillary pouch.

The IGHL complex clearly plays an important role in shoulder stability as it often becomes disrupted following anterior dislocation. The relative location of the IGHLC changes with respect to

arm position. When the shoulder is internally rotated, the complex moves posteriorly, preventing excessive posterior translation. Conversely, the complex moves anteriorly during external rotation to limit anterior displacement. During abduction, the complex is located inferior to the humeral head and becomes taut, thereby limiting inferior translation. The anterior and posterior components of the complex variably tighten during forward flexion or extension to limit anteroposterior displacement.[21,22] Therefore, the IGHLC makes up a net that captures the humeral head to limit its translation on the glenoid fossa throughout much of normal shoulder motion.

Rotator Cuff

The labrum and glenohumeral ligaments are regarded as static stabilizers because each of these structures provides a unidirectional limitation to translation in any given shoulder position. By contrast, the rotator cuff is perfectly positioned to dynamically stabilize the joint throughout its range of motion.[23] Active contraction of the rotator cuff imparts stability via 2 mechanisms: (1) active joint compression of the humeral head into the glenoid, and (2) glenohumeral ligament dynamization through direct attachments to the rotator cuff.

Biomechanical studies by Lippitt and Matsen[24] showed that the magnitude of tangential forces needed to dislocate the shoulder increased as more compression forces were applied across the joint. Lippitt and Matsen described the concept as "concavity-compression" and noted that given an intact labrum, the joint could sustain tangential forces up to 60% of the compressive force. Bowen and colleagues[25] showed that even when three-fourths of the joint capsule had been sectioned, a compressive force of 111 N could prevent dislocation in the face of a 50-N tangential force. Synchronous rotator cuff contraction is needed to center and contain the humeral head on the glenoid, thus providing a stable fulcrum for humeral elevation. Deficiencies in rotator cuff musculature result in superior migration of the humeral head. The degree of migration is directly related to the magnitude of cuff deficiency.[26] In overhead throwing athletes who have instability related to overuse injury, Warner and colleagues[16] showed that symptomatic patients had altered rotator cuff strength patterns predisposing them to injury of the GHL and capsule.

Intraoperative arthroscopic observation indicates that the various glenohumeral ligaments are intimately related to the rotator cuff tendons, and anatomic studies have confirmed that in many locations the ligaments are directly attached to the cuff.[27,28] Furthermore, the joint capsule is in contact with the cuff in all locations except in the RI. Therefore, it is postulated that with active joint motion, the rotator cuff will dynamize the attached capsuloligamentous structures, further enhancing their ability to maintain physiologic extents of humeral translation. Further studies are needed to elucidate the direct effect of dynamic cuff contraction on each ligamentous structure during shoulder range of motion.

Biceps Tendon

The LHBT originates from the supraglenoid tubercle and superior labrum and courses through the joint to pierce the apex of the RI, becoming extra-articular as it enters the bicipital groove. Using a dynamic cadaveric model, Rodosky and colleagues[29] showed that detachment of the superior glenoid labrum increased anterior shoulder instability and placed greater strain in the IGHL complex during torsional loading in the abducted, externally rotated position. Pagnani and colleagues[30] showed that a superior labral lesion that disrupted the supraglenoid biceps origin resulted in increased glenohumeral translation in anteroposterior and superoinferior directions. In an electromyographic analysis of biceps muscle function in patients with anterior instability, Kim and colleagues[31] found that the voltage of the biceps was significantly greater in affected individuals than in matched controls, especially with the shoulder in abduction or external rotation. These

studies support the concept that the biceps play a compensatory role as a dynamic stabilizer when the rotator cuff and static stabilizers are deficient, as in patients with recurrent instability or at the extremes of shoulder motion in overhead athletes.

NORMAL VARIANTS

Although the various anatomic structures all have a defined role in maintaining shoulder stability, there are many variations in normal anatomy that must be recognized at arthroscopy so they are not mistaken for pathologic lesions.

Sublabral Foramen and the Buford Complex

As described previously, the superior half of the labrum is more loosely and variably attached to the glenoid than the inferior hemisphere. The result is the presence of sublabral foramen, either in isolation or in conjunction with other variant anatomy, in a significant percentage of patients undergoing arthroscopy (**Fig. 5**). The anterosuperior quadrant is the most common location for sublabral foramen, with incidence of 11.9% to 18.5% in shoulders undergoing arthroscopy in recent series.[32,33] These observational studies found that sublabral foramens are not independent contributors to instability, and validated the prevailing practice of ignoring them during arthroscopy, especially if they occur above the glenoid equator and are in isolation.

The Buford complex is a rare but widely recognized normal variant defined by a large anterosuperior sublabral foramen occurring in conjunction with

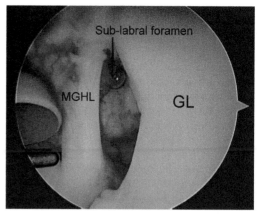

Fig. 5. Posterior viewing portal of a sublabral foramen (LEFT shoulder Beach chair position: GL, glenoid; MGHL, middle glenohumeral ligament; *arrow* points to sublabral foramen). (*Courtesy of* Center for Shoulder, Elbow and Sports Medicine, Columbia University.)

a thickened, cordlike MGHL.[34] The Buford complex can be mistaken for an anterior labral avulsion or superior labral tear when interpreted on magnetic resonance imaging (MRI), but is readily recognizable during arthroscopy because of its characteristic appearance. In 3 recent series of patients undergoing arthroscopy, the incidence of the Buford complex was noted to be 6.5% to 10.2%,[32,33,35] although a cadaveric series of 84 shoulders found the incidence to be 1.3%.[36] Most investigators agree that the Buford complex in isolation does not necessitate arthroscopic repair, but there is some evidence that this variant may occur with greater frequency in patients with superior labral anterior posterior (SLAP) tears.[37]

MGHL Variations

The MGHL is highly variable in appearance and can be absent in up to 30% to 40% of shoulders.[28,38] MGHL can originate from the anterosuperior labrum, the suprageloid tubercle, or the scapular neck. The 2 most common versions of the MGHL are the cordlike appearance with foraminal separation between it and the IGHL (**Fig. 6**) or the sheetlike variant that blends in with the anterior band of the IGHL.[13,19] The MGHL can often be detached along with the IGHL during anterior dislocation as part of the Bankart lesion. This pathologic detachment of the MGHL must be differentiated from the anatomic sublabral foramen that often occurs in close proximity to this ligament.

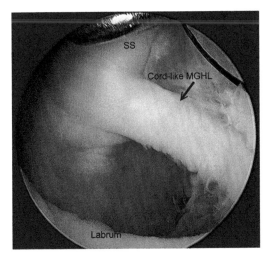

Fig. 6. Posterior viewing portal of a cordlike MGHL (LEFT Shoulder lateral decubitus position: SS, subscapularis). (*Courtesy of* Center for Shoulder, Elbow and Sports Medicine, Columbia University.)

Superior Labral Variants

The superior labrum can have great anatomic variability owing to its loose glenoid attachment and its relationship with the LHBT. Vangness and colleagues[39] described the highly variable origin of the LHBT from the superior labrum and scapula, noting 4 main types of biceps insertion that each occurred with significant frequency (the rarest type was a primarily anterior origin that occurred in 8%). The presence of a synovial recess between the biceps tendon and the superior labrum should not be mistaken for a SLAP tear, because arthroscopic inspection will reveal a firm biceps insertion.[40] Finally, a meniscoid superior labrum is a normal variant that is not associated with shoulder symptoms.[8,41]

PATHOLOGIC LESIONS
Bankart Lesion

In 1923, Bankart published his observation of labral detachment in 4 patients with recurrent instability and called this the "essential lesion."[42] More than a decade later he reported successful results on 27 patients who underwent labral reattachment.[43] The Bankart lesion now commonly refers to the detachment of the anteroinferior labrum with its attached IGHL (anterior band). The Bankart lesion can be found in up to 85% of patients with traumatic anterior shoulder dislocation, and occurs nearly 100% of the time in patients younger than 30 years.[44] There is clear experimental and clinical evidence that detachment of the anteroinferior labrum and capsule causes increased anterior humeral translation.[45]

Although the Bankart lesion cannot be directly observed on plain films, any shoulder series showing anterior dislocation should raise concern for its presence. Evaluation with MRI will demonstrate abnormal signal intensity in the inferior labrum, fraying or irregularity of the labral surface, and possibly frank displacement from the anterior glenoid rim (**Fig. 7**).[46] MRI may also reveal concomitant tears in the rotator cuff, which can occur in 80% of patients older than 60 years who suffer dislocation.[44]

At arthroscopy, detachment of the labrum from 3 to 6 o'clock (right shoulder) or 6 to 9 o'clock (left shoulder) is always pathognomonic for a Bankart lesion (**Fig. 8**).

Anterior Labroligamentous Periosteal Sleeve Avulsion

Although it has long been recognized as a distinct intra-articular lesion associated with anterior shoulder instability,[47,48] the anterior labroligamentous

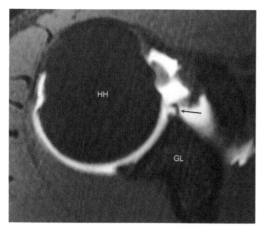

Fig. 7. Axial MRI arthrogram showing gadolinium interposed between the labrum and the glenoid indicating an anterior labral tear (HH, humeral head; GL, glenoid; *arrow* points to detached anterior labrum; note interposed gadolinium between detached labrum and glenoid). (*Courtesy of* Center for Shoulder, Elbow and Sports Medicine, Columbia University.)

periosteal sleeve avulsion (ALPSA) lesion was brought to clinical attention by Neviaser in 1993.[49] Like the classic Bankart lesion, the ALPSA lesion also involves disruption of the capsulolabral attachments at the anteroinferior glenoid. However, it is distinguished from the Bankart lesion by the presence of an intact sleeve of anterior scapular periosteum. During forceful anterior translation of the humeral head, the labrum, IGHL, and anterior scapular periosteum are stripped off their bony attachments as one sleeve-like unit, with the resulting potential space extending medially along the glenoid neck. The detached labrum becomes medially displaced and inferiorly rotated, and can be seen lying against the glenoid neck, which distinguishes it from the Bankart lesion where the detached labrum would seem to be "floating" with an obvious space between the labrum and the glenoid rim (**Fig. 9**).

Chronic ALPSA lesions are encountered in patients with recurrent instability. In these patients the displaced labrum has become adherent to the glenoid neck due to a covering of fibrous tissue that undergoes synovial transformation over time. The space between the glenoid border and the fibrosed labrum is marked by a crease that may have a variable appearance on arthroscopy. This crease must be identified because it represents the starting point for dissection of the labrum during the repair procedure.

Acute ALPSA lesions can be seen on T2 MRI coronal and axial sections, where joint fluid has appeared in the space between the detached labral-periosteal complex and the surface of the scapula. The chronic ALSPA lesion has a different appearance. On axial T2 sequences, the apparently detached labrum has become medialized on the scapular neck.[46]

A recent report by Ozbaydar and colleagues[50] suggests that ALPSA lesions may be associated with a higher risk of recurrent dislocation than Bankart lesions. In their series of 93 shoulders, the failure rate after arthroscopic repair was higher in the ALPSA group than the Bankart group. These

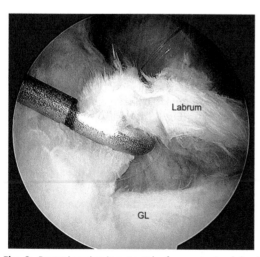

Fig. 8. Posterior viewing portal of an anterior labral tear (RIGHT shoulder lateral decubitus position: GL, glenoid; note probe pulling labral tear away from the glenoid). (*Courtesy of* Center for Shoulder, Elbow and Sports Medicine, Columbia University.)

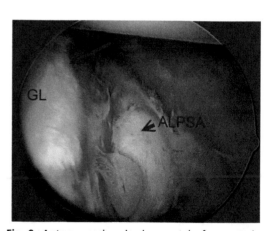

Fig. 9. Anterosuperior viewing portal of an anterior periosteal sleeve avulsion (ALPSA) injury (LEFT shoulder lateral decubitus position: GL, glenoid; ALPSA denoted by *short arrow*; *long arrow* shows position that labrum should be attached to the glenoid). (*Courtesy of* Center for Shoulder, Elbow and Sports Medicine, Columbia University.)

findings emphasize the importance of correctly identifying and treating these destabilizing lesions.

The Bony Bankart and Glenoid Bone Loss

The bony Bankart is the classic lesion plus avulsion of a portion of the anterior glenoid rim. Glenoid bone loss can also result from compression-type bony erosion seen in chronically dislocated or subluxated shoulders.[44] Either mechanism can lead to an inverted pear-shaped glenoid, which greatly predisposes to recurrent dislocation.[51] Plain films of a bony Bankart lesion will reveal a bony fragment along the inferior half of the glenoid (**Fig. 10**). Computed tomography (CT) with fine axial cuts can be used to determine the degree of glenoid bone loss, and 3-dimensional CT scanning is often obtained to better define the lesion (**Fig. 11**). The percentage of anterior glenoid bone loss can also be calculated arthroscopically by using the bare area as a central reference point.[52] Although the indications for no repair versus arthroscopic or open reconstruction are somewhat dependent on patient factors and preinjury function, a recent review suggests that most defects greater than 15% of the glenoid surface can be addressed arthroscopically while those more than 30% would probably benefit from open bony augmentation.[53]

The Hill-Sachs Lesion and Humeral Bone Loss

During anterior dislocation, a bony defect, known as a Hill-Sachs lesion, may occur on the posterolateral humeral head. The Hill-Sachs lesion is

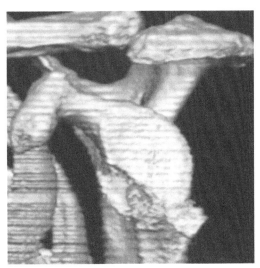

Fig. 11. 3-Dimensional sagittal CT scan of same patient from **Fig. 10** demonstrating comminuted displaced bony Bankart lesion. (*Courtesy of* Center for Shoulder, Elbow and Sports Medicine, Columbia University.)

present in more than 80% of anterior dislocations, and is nearly always found in patients undergoing arthroscopy for recurrent anterior instability.[3,54] Although a small lesion has minimal clinical significance, a Hill-Sachs lesion involving more than 30% of the humeral articular surface may contribute to recurrent anterior instability.[55] Large Hill-Sachs lesions cause recurrent dislocation when the arm is in an externally rotated position, rotating the posterior humeral impression anteriorly and thereby allowing it to engage the glenoid rim as it did during initial dislocation. The lesion may be readily viewed on plain films with the axillary view. Visualization with CT scan, however, is most useful for quantifying the size of the Hill-Sachs lesion, which is expressed as a percentage of the humeral articular surface (**Fig. 12**).

Small lesions can often be ignored and the instability managed arthroscopically. Large lesions, however, may require reconstruction with allograft bony augmentation, partial resurfacing arthroplasty, or humeral head replacement.[56,57]

Humeral Avulsion of the Glenohumeral Ligaments

In 1942 Nicola[58] first described capsular avulsion from the neck of the humerus in 4 out of 5 cases of acute dislocation. Bach and colleagues[59] confirmed the presence of humeral-sided ligament disruption in patients with recurrent dislocation and suggested that this injury should be

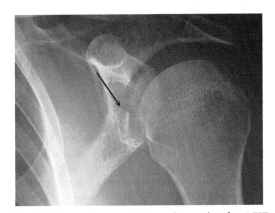

Fig. 10. True anteroposterior radiograph of a LEFT shoulder demonstrates bony Bankart lesion (Ideberg 1A) in a man aged 25 years following a bicycle accident (*arrow* indicates displaced fracture). (*Courtesy of* Center for Shoulder, Elbow and Sports Medicine, Columbia University.)

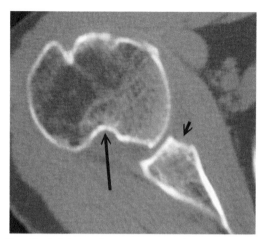

Fig. 12. Axial CT of a woman aged 67 years who suffered a first-time dislocation, and has a large Hill-Sachs deformity (*long arrow*) and a displaced bony Bankart lesion (*short arrow*). (*Courtesy of* Center for Shoulder, Elbow and Sports Medicine, Columbia University.)

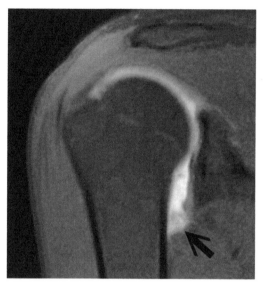

Fig. 13. Coronal T2 RIGHT shoulder of a man aged 23 years with recurrent anterior instability demonstrates an HAGL (humeral avulsion of glenohumeral ligament) lesion (*arrow*). (*Courtesy of* Center for Shoulder, Elbow and Sports Medicine, Columbia University.)

suspected in shoulders with minimal injury to the glenoid labrum. Bigliani and colleagues[60] demonstrated this lesion in the laboratory and found that failure occurred at the humeral insertion site 25% of the time.

In a larger case series of 64 shoulders, Wolf and colleagues[61] noted 6 patients with humeral capsular avulsions, all of whom underwent surgical repair (2 open, 4 arthroscopically) with resolution of instability and return to full range of shoulder motion. Wolf and colleagues coined the humeral avulsion of the glenohumeral ligaments (HAGL) lesion, and noted that it involved the humeral insertion of the IGHL with possible extension into a portion of the MGHL. The 2 largest case series in the literature report the incidence of HAGL lesions in shoulders with instability to be 7.8% to 9.3%, making it necessary to routinely evaluate for this lesion during diagnostic arthroscopy.[61,62] The HAGL lesion can occur in isolation or in combination with other intra-articular pathologic conditions, including Bankart and Hill-Sachs lesions, rotator cuff tears, and subscapularis tears.[63–67]

MRI coronal sequences will reveal markedly increased T2 signal intensity between the capsule and humeral neck, with the humeral insertion of the IGHL detached and floating freely in a pool of joint fluid and edema (**Fig. 13**).[46]

Superior Labrum Anterior and Posterior Lesions

The earliest report of superior labral tears was made by Andrews and colleagues[68] in 1985 in a series of 73 overhead throwing athletes. In 1990, Snyder and colleagues[69] classified these lesions into 4 types and coined the term SLAP for superior labral lesions that began posteriorly and extended anteriorly to include the origin of the long head of the biceps. The incidence of SLAP lesions was only 1.2% of 585 consecutive patients in a 3-year period in Warner's series, and was less than 4% in Snyder's original series.[69,70] However, the SLAP lesion is more common among patients with chronic shoulder instability and can occur in conjunction with other capsulolabral lesions, especially the Bankart lesion.[71,72] This led Maffet and colleagues[73] to extend the classification system to include 3 more types, the most common of which was type V, representing a SLAP tear in continuity with a Bankart lesion.

Oblique coronal MRI sections best visualize the superior labrum and biceps origin. Various signal abnormalities can include fraying or irregularity of the labral surface, high signal intensity within the labrum, and avulsion of the labrum away from the glenoid. Higher-grade lesions may reveal displacement of the labral fragment or extension of abnormal signal into the biceps anchor (**Fig. 14**). MRI findings can be roughly correlated with the different types of SLAP lesions.[46]

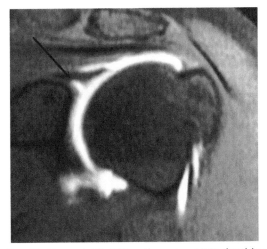

Fig. 14. Coronal T2 MRI arthrogram LEFT shoulder demonstrates a SLAP tear (*arrow*). Note the dye "turning the corner," indicating pathologic displacement of the superior labrum from the glenoid. (*Courtesy of* Center for Shoulder, Elbow and Sports Medicine, Columbia University.)

Glenolabral Articular Disruption Lesions

Coined by Neviaser in 1993,[74] the glenolabral articular disruption (GLAD) lesion is caused by a forced adduction injury to the shoulder from an abducted and externally rotated position. Neviaser observed that all 5 patients had normal arthrograms and no clinical evidence of anterior instability, yet all complained primarily of anterior

shoulder pain. Some patients had evidence of labral tears with CT or MRI. Arthroscopic findings were significant for a superficial anteroinferior labral tear, while the deep fibers of the anterior IGHL remained strongly attached to the labrum and glenoid, thus explaining the lack of anterior instability. There was a varying degree of glenoid articular cartilage damage in the anteroinferior quadrant, down to subchondral bone in the most severe case (**Fig. 15**). All patients in his series were successfully treated with arthroscopic debridement of the labrum and chondral defect.[74]

SUMMARY

The management of shoulder instability requires a thorough knowledge of the normal anatomic structures that maintain stability. Normal variants must not be confused with pathologic entities during arthroscopic examination. Various pathologic lesions can predispose the patient to recurrent instability, and these must be addressed during arthroscopic stabilization to maximize the chances of reestablishing preinjury shoulder function. Large bony defects on the glenoid or humeral side should be diagnosed and quantified preoperatively, because arthroscopic soft tissue procedures may not be sufficient to prevent recurrent instability.

REFERENCES

1. Mok DW, Fogg AJ, Hokan R, et al. The diagnostic value of arthroscopy in glenohumeral instability. J Bone Joint Surg Br 1990;72(4):698–700.
2. Hintermann B, Gachter A. Arthroscopic findings after shoulder dislocation. Am J Sports Med 1995; 23(5):545–51.
3. Norlin R. Intraarticular pathology in acute, first-time anterior shoulder dislocation: an arthroscopic study. Arthroscopy 1993;9(5):546–9.
4. Baker CL, Uribe JW, Whitman C. Arthroscopic evaluation of acute initial anterior shoulder dislocations. Am J Sports Med 1990;18(1):25–8.
5. Hovelius L, Augustini BG, Fredin H, et al. Primary anterior dislocation of the shoulder in young patients. A ten-year prospective study. J Bone Joint Surg Am 1996;78(11):1677–84.
6. Kralinger FS, Golser K, Wischatta R, et al. Predicting recurrence after primary anterior shoulder dislocation. Am J Sports Med 2002;30(1):116–20.
7. Robinson CM, Jenkins PJ, White TO, et al. Primary arthroscopic stabilization for a first-time anterior dislocation of the shoulder. A randomized, double-blind trial. J Bone Joint Surg Am 2008; 90(4):708–21.

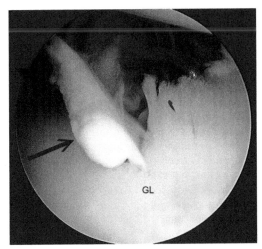

Fig. 15. Posterior viewing portal of a GLAD (glenolabral articular disruption) lesion (*arrow* indicates disrupted articular cartilage) (RIGHT shoulder lateral decubitus position). (*Courtesy of* Center for Shoulder, Elbow and Sports Medicine, Columbia University.)

8. O'brien SJ, Arnoczky SP, Warren RF, et al. Developmental anatomy of the shoulder and anatomy of the glenohumeral joint. In: Rockwood CA, Matsen FA, editors. The shoulder. Philadelphia: Saunders; 1990. p. 1–33.

9. Cooper DE, Arnoczky SP, O'brien SJ, et al. Anatomy, histology, and vascularity of the glenoid labrum. An anatomical study. J Bone Joint Surg Am 1992; 74(1):46–52.

10. Howell SM, Galinat BJ. The glenoid-labral socket. A constrained articular surface. Clin Orthop Relat Res 1989;243:122–5.

11. Soslowsky LJ, Flatow EL, Bigliani LU, et al. Quantitation of in situ contact areas at the glenohumeral joint: a biomechanical study. J Orthop Res 1992;10(4): 524–34.

12. Harryman DT 2nd, Sidles JA, Harris SL, et al. The role of the rotator interval capsule in passive motion and stability of the shoulder. J Bone Joint Surg Am 1992;74(1):53–66.

13. Cole BJ, Rios CG, Mazzocca AD, et al. Anatomy, biomechanics, and pathophysiology of glenohumeral instability. In: Iannotti JP, Williams GR, editors. Disorders of the shoulder: diagnosis & management. 2nd edition. Philadelphia: Lippincott Williams & Wilkins; 2007. p. 289.

14. Harryman DT 2nd, Sidles JA, Clark JM, et al. Translation of the humeral head on the glenoid with passive glenohumeral motion. J Bone Joint Surg Am 1990;72(9):1334–43.

15. Basmajian JV, Bazant FJ. Factors preventing downward dislocation of the adducted shoulder joint. An electromyographic and morphological study. J Bone Joint Surg Am 1959;41:1182–6.

16. Warner JJ, Micheli LJ, Arslanian LE, et al. Patterns of flexibility, laxity, and strength in normal shoulders and shoulders with instability and impingement. Am J Sports Med 1990;18(4):366–75.

17. Turkel SJ, Panio MW, Marshall JL, et al. Stabilizing mechanisms preventing anterior dislocation of the glenohumeral joint. J Bone Joint Surg Am 1981; 63(8):1208–17.

18. O'connell PW, Nuber GW, Mileski RA, et al. The contribution of the glenohumeral ligaments to anterior stability of the shoulder joint. Am J Sports Med 1990;18(6):579–84.

19. O'Brien SJ, Neves MC, Arnoczky SP, et al. The anatomy and histology of the inferior glenohumeral ligament complex of the shoulder. Am J Sports Med 1990;18(5):449–56.

20. Ticker JB, Bigliani LU, Soslowsky LJ, et al. Inferior glenohumeral ligament: geometric and strain-rate dependent properties. J Shoulder Elbow Surg 1996;5(4):269–79.

21. Warner JJ, Deng XH, Warren RF, et al. Static capsuloligamentous restraints to superior-inferior translation of the glenohumeral joint. Am J Sports Med 1992;20(6):675–85.

22. O'brien SJ, Schwartz RS, Warren RF, et al. Capsular restraints to anterior-posterior motion of the abducted shoulder: a biomechanical study. J Shoulder Elbow Surg 1995;4(4):298–308.

23. Bigliani LU, Kelkar R, Flatow EL, et al. Glenohumeral stability. Biomechanical properties of passive and active stabilizers. Clin Orthop Relat Res 1996;330: 13–30.

24. Lippitt S, Matsen F. Mechanisms of glenohumeral joint stability. Clin Orthop Relat Res 1993;291:20–8.

25. Bowen M, Deng X, Warner J, et al. The effect of joint compression on stability of the glenohumeral joint. Trans Orthop Res Soc 1992;38:289.

26. Hsu HC, Luo ZP, Cofield RH, et al. Influence of rotator cuff tearing on glenohumeral stability. J Shoulder Elbow Surg 1997;6(5):413–22.

27. Clark J, Sidles JA, Matsen FA. The relationship of the glenohumeral joint capsule to the rotator cuff. Clin Orthop Relat Res 1990;254:29–34.

28. Ferrari DA. Capsular ligaments of the shoulder. Anatomical and functional study of the anterior superior capsule. Am J Sports Med 1990;18(1):20–4.

29. Rodosky MW, Harner CD, Fu FH. The role of the long head of the biceps muscle and superior glenoid labrum in anterior stability of the shoulder. Am J Sports Med 1994;22(1):121–30.

30. Pagnani MJ, Deng XH, Warren RF, et al. Effect of lesions of the superior portion of the glenoid labrum on glenohumeral translation. J Bone Joint Surg Am 1995;77(7):1003–10.

31. Kim SH, Ha KI, Kim HS, et al. Electromyographic activity of the biceps brachii muscle in shoulders with anterior instability. Arthroscopy 2001;17(8): 864–8.

32. Rao AG, Kim TK, Chronopoulos E, et al. Anatomical variants in the anterosuperior aspect of the glenoid labrum: a statistical analysis of seventy-three cases. J Bone Joint Surg Am 2003;85(4):653–9.

33. Ilahi OA, Labbe MR, Cosculluela P. Variants of the anterosuperior glenoid labrum and associated pathology. Arthroscopy 2002;18(8):882–6.

34. Williams MM, Snyder SJ, Buford D Jr. The Buford complex—the "cord-like" middle glenohumeral ligament and absent anterosuperior labrum complex: a normal anatomic capsulolabral variant. Arthroscopy 1994;10(3):241–7.

35. Ilahi OA, Cosculluela PE, Ho DM. Classification of anterosuperior glenoid labrum variants and their association with shoulder pathology. Orthopedics 2008;31(3):226.

36. Ide J, Maeda S, Takagi K. Normal variations of the glenohumeral ligament complex: an anatomic study for arthroscopic Bankart repair. Arthroscopy 2004; 20(2):164–8.

37. Bents RT, Skeete KD. The correlation of the Buford complex and slap lesions. J Shoulder Elbow Surg 2005;14(6):565–9.

38. Plausinis D, Jazrawi LM, Zuckerman JD, et al. Anatomy and biomechanics of the shoulder. In: Schepsis AA, Busconi BD, editors. Sports medicine. Philadelphia: Lippincott Williams and Wilkins; 2006. p. 180.

39. Vangsness CT, Jorgenson SS, Watson T, et al. The origin of the long head of the biceps from the scapula and glenoid labrum. An anatomical study of 100 shoulders. J Bone Joint Surg Br 1994;76(6): 951–4.

40. Levine WN, Flatow EL. The pathophysiology of shoulder instability. Am J Sports Med 2000;28(6): 910–7.

41. Lee SB, Harryman DT 2nd. Superior detachment of a glenoid labrum variant resembling an incomplete discoid meniscus in a wheelchair ambulator. Arthroscopy 1997;13(4):511–4.

42. Bankart ASB. Recurrent or habitual dislocation of the shoulder-joint. Br Med J 1923;II:1132–3.

43. Bankart ASB. The pathology and treatment of recurrent dislocation of the shoulder joint. Br J Surg 1938; 26(26):23–9.

44. Bicos J, Mazzocca AD, Arciero RA. Anterior instability of the shoulder. In: Schepsis AA, Busconi BD, editors. Sports medicine. Philadelphia: Lippincott Williams and Wilkins; 2006. p. 215, 218.

45. Matsen FA, Thomas SC, Rockwood CA. Glenohumeral instability. In: Rockwood CA, Matsen FA, editors. The shoulder. 2nd edition. Philadelphia: Saunders; 1990. p. 633–9.

46. Sanders TG, Miller MD. A systematic approach to magnetic resonance imaging interpretation of sports medicine injuries of the shoulder. Am J Sports Med 2005;33(7):1088–105.

47. Broca A, Hartmann H. Contribution à l'étude des luxations de l'épaule (luxations dites incomplètes, décollements periostiques, luxations directes et luxations indirections). Bull Soc Anat Paris 1890;4: 312–36.

48. Mclaughlin H. Recurrent anterior dislocation of the shoulder. Am J Surg 1960;99:628–32.

49. Neviaser TJ. The anterior labroligamentous periosteal sleeve avulsion lesion: a cause of anterior instability of the shoulder. Arthroscopy 1993;9(1):17–21.

50. Ozbaydar M, Elhassan B, Diller D, et al. Results of arthroscopic capsulolabral repair: Bankart lesion versus anterior labroligamentous periosteal sleeve avulsion lesion. Arthroscopy 2008;24(11): 1277–83.

51. Burkhart SS, De Beer JF. Traumatic glenohumeral bone defects and their relationship to failure of arthroscopic Bankart repairs: significance of the inverted-pear glenoid and the humeral engaging Hill-Sachs lesion. Arthroscopy 2000;16(7):677–94.

52. Lo IK, Parten PM, Burkhart SS. The inverted pear glenoid: an indicator of significant glenoid bone loss. Arthroscopy 2004;20(2):169–74.

53. Piasecki DP, Verma NN, Romeo AA, et al. Glenoid bone deficiency in recurrent anterior shoulder instability: diagnosis and management. J Am Acad Orthop Surg 2009;17(8):482–93.

54. Calandra JJ, Baker CL, Uribe J. The incidence of Hill-Sachs lesions in initial anterior shoulder dislocations. Arthroscopy 1989;5(4):254–7.

55. Rowe CR, Sakellarides HT. Factors related to recurrences of anterior dislocations of the shoulder. Clin Orthop 1961;20:40–8.

56. Gerber C, Lambert SM. Allograft reconstruction of segmental defects of the humeral head for the treatment of chronic locked posterior dislocation of the shoulder. J Bone Joint Surg Am 1996; 78(3):376–82.

57. Weber BG, Simpson LA, Hardegger F. Rotational humeral osteotomy for recurrent anterior dislocation of the shoulder associated with a large Hill-Sachs lesion. J Bone Joint Surg Am 1984;66(9): 1443–50.

58. Nicola T. Anterior dislocation of the shoulder: the role of the articular capsule. J Bone Joint Surg Am 1942; 25:614–6.

59. Bach BR, Warren RF, Fronek J. Disruption of the lateral capsule of the shoulder. a cause of recurrent dislocation. J Bone Joint Surg Br 1988;70(2): 274–6.

60. Bigliani LU, Pollock RG, Soslowsky LJ, et al. Tensile properties of the inferior glenohumeral ligament. J Orthop Res 1992;10(2):187–97.

61. Wolf EM, Cheng JC, Dickson K. Humeral avulsion of glenohumeral ligaments as a cause of anterior shoulder instability. Arthroscopy 1995; 11(5):600–7.

62. Bokor DJ, Conboy VB, Olson C. Anterior instability of the glenohumeral joint with humeral avulsion of the glenohumeral ligament. A review of 41 cases. J Bone Joint Surg Br 1999;81(1):93–6.

63. Rhee YG, Cho NS. Anterior shoulder instability with humeral avulsion of the glenohumeral ligament lesion. J Shoulder Elbow Surg 2007; 16(2):188–92.

64. Bui-Mansfield LT, Banks KP, Taylor DC. Humeral avulsion of the glenohumeral ligaments: the Hagl lesion. Am J Sports Med 2007;35(11):1960–6.

65. Schippinger G, Vasiu PS, Fankhauser F, et al. Hagl lesion occurring after successful arthroscopic Bankart repair. Arthroscopy 2001;17(2):206–8.

66. Warner JJ, Beim GM. Combined Bankart and Hagl lesion associated with anterior shoulder instability. Arthroscopy 1997;13(6):749–52.

67. Field LD, Bokor DJ, Savoie FH 3rd. Humeral and glenoid detachment of the anterior inferior

glenohumeral ligament: a cause of anterior shoulder instability. J Shoulder Elbow Surg 1997; 6(1):6–10.

68. Andrews JR, Carson WG Jr, McLeod WD. Glenoid labrum tears related to the long head of the biceps. Am J Sports Med 1985;13(5):337–41.

69. Snyder SJ, Karzel RP, Del Pizzo W, et al. Slap lesions of the shoulder. Arthroscopy 1990;6(4):274–9.

70. Warner JJ, Kann S, Marks P. Arthroscopic repair of combined Bankart and superior labral detachment anterior and posterior lesions: technique and preliminary results. Arthroscopy 1994;10(4):383–91.

71. Yiannakopoulos CK, Mataragas E, Antonogiannakis E. A comparison of the spectrum of intra-articular lesions in acute and chronic anterior shoulder instability. Arthroscopy 2007;23(9):985–90.

72. Snyder SJ, Banas MP, Karzel RP. An analysis of 140 injuries to the superior glenoid labrum. J Shoulder Elbow Surg 1995;4(4):243–8.

73. Maffet MW, Gartsman GM, Moseley B. Superior labrum-biceps tendon complex lesions of the shoulder. Am J Sports Med 1995;23(1):93–8.

74. Neviaser TJ. The glad lesion: another cause of anterior shoulder pain. Arthroscopy 1993;9(1):22–3.

Management of the Throwing Shoulder: Cuff, Labrum and Internal Impingement

R. Michael Greiwe, MD[a], Christopher S. Ahmad, MD[a],*

KEYWORDS

- Shoulder • Throwing-related injury
- Glenohumeral ligament • Cuff impingement
- Labrum impingement • Internal impingement

Repetitive throwing places the shoulder in extreme positions in combination with tremendous stresses. In fact, professional pitchers generate up to 92 N·m of humeral rotation torque, greater than the torsional failure limit in human cadaveric shoulders.[1] Throwers are therefore constantly at risk for injury.

Preventing injury begins with maintenance of the "kinetic chain" that coordinates transmission of force from the legs and trunk to the upper extremity. Studies show that muscle imbalances in the "kinetic chain" are common in shoulder impingement,[2–4] rotator cuff tears,[4,5] and instability.[5,6] One study reported that throwers with labral tears commonly have back inflexibility, infraspinatus and teres minor weakness, and core weakness.[7] Injuries to the foot and ankle, tightness of the muscles crossing the hip and knee, weakness of hip abductors and trunk stabilizers, and conditions altering spine alignment influence kinetic chain transmission.

Kinetic chain abnormalities can cause the shoulder to assume a hyperabducted, externally rotated position that moves the arm out of the "safe zone" of glenohumeral angulation described by Pink and Perry.[8] Violent acceleration from hyperabduction increases compressive and shear forces on the glenoid, capsulolabral complex, and rotator cuff. This motion can injure the posterior capsule, damage and peel the labrum off the glenoid, tear and delaminate the rotator cuff, and tear and stretch the anterior restraints.

The phases of the baseball pitch have been extensively studied (**Fig. 1**). During wind-up, hip stability allows proper balance in preparation for the early cocking, when the hips drive toward home plate. Early cocking ends as the lead foot lands and decelerates the driving lower extremity and trunk. Flaws during this stage include opening up, or abduction of the lead leg, causing poor pelvis rotation with consequent loss of velocity and increased anterior shoulder strain.[9,10] Most injured pitchers experience pain during the late cocking phase, when the throwing humerus externally rotates from roughly 45° to 170°. During this time, the periscapular muscles, including the trapezius, rhomboids, levator scapula, and serratus anterior, stabilize the scapula, which functions as a fulcrum for energy transfer from the lower extremity and trunk to the humerus.

Periscapular muscle weakness also contributes to shoulder injury.[11] To compensate for diminished serratus anterior strength, the thrower may drop the elbow, thus decreasing the degree of scapular rotation and elevation needed. If the pathologic process continues, the player may attempt to compensate further by moving the humerus behind the scapular plane worsening

[a] Department of Orthopaedic Surgery, Center for Shoulder, Elbow, and Sports Medicine, Columbia-Presbyterian Hospital, Columbia University, 622 West 168th Street, PH-11-Center, New York, NY 10032, USA
* Corresponding author.
E-mail address: csa4@columbia.edu

Orthop Clin N Am 41 (2010) 309–323
doi:10.1016/j.ocl.2010.03.001
0030-5898/10/$ – see front matter © 2010 Elsevier Inc. All rights reserved.

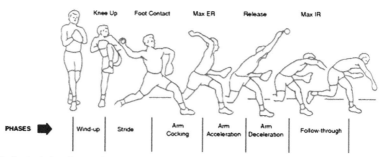

Fig. 1. The baseball pitch has been divided into six phases: wind-up, early cocking, late cocking, acceleration, deceleration, and follow-through. (*From* DiGiovine NM, Jobe FW, Pink M, et al. An electromyographic analysis of the upper extremity in pitching. J Shoulder Elbow Surg 1992;1(1):16; with permission.)

hyperabduction. Eccentric contraction of the subscapularis muscle then decelerates the externally rotating humerus, preparing it for acceleration.

In acceleration, the humerus reaches maximal external rotation and the lower extremity and trunk energy is transferred through the shoulder to the elbow and wrist as the body falls forward. Just before ball release, the arm internally rotates 80°, reaching peak angular velocities near 7000° per second. Within 0.05 seconds, the ball is released with speeds exceeding 90 mph.[12] If the thrower opens up too quickly, positioning the elbow behind the plane of the scapula, the glenohumeral joint hyperangulates, resulting in more pronounced internal impingement.

In deceleration and follow-through in a right-hander, the ball is released and the right hip rises up and over the left leg. During this phase, the teres minor, infraspinatus, and scapular rotator muscles eccentrically contract, dissipating unused kinetic energy. The glenohumeral distraction force absorbed by the capsule and posterior rotator cuff reaches 1 to 1.5 times the thrower's body weight.[13] Eccentric contraction by the scapular rotators continue to decelerate the arm, and the posterior capsule experiences tension as the arm adducts.

ASYMPTOMATIC THROWING SHOULDER ADAPTATION
Overall Motion

The dominant shoulder of a thrower exhibits increased external rotation and diminished internal rotation compared with the contralateral arm.[14–21] In asymptomatic throwers, the total arc of shoulder motion is maintained but shifted by 10° into external rotation.[22–24]

Adaptations in bone and soft tissue are responsible for increased external rotation. Crockett and colleagues[25] showed that professional pitchers show 17° greater humeral retroversion in their throwing shoulder compared with their

nondominant shoulder. During development, humeral retroversion decreases from 78° to 30°, and repetitive throwing during growth is hypothesized to restrict this physiologic derotation.[26–29] Soft tissue adaptations also occur. The anterior capsule and glenohumeral ligaments become lax, whereas the posterior capsule and glenohumeral ligaments stiffen. Repetitive microtrauma to the anterior capsule, particularly during the cocking phase of throwing, leads to anterior laxity and more external rotation.[16–18]

Injury Patterns

The typical motions and forces around the glenohumeral joint during throwing lead to predictable injury patterns. Superior labral tears are frequent and commonly extend into the posterosuperior labrum. The posterior supraspinatus and anterior infraspinatus are usually partially torn with occasional intratendinous delamination. Andrews and colleagues[30] noted that labral tears were present in 100% of 36 competitive athletes with articular-sided partial-thickness rotator cuff tears, of whom 64% were baseball pitchers. In addition, the anterior capsule may become pathologically lax and the posterior capsule pathologically contracted.

Although the injury patterns are consistent, the exact mechanism is debated. Andrews and colleagues[30] originally theorized that articular-sided tears resulted from repetitive large eccentric forces to the supraspinatus and infraspinatus tendons during the deceleration phase of throwing. Davidson and colleagues[31] hypothesized that repetitive contact between the articular side of the rotator cuff and the posterosuperior glenoid in late cocking caused tears. This pathology is aggravated by anterior subluxation and instability, particularly when dynamic stabilizers fatigue. Burkhart and colleagues[32] proposed that the primary cause of rotator cuff and labral lesions was posterior capsular contracture, leading to posterosuperior migration of the humeral head. This article describes the leading theories.

Internal impingement theory

Walch and colleagues[33] initially described internal impingement as occurring in the 90° abducted and 90° externally rotated position. In this position, the posterosuperior rotator cuff contacts the posterosuperior glenoid labrum and can be pinched between the labrum and greater tuberosity (**Fig. 2**). Although physiologic in a static position, forceful and repeated contact of the undersurface of the rotator cuff and the superior labrum during overhead activity can explain the development of partial-thickness rotator cuff tears and superior labrum anterior posterior (SLAP) lesions,[17,31,33–35] which commonly coexist in throwers. In addition, kinetic chain abnormalities previously described can exacerbate this process when throwers compensate for poor mechanics through "opening up" or hyperangulating the arm.

Posterior capsular contracture theory

Burkhart and colleagues[36] proposed posterior capsular contracture as a consequence of throwing. They reasoned that the posterior capsule must withstand tensile forces of up to 750 N during the deceleration and follow-through phases of throwing. These posterior tensile forces are resisted by both the eccentric contraction of the rotator cuff, primarily the infraspinatus, and the posteroinferior capsule (posterior band of the inferior glenohumeral ligament [IGHL]). With repetitive infraspinatus eccentric contraction, the muscle and the posteroinferior capsule become

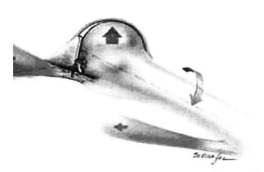

Fig. 2. Internal impingement results in the 90° abducted, 90° externally rotated position when the posterosuperior rotator cuff presses against the posterosuperior glenoid labrum. (*From* Jobe CM, Pink M, Jobe FW, et al. Anterior shoulder instability, impingement, and rotator cuff tear. In: Jobe FW, Pink MM, Glousman RE, et al, editors. Operative techniques in upper extremity sports injuries. St Louis (MO): Mosby; 1996. p. 170 with permission.)

hypertrophied and stiff. The posterior contracture shifts the center of rotation of the shoulder to a more posterosuperior location, creating posterosuperior instability with shoulder in abduction and external rotation, which has been supported by biomechanical cadaver research.[37] The humeral head can consequently externally hyperrotate, producing increased shear in the rotator cuff tendon and more pronounced internal impingement. In addition, a peel-back phenomenon occurring during late cocking, consisting of a torsional force applied to the biceps anchor, contributes to SLAP lesion development.[38]

Scapulothoracic function

The scapula plays a critical role in energy transfer from the trunk to the humerus. In the asymptomatic thrower, adaptive scapulothoracic changes leading to scapular asymmetry have been described.[21,39–42] Altered static and dynamic scapular mechanics arise from overuse and weakness of scapular stabilizers and posterior rotator cuff muscles.[13] With the arm hanging at the side, the throwing shoulder's scapula has increased upward rotation (abduction), internal rotation (protraction), antetilting in the sagittal plane and inferior translation. During cocking, when the humerus is terminally externally rotated and abducted, upward scapular rotation helps maintain glenohumeral articular congruency.[42] Weakness, inflexibility, or imbalance of the periscapular and posterior rotator cuff muscles disturb the normal anatomic static and dynamic relationships of the scapula. Aberrant scapulothoracic motion has been called *scapular dyskenesis*.[39,43] The abnormally positioned thrower's scapula has been labeled SICK (scapular malposition, inferior medial border prominence, coracoid pain, and dyskinesis of scapular movement) scapula by Burkhart and colleagues.[44]

The SICK scapula predisposes the shoulder to labral and rotator cuff tears because the scapula sits in a protracted and upwardly tilted position, causing the glenoid to face anterior and superior. This position leads to three developments: anterior tension, posterior compression, and increased glenohumeral angulation. First, with glenoid protraction, the anterior band of the IGHL tightens, limiting anterior translation of the humeral head and, over time, becoming susceptible to chronic strain.[6] Second, simultaneously, the posterior edge of the glenoid is brought toward the humerus, placing the posterosuperior labrum and rotator cuff at risk for injury. Finally, excessive protraction increases glenohumeral angulation. The thrower with increased glenohumeral angulation will find that the "arm lags behind the body." Excessive external rotation in this setting has two harmful consequences. One, it exacerbates the aforementioned biceps peel back effect.[44] Two, with preexisting scapular protraction, external rotation and abduction produce posterosuperior glenoid impingement.[39,40]

A cascade of pathologic entities explain injuries associated with the SICK scapula: coracoid pain from pectoralis minor contracture and tendinopathy, superior medial angle scapular pain from levator scapula insertional tendinopathy, subacromial origin pain from acromial malposition and decreased subacromial space from upward tilting, acromioclavicular joint pain caused by anterior joint incongruity, sternoclavicular pain, thoracic outlet syndrome radicular pain, and subclavian vascular problems such as arterial pseudoaneurysm or venous thrombosis.[13]

In summary, anterior instability, posterior capsular contracture, and internal impingement in throwers are influenced by alterations in the kinetic chain and scapulothoracic thoracic function. Shoulder pathology should be viewed as a syndrome because the injury cascade is a continuum of interrelated pathomechanics. Although when viewed independently some of the current popular theories on the cause of specific throwing-related shoulder injuries may conflict, they complement each other when they are considered elements of a pathologic continuum.

EVALUATION OF THE OVERHEAD ATHLETE
History

A wide variety of disorders may present in the thrower, including those that affect the kinetic chain such as the hip, core, and low back. The goal should be to accurately diagnose and efficiently direct treatment. Initial symptoms may be vague, such as loss of control, velocity, or difficulty warming up. Typical shoulder-related symptoms include anterosuperior or posterosuperior shoulder pain in the late cocking phase. Popping, locking, and snapping may occur with unstable labral tears. Instability symptoms may be related to rotator cuff dysfunction and excessive anterior capsular laxity.

Physical Examination

A systematic physical examination should be performed to assess the knee, hip, and low back. Functional movement may be assessed with single leg squats for hip and trunk control, muscle imbalance, and inflexibilities.

Muscular atrophy and scapular winging should be noted. Tenderness should be assessed at glenohumeral joint lines, the acromioclavicular joint, the long head of the biceps tendon, and the coracoid process. Tenderness over the long head of the biceps tendon suggests tendonitis or a SLAP tear. Coracoid process tenderness suggests pectoralis minor tendonitis or tightness, which has been correlated with scapular protraction and dyskenesis.[44]

Active and passive range of motion of the glenohumeral and scapulothoracic joints are measured. Forward elevation in the plane of the scapula, external rotation, and internal rotation (in 0° of abduction, this is the highest spinal level the patient can reach with thumb behind the back) in both 0° and 90° of abduction should be documented. Kibler[39] measured scapular asymmetry through comparing the distance from the inferior angle of the scapula to the spinous process of the thoracic vertebra in the same horizontal plane (the reference vertebra) in three test positions. In position one, the arm is at the side. In position two, the humerus is internally rotated and abducted 45°, as the hands are placed on the hips. In position three, the shoulder is abducted further to 90°. An asymmetrical difference of greater than 1.5 cm determines a positive lateral scapular slide test (LSST).[39]

With the scapular assistance test, scapular upward rotation is assisted through manually stabilizing the upper medial scapular border and rotating the inferomedial border as the arm is abducted. A positive test will relieve symptoms of impingement, clicking, or rotator cuff weakness present without the manual assistance. The scapular retraction test is performed through manually stabilizing the medial border of the scapula. When manual stabilization increases strength in patients with apparent rotator cuff weakness and a protracted scapula, scapular dyskenesia is present.

Manual muscle strength testing should aim to isolate the muscle being tested and compare the injured with the contralateral, uninjured side. The supraspinatus can be isolated in the "empty can" position. The subscapularis is best assessed using the "lift off" test,[45] or the internal rotation lag sign, which is more sentsitive.[46]

A proper examination assesses range of motion of both shoulders in both adduction and 90° of abduction. An overhead athlete will typically have reduced internal rotation and increased external rotation. The Jobe's relocation test is also a provocative maneuver that reproduces the symptoms of internal impingement. In this test, the patient is supine and the arm is placed into 90° of abduction and 10° of forward flexion, and the shoulder is forced anteriorly. Pain represents a positive test. Pain subsequently subsides with a posteriorly directed force.[17]

Many tests have been described to assist in diagnosing SLAP lesions. The active compression test has good sensitivity and specificity for type II SLAP lesions.[47] The arm is positioned in 15° of adduction and 90° of forward elevation. The examiner applies downward force on the forearm while the hand is both pronated and supinated, and compares the resulting pain and weakness. A positive test occurs when the patient reports pain that is worse in the pronated position. The compression–rotation test is similar to McMurray's test of the knee.[48] It is performed through compressing the glenohumeral joint and then rotating the humerus in an attempt to trap the labrum in the joint. This test should be performed in the supine position, so that the patient is more relaxed.

Speed's biceps tension test is also sensitive for SLAP lesions.[49,50] This test is performed through having the patient resist downward pressure with the arm in 90° of forward elevation, with the elbow extended and the forearm supinated. Although this test is more suggestive of biceps tendon damage, an unstable biceps anchor will cause the test to elicit pain. A positive apprehension relocation sign for posterior shoulder pain may suggest a SLAP lesion in the posterior labrum as part of a spectrum of internal impingement.

Many other tests have been described, but the authors have found them to be less useful.[51–53] Finally, external impingement should be assessed with impingement tests such as the Neer and Hawkins tests.

Imaging

Radiographic evaluation includes the standard three views of the shoulder (anteroposterior, axillary, and outlet views) to help exclude other bony abnormalities. MRI-enhanced arthrography outperforms plain MRI when diagnosing SLAP lesions with sensitivity of 89%, a specificity of 91%, and an accuracy of 90%.[54] The diagnostic feature of the MR arthrogram is contrast between the superior labrum and the glenoid that extends around and under the biceps anchor on the coronal oblique view (**Fig. 3**). The axial views visualize possible extension into the anterior and or posterior labrum. Partial thickness rotator cuff tears will also be identified (see **Fig. 3**).

Some experts have recommended MRI with the shoulder in both the abducted and abducted and externally rotated position.[55] These views may further enhance visualization of the articular side of the rotator cuff and superior glenoid, and may

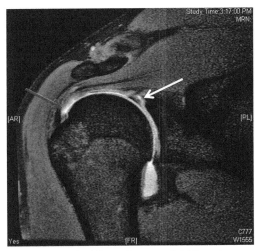

Fig. 3. Coronal oblique image of MRI arthrogram showing a superior labral tear (*white arrow*) with dye tracking into the space between glenoid and labrum, and a partial-thickness rotator cuff tear (*red arrow*). (*Courtesy of* Columbia University, Department of Orthopaedic Surgery, New York, NY; with permission.)

be helpful in diagnosing delaminating tears of the rotator cuff.[56] Up to 40% of professional pitchers have completely asymptomatic partial articular-sided supraspinatus tendon avulsion (PASTA) lesions.[57]

MANAGEMENT OF SPECIFIC SHOULDER CONDITIONS IN ATHLETES
Nonoperative Treatment

Nonoperative treatment is directed at all observed pathology, such as correcting lower extremity, hip, core, and low back disorders, in addition to scapular function, restoring shoulder range of motion, strength, and flexibility. Several phases of rehabilitation can be used, progressing from inflammation reduction, to range of motion restoration, muscle strengthening, and soft tissue flexibility, and finishing with proprioception and neuromuscular control and a comprehensive return to throwing program. Although nonoperative treatment strategies have been presented comprehensively in other sources,[21,58] the following discussion focuses on several important pathologic features.

Correction of pathologic posterior capsular contracture is critical. Nonoperative management has proved successful in the management of glenohumeral internal rotation deficit, reported as greater than 20°.[59] Some authors have detailed a series of exercises that, theoretically, improve posterior capsular contracture and fairly reliably decrease glenohumeral internal rotation deficit.[21,60] These exercises include "sleeper stretches," which require athletes to lie on their side with the shoulder in 90° of flexion, in neutral rotation, with the elbow also in 90° of flexion. The shoulder is then passively internally rotated by pushing the forearm toward the table around the fixed point of the elbow.[44] In the horizontal adduction stretch, the arm is horizontally adducted while the scapula is stabilized. The pectoralis minor should also be stretched, which can be performed by placing a rolled towel between the shoulder blades while the patient is supine, and steadily pushing posteriorly on the shoulders.

Treatment for SICK scapula consists of scapular stabilizer muscular strengthening, and re-education.[13,44,61–63] The involved side is addressed first, using closed chain exercises followed by open chain exercises. The kinetic chain is incorporated into the rehabilitation. Scapular rehabilitation has been successful in returning patients with SICK scapula to their previous level of competitive play.

For patients with an acute injury, such as a development of a SLAP and or partial thickness rotator cuff tear, initial treatment is directed at eliminating pain, restoring motion, correcting strength deficits, and restoring normal synchronous muscle activity. Initial treatment involves rest from provocative activities, anti-inflammatory medication, and therapeutic modalities. Strengthening is initiated once pain is resolved. For throwing athletes, a gradual return to throwing may begin as muscular balance and range of motion are restored. Failure of a nonoperative program, early suspicion of significant mechanical dysfunction, or seasonal timing may direct treatment toward surgical intervention.

Classic subacromial bursitis symptoms and external impingement may also be present and can be treated with nonsteroidal anti-inflammatory drugs or subacromial corticosteroid injection. Rotator cuff strengthening may proceed only after proper capsular elasticity and scapular dynamics have been restored.

Examination Under Anesthesia and Arthroscopic Evaluation

When the decision is made for surgery, the shoulder should be tested for translation and range of motion under anesthesia because it provides useful laxity measurements. Often, the office examination may be clouded by patient apprehension, muscle tightness, or pain. Examination under anesthesia provides an unobstructed examination and can provide useful preoperative information.

The shoulder should be tested for translation in multiple planes. The arm should be positioned in 90° of abduction and 30° of forward flexion. An axial load should be applied along the humeral shaft, and the humerus is translated in all planes. Translation is graded based on the amount of humeral head translation relative to the glenoid. Grade 1 represents mild translation, grade 2 translates to the glenoid rim, grade 3 translation produces a dislocation that spontaneously reduces, and grade 4 represents translation that results in a fixed dislocation. Range of motion should also be evaluated in all planes, and comparison is ideally made to the contralateral limb.

The diagnosis of SLAP lesions ultimately relies on arthroscopic evaluation.[64] Types I, III, and IV lesions are obvious when fraying or splitting of the labrum is noted. Viewing the joint from both the anterior and posterior portals is mandatory to entirely assess the degree of involvement. Diagnosis of type II lesions is more difficult. The normal superior labrum often has a small cleft between it and the glenoid, especially in the setting of a meniscoid labrum. The stability of the biceps anchor is determined through probing and attempting to elevate the labrum and biceps. The glenoid articular cartilage usually extends medially over the superior corner of the glenoid. Absence of cartilage in this region indicates labral detachment. Traction on the biceps tendon will show any loss of integrity at the superior labral attachment.

Burkhart and Morgan[38] described the arthroscopic examination for peel-back. The arm is placed in a throwing position and, with humeral external rotation, the labrum peels away from the posterosuperior glenoid.

A comprehensive and methodical diagnostic arthroscopy is performed visualizing the entirety of the joint with the assistance of a probe. Typically, two portals are used for the diagnostic arthroscopy: a posterior portal and a rotator interval portal. When planning a SLAP repair, both portals should be made relatively laterally to allow access to the glenoid rim.

Depending on the nature of the expected pathology, the patient is placed into the beach chair position for rotator cuff and external impingement, or the lateral decubitus position for labral tears and capsular laxity. First, the glenoid and humeral head are evaluated for any chondral wear. Next, the biceps is evaluated at its superior attachment and throughout its course in the rotator interval. The probe is used to pull the tendon into the joint and evaluate for synovitis or fraying. Next, the superior and anterior labrum is evaluated from 12 o'clock to 6 o'clock. The arthroscope is then placed in the axillary pouch and the recess evaluated for hemosiderin deposits, synovitis, or excessive volume. At this time, the posterior labrum can be visualized and probed.

Visualization through the anterior portal improves visualization of the posterior labrum and posterior IGHL, and should be performed when any posterior labral pathology is suspected. The arm may be brought into 90° of abduction and maximal external rotation, with the camera in the posterior viewing portal, and abnormal impingement of the rotator cuff and posterosuperior labrum visualized. Evidence of peel-back may also be seen. Finally, the capsule and anterior glenohumeral ligaments can be fully assessed, and the degree of capsular laxity or tears determined. Finally, the subscapularis tendon is evaluated for its integrity in internal and external rotation.

The rotator cuff should be carefully evaluated. In the thrower, special attention should be given to the undersurface of the rotator cuff at the junction between the supraspinatus and infraspinatus tendons. Tears of the rotator cuff at this location are common and care should be taken to evaluate for intratendinous delamination.

The subacromial space should be entered and examined carefully for bursitis and evidence of external impingement, such as fraying or ossification of the coracoacromial ligament or inflammation of the bursa. Once a careful examination under anesthesia and an arthroscopic evaluation is performed, the surgeon may proceed with operative fixation of the pathology at hand.

OPERATIVE TREATMENT
Anterior Capsular Laxity with Instability

Nonoperative treatment is usually successful for isolated anterior instability. Surgical intervention is commonly considered after no improvement occurs with nonoperative treatment after 3 months, or the patient fails to return to sport by 6 months. Open capsular procedures have been described that have had reasonable results in throwers but are associated with risk for morbidity to the subscapularis.

Thermal-assisted capsular shrinkage is advocated by some authors for treating arthroscopic microinstability in throwers.[65,66] However, several studies have reported unpredictable outcomes and this technique is associated with the potential for serious complications, so the authors do not recommend this treatment currently. They prefer to perform arthroscopic capsulorrhaphy. A rasp is used to abrade the capsule to stimulate healing. A curved suture passer is used to penetrate capsule laterally and then advance the capsule onto the labrum. A nonabsorbable suture is passed and tied with the suture knot away from the glenoid. The plication sutures are repeated as necessary. Care must be taken to avoid overtightening the capsule. Range of motion should be assessed at the end of the procedure.

Posterior Capsular Contracture

Operative management should only be offered to those for whom aggressive rehabilitation fails to provide relief. For the rare patients for whom nonoperative treatment fails, arthroscopic posteroinferior quadrant capsulotomy is recommended, from 6 o'clock to 3 or 9 o'clock. The capsule should be incised until the muscle belly of the external rotators can be visualized.

Morgan[13] found an average 62° (55°–68°) increase in internal rotation after the capsulotomy. Yoneda and colleagues[67] performed posterior capsular releases on 16 patients and reported that 11, including all 4 who had no other concomitant lesions, returned to their preinjury level of performance.

Superior Labrum Anterior Posterior Lesions

Appreciating the normal anatomic variants of the superior labrum and biceps insertion is critical to recognizing abnormal pathology. First, although the labrum located inferior to the glenoid equator is a constant fibrous structure continuous with the articular cartilage, the anterior superior labrum has a high degree of normal variation. Typically, it is either rounded or meniscoid, with the meniscal component overlying but not attached to the glenoid articular surface. Soft tissue variants exist and include a cord-like middle glenohumeral ligament. The Buford complex is a normal variant consisting of a cord-like middle glenohumeral ligament that originates directly from the superior labrum at the base of the biceps tendon. As a result, there is an absence of anterosuperior labral tissue. Inappropriate surgical attachment of the cord-like middle glenohumeral ligament on the anterosuperior glenoid results in painful restriction of external rotation and elevation.

Snyder and colleagues[68] originally described four types of SLAP lesions. Type I lesions consist of fraying and degeneration of the superior labrum without instability of the long head of biceps attachment. Type II lesions consist of detachment of the biceps tendon anchor from the superior glenoid tubercle. Type III lesions consist of a bucket-handle tear of a meniscoid superior labrum with an intact biceps tendon anchor. Type IV lesions consist of a superior labral tear that extends into the biceps tendon. Different SLAP types may coexist. Typically, type III or IV lesions will present in conjunction with a significantly detached biceps anchor (type II lesions). If this scenario presents, the lesions are classified as complex SLAP type II and III or type II and IV.

Maffet and colleagues[69] expanded this classification to include (1) anteroinferior Bankart-type labral lesions in continuity with SLAP lesions, (2) biceps tendon separation with an unstable flap tear of the labrum, and (3) extension of the superior labrum–biceps tendon separation to just beneath the insertion of the middle glenohumeral ligament.

Type I SLAP lesions are treated with debridement alone. Type II SLAP lesions are repaired back to the glenoid rim using suture anchors. In the case of type III SLAP lesions, if the unstable bucket-handle fragment is small, simple resection suffices. If the unstable fragment is large, it should be repaired. Type IV SLAP lesions are treated similarly to type III lesions, and the tendon split is managed with tenotomy, tenodesis, or repair. Biceps tendon management depends on the age and activity level of the patient and the condition of the tendon.

Although labral repairs can be performed in the beach chair or the lateral decubitus position, the authors prefer the lateral decubitus position, with traction to improve visualization and access the posterior labrum. The patient is positioned in 20° of reverse Trendelenberg and tilted slightly posteriorly. Typically, 10 lb of traction are applied to the arm with a modular joint distractor or a hydraulic positioner. Traditionally, three portals are used for labral repair in the lateral decubitus position (**Fig. 4**). The anterior and posterior portals are made to create an appropriate angle to the face of the glenoid for anchor placement. The transrotator cuff portal is made at the junction between the middle and posterior one third of acromion just off the lateral edge. Diagnostic arthroscopy begins and the superior labrum is probed.

True avulsion of the superior labrum is indicated through fraying and irregularity of the labral undersurface and visible chondromalacia of the normally smooth hyaline cartilage of the underlying superior glenoid rim. Arthroscopic examination should include placing the shoulder in the late-cocking position of throwing and observing the posterosuperior labrum for peel-back. Hypermobility of the posterosuperior labrum and traction of the posterior capsule will cause the biceps labral complex to move medially and off the articular edge of the glenoid. The articular surface of the rotator cuff is also examined in this position for injury.

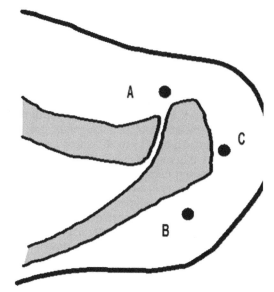

Fig. 4. Location of portals used for labral repair include the (*A*) anterior and (*B*) posterior, and (*C*) the portal of Wilmington. (*Courtesy of* Columbia University, Department of Orthopaedics, New York, NY; with permission.)

Degenerative tissue is debrided from the labrum, biceps, and articular surface of the rotator cuff. In cases requiring multiple sites of repair, the authors' preferred order of repair is as follows: (1) anterior inferior labrum proceeding superiorly along the anterior glenoid to the glenoid sulcus, (2) posterior inferior labrum proceeding from inferior to superior, (3) anterior superior labrum, and (4) rotator cuff. Care should be taken not to overtighten the joint or constrain the biceps. Significant decrease in rotation can result, precluding return to competitive throwing. Sutures should be placed, including in the labrum and only enough of the capsular reflection necessary for tissue integrity. Likewise, anchors and sutures should not be placed directly at the biceps–labral base so as to preserve maximal biceps excursion with external and internal rotation.

A type II SLAP repair is illustrated in **Fig. 5**. For a reparable lesion, a motorized shaver is introduced through the anterior working portal and used to prepare the superior neck of the glenoid beneath the detached labrum. The soft tissues are debrided and the bone abraded to enhance healing.

Because SLAP lesions often coexist with partial articular-sided supraspinatus tears and rotator cuff function is critical in throwers, the authors use a percutaneous technique that minimizes morbidity to the supraspinatus. A spinal needle is used to find a position at the desired angle on

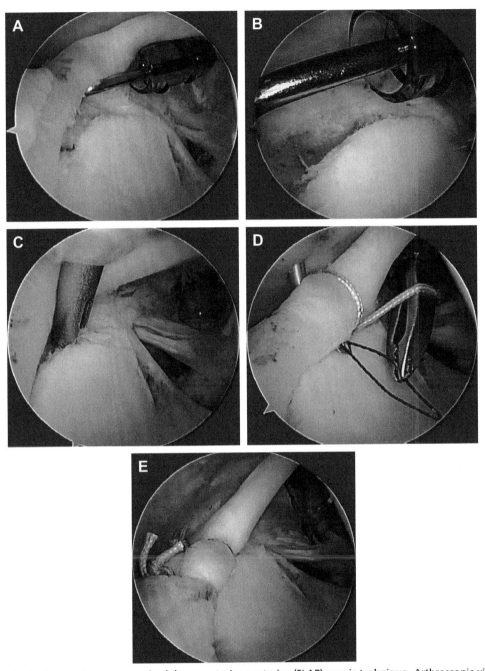

Fig. 5. Author's percutaneous superior labrum anterior posterior (SLAP) repair technique. Arthroscopic view of a right shoulder in the lateral decubitus position. (*A*) A motorized shaver is introduced through the anterior working portal and used to prepare the superior neck of the glenoid beneath the detached labrum of a type II SLAP tear. (*B*) The superior labrum is debrided and the bone is abraded to a cancellous surface. (*C*) Anchor guide in position on the superior aspect of the glenoid. (*D*) Percutaneous suture passage demonstrated using a suture shuttling device (*E*) Completed repair demonstrating anatomic restoration of the superior labrum. Note secure fixation with knots medial to the glenohumeral articulation. (*Courtesy of* Columbia University, Department of Orthopaedics, New York, NY; with permission.)

the glenoid at the location of the Wilmington portal, posterior to the biceps. A small stab incision allows introduction of the drill guide that penetrates the supraspinatus The anchor is placed and the suture limb that will be passed through the labrum is retrieved through the anterior cannula. A 90° suture lasso (Arthrex, Inc, Naples FL, USA) is inserted percutaneously, through the supraspinatus, and then passed through the labrum. Both suture limbs are then retrieved out the anterior cannula, with the cannula placed posterior to the biceps to facilitate knot tying. In meniscoid-type labrums, sutures may be placed in a vertical fashion to achieve a more anatomic repair. Knot tying is performed with the goal of keeping the knots away from the glenohumeral articulation.

Rehabilitation

Postoperatively, the shoulder is protected in a sling for 3 weeks to avoid undue stress on the biceps tendon. The patient begins elbow, wrist, and hand exercises immediately, and gentle pendulum exercises in 1 week. Strengthening exercises for the rotator cuff, scapular stabilizers, and deltoid are initiated with the goal of restoring full range of motion at 6 weeks. Biceps strengthening is begun 8 weeks postoperatively. Strenuous lifting activities are implemented after 3 months. At 4 months, throwing athletes begin an interval throwing program on a level surface. They continue a stretching and strengthening program, with particular emphasis on posteroinferior capsular stretching. At 6 months, pitchers may begin throwing full-speed, and at 7 months pitchers are allowed to throw from the mound at maximal effort.

Outcomes

For unstable SLAP lesions, simple debridement has yielded poor results.[70] Surgical repair has achieved improved results as fixation techniques have evolved. Stapling[71] and absorbable tack devices[72–74] initially were superior to debridement alone, but concerns developed, including synovitis, foreign body reaction, adhesive capsulitis, and breakage of the tack devices.[72,75,76]

Transglenoid sutures have also been used to repair SLAP lesions with good results but with substantial technical difficulty.[49] More recently, suture anchors have achieved more reliable results than previous devices.[77–80] Kim and colleagues[78] reported 94% satisfactory results after repair with suture anchors in 34 patients with isolated SLAP lesions, with 91% regaining their preinjury level of shoulder function. Similarly, Morgan and colleagues[79] were able to return 87% of throwing

athletes in their study to preinjury levels of throwing after suture anchor repair.

Conway described results of SLAP repair in nine baseball players. At 1 year, eight were able to return to play at the same or a higher level.[56] A study by Ide and colleagues with 3-year follow-up showed a 90% return to sports competition after type II SLAP repair in 40 overhead athletes. Within a group of baseball players, 18 of 19 returned to play, but 5 could not return to their previous level of competition.[81]

Brockmeier and colleagues[82] reported on 61 patients with isolated type II SLAP repairs. Of these, 12 of 16 baseball or softball players returned to their previous level of competition. Because of the professional requirements of pitchers, including velocity, control, and endurance, return to play can be challenging.

Partial Articular-sided Supraspinatus Tendon Avulsion Lesion Management

Partial rotator cuff tears can be bursal-sided, instrasubstance, or articular-sided. In athletes, articular-sided tears predominate and have been referred to as PASTA lesions by Snyder.[83] Conway[56] further described (PAINT) in throwers, in whom the tear extends into the middle layers of the infraspinatus tendon. Surgical treatment is reserved for patients for whom nonsurgical management fails. Diagnostic arthroscopy often shows concomitant pathology that may be the primary cause of the patient's symptoms.

Many surgical options exist for managing PASTA lesions, including debridement of rotator cuff tear, subacromial decompression, arthroscopic in situ repair, or completion of the tear followed by open, mini-open, or all arthroscopic repair. Tears are classified according to percent of thickness of tear, number of tendons involved, and whether it involves the bursal or articular side. Weber found that tears greater than 50% of tendon insertion width in a medial to lateral direction did better with repair.[84] Mazzocca and colleagues[85] found in a cadaver model that articular-sided partial tears with 50% of depth or greater significantly increased strain in the remaining intact bursal tendon fibers.

Although a consensus has not been established for treatment, the authors' guidelines are consistent with those of others.[86] The normal footprint of the supraspinatus insertion ranges from approximately 12 to 21 mm in width. Therefore, the percentage that the partial-thickness tear involves can be calculated. If 25% of cuff is torn, rotator cuff debridement and subacromial debridement is performed. If 50% of the cuff is torn, an in situ all-arthroscopic repair to the footprint is performed without completing the tear. If 75% or greater of cuff is torn, the tear is completed and an all-arthroscopic rotator cuff repair is performed. Bursal-sided tears have superior results when an acromioplasty is concurrently performed. For intratendinous laminar tears, intratendinous repair is performed. In younger throwing athletes, intratendinous repairs are preferable and acromioplasty should be avoided if no bursal-sided damage is present.

The normal bare area that exists between the articular margin and the posterior rotator cuff insertion is important to recognize. In throwing athletes, repairs must be avoided in this area because it makes normal contact with the posterosuperior glenoid. Occasionally, anterior rotator cuff detachments are repaired to bone in the most anterior aspect of the rotator cuff footprint because this area has less normal internal impingement contact in throwing athletes.

Rotator Cuff Repair

Managing rotator cuff tears that have failed nonoperative treatment is a challenge in overhead throwers. For many throwers, rotator cuff footprint contact on the glenoid from internal impingement is expected, and therefore repair into those insertional regions is subject to failure. The various tear types require different repair techniques.

Intratendinous Tears

Tears with intralaminar extension are commonly observed and repair can prevent propagation. An intratendinous repair technique is illustrated in **Fig. 6**. Glenohumeral arthroscopy shows what is typically a frayed and degenerated undersurface of the supraspinatus and infraspinatus. The magnitude and mobility of the lamination is appreciated using a grasper. The inside of the lamination is abraded with a shaver or rasp to enhance healing. If the tear is retracted posteriorly but reduces anatomically when pulled anterior, the sutures are passed first through the posterior aspect and then through the anterior aspect of the lamina.

Before repairing the tear, the subacromial space is inspected and a complete bursectomy is performed to enhance visualization. Mattress sutures are then placed from outside (bursal surface) to inside using a spinal needle and #2 nonabsorbable sutures. The spinal needle is introduced percutaneously just lateral to the acromion to penetrate the intact bursal lamina. The needle is maneuvered to penetrate the articular lamina at the desired location. A monofilament suture is passed through the needle and retrieved out the anterior cannula.

A needle meniscal repair device with a wire shuttle is used to retrieve the suture. Alternatively, another monofilament suture is passed and retrieved out the anterior cannulae and tied to the first. A #2 nonabsorbable suture is then shuttled through the rotator cuff to create a mattress suture. These steps are repeated to create the necessary number of mattress sutures. The camera is then placed in the subacromial space and the sutures tied through a standard lateral working portal. The camera is then placed back in the glenohumeral joint and the repair is evaluated.

Outcomes

Ide and colleagues[87] presented a transtendinous suture anchor technique in a series of 17 patients, including 6 participating in overhead-throwing sports. They noted excellent outcomes in 16 patients, but only 2 of the 6 overhead-throwing athletes were able to resume sports at their previous level of competition. Conway[56] used a suture shuttling technique and found that of 14 baseball players (average age, 16 years) treated with repair of intratendinous rotator cuff tears and concurrent pathology (labral tears, SLAP tears), 89% percent were able to return at the same or higher level at 16-month follow-up.

Complete Tears

Near complete tears are treated with tear completion and arthroscopic repair. Complete tears are also treated with repair. The authors prefer double-row transosseous-equivalent repair techniques to create tissue compression against the tuberosity to enhance healing.[88] These new techniques have also been referred to as suture bridge techniques.

Research studies have shown that transosseous equivalent repair techniques provide improved footprint coverage,[89] pressurized contact area at the footprint,[90] and reduced motion at the footprint tendon–bone interface compared with standard double-row fixation.[91] Experts believe that improved contact characteristics will help maximize healing potential between repaired tendons and the greater tuberosity.

Outcomes

Full-thickness tears have a poor prognosis in elite throwers. Mazoué and Andrews[92] reported the results after a mini-open repair of a full-thickness rotator cuff tear in 16 professional baseball players. Among these patients, 12 were pitchers with injury to their dominant shoulders, 4s were position players, 2 had injuries involving their dominant shoulders, and 2 had injuries to their nondominant shoulders. Only 1 player (8%) with

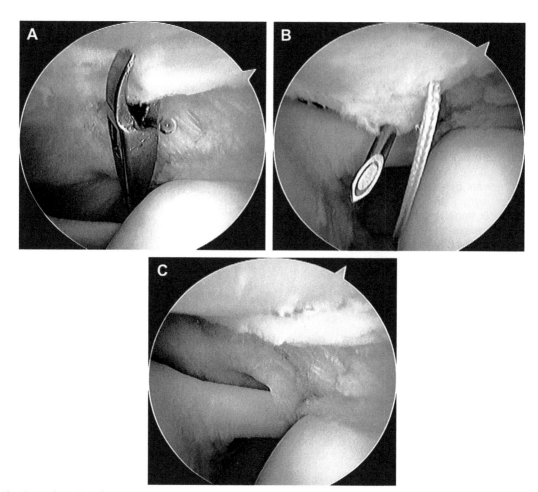

Fig. 6. Author's intralaminar tear repair technique. Arthroscopic view of a right shoulder in beach chair position. (*A*) An intratendinous partial-thickness tear with retraction. The tear is grasped to determine mobility and its anatomic repair site. (*B*) Spinal needle placement through both laminations of the tear, and sutures are passed. (*C*) Completion of the repair as visualized from the glenohumeral joint. (*Courtesy of* Columbia University, Department of Orthopaedics, New York, NY; with permission.)

a dominant arm repair returned to a high competitive level of baseball with no significant shoulder problems. The authors concluded that it is uncommon for a professional baseball pitcher to return to a competitive level of pitching after a full-thickness rotator cuff repair with a mini-open approach.

Postoperative Rehabilitation

The postoperative rehabilitation protocol after transtendon or laminar rotator cuff repair is similar to that for full-thickness rotator cuff repair techniques. After the procedure, the treated arm is placed at the side in a sling with a small pillow. The sling is worn continuously for 6 weeks, except during bathing and exercises. Active elbow flexion and extension are encouraged. Patients may begin passive external rotation exercises immediately postoperatively; however, overhead stretching is avoided until after 6 weeks to avoid stressing the repair. At 6 weeks, the sling is discontinued and overhead stretches with a rope and pulley and internal rotation stretches are commenced. Isotonic strengthening is not begun until 10 to 12 weeks after surgery, at which point the authors begin rehabilitation of the rotator cuff, deltoid, and scapular stabilizers. Progressive activities are incorporated as strength allows, and unrestricted activities are usually resumed 6 to 12 months after surgery.

SUMMARY

Shoulder injuries in athletes are highly prevalent and debilitating. The treating orthopedic surgeon must pay special attention to the acuity and severity of the injury with particular focus on the specific biomechanics of the sport in question. New understanding of the pathophysiology and management of shoulder injuries in various sports has improved outcomes. Nonoperative rehabilitation and arthroscopic and open techniques, applied judiciously, can improve shoulder biomechanics and return athletes to the sports arena as quickly and as wholly as possible.

REFERENCES

1. Sabick MB, Torry MR, Kim YK, et al. Humeral torque in professional baseball pitchers. Am J Sports Med 2004;32(4):892–8.
2. McQuade KJ, Dawson J, Smidt GL. Scapulothoracic muscle fatigue associated with alterations in scapulohumeral rhythm kinematics during maximum resistive shoulder elevation. J Orthop Sports Phys Ther 1998;28(2):74–80.
3. Tyler TF, Nicholas SJ, Roy T, et al. Quantification of posterior capsule tightness and motion loss in patients with shoulder impingement [comment]. Am J Sports Med 2000;28(5):668–73.
4. Warner JJ, Micheli LJ, Arslanian LE, et al. Scapulothoracic motion in normal shoulders and shoulders with glenohumeral instability and impingement syndrome. A study using Moire topographic analysis. Clin Orthop Relat Res 1992;285:191–9.
5. Paletta GA Jr, Warner JJ, Warren RF, et al. Shoulder kinematics with two-plane x-ray evaluation in patients with anterior instability or rotator cuff tearing. J Shoulder Elbow Surg 1997;6(6):516–27.
6. Weiser WM, Lee TQ, McMaster WC, et al. Effects of simulated scapular protraction on anterior glenohumeral stability. Am J Sports Med 1999;27(6):801–5.
7. Burkhart SS, Morgan CD, Kibler WB. Shoulder injuries in overhead athletes. The "dead arm" revisited. Clin Sports Med 2000;19(1):125–58.
8. Pink M, Perry J. Biomechanics of the shoulder. In: Jobe FW, Pink MM, Glousman RE, et al, editors. Operative techniques in upper extremity sports injuries. St. Louis (MO): Mosby; 1996. p. 109–24.
9. Fleisig G. The biomechanics of baseball pitching [dissertation]. Birmingham (AL): University of Alabama at Birmingham; 1994.
10. Fleisig GS, Andrews JR, Dillman CJ, et al. Kinetics of baseball pitching with implications about injury mechanisms. Am J Sports Med 1995;23(2):233–9.
11. Glousman R, Jobe F, Tibone J, et al. Dynamic electromyographic analysis of the throwing shoulder with glenohumeral instability. J Bone Joint Surg Am 1988;70(2):220–6.
12. Dillman CJ, Fleisig GS, Andrews JR. Biomechanics of pitching with emphasis upon shoulder kinematics. J Orthop Sports Phys Ther 1993;18(2):402–8.
13. Burkhart SS, Morgan CD, Kibler WB, et al. The disabled throwing shoulder: spectrum of pathology Part II: evaluation and treatment of SLAP lesions in throwers. Arthroscopy 2003;19(5):531–9.
14. Bigliani LU, Codd TP, Connor PM, et al. Shoulder motion and laxity in the professional baseball player. Am J Sports Med 1997;25(5):609–13.
15. Brown LP, Niehues SL, Harrah A, et al. Upper extremity range of motion and isokinetic strength of the internal and external shoulder rotators in major league baseball players. Am J Sports Med 1988;16(6):577–85.
16. Garth WP Jr, Allman FL Jr, Armstrong WS. Occult anterior subluxations of the shoulder in noncontact sports. Am J Sports Med 1987;15(6):579–85.
17. Jobe CM. Posterior superior glenoid impingement: expanded spectrum. Arthroscopy 1995;11(5):530–6.
18. Jobe FW, Giangarra CE, Kvitne RS, et al. Anterior capsulolabral reconstruction of the shoulder in athletes in overhand sports. Am J Sports Med 1991;19(5):428–34.
19. Johnson L. Patterns of shoulder flexibility among college baseball players. J Athl Train 1992;27(1):44–9.
20. Wilk KE, Arrigo C. Current concepts in the rehabilitation of the athletic shoulder. J Orthop Sports Phys Ther 1993;18(1):365–78.
21. Wilk KE, Meister K, Andrews JR. Current concepts in the rehabilitation of the overhead throwing athlete. Am J Sports Med 2002;30(1):136–51.
22. Meister K, Day T, Horodyski M, et al. Rotational motion changes in the glenohumeral joint of the adolescent/little league baseball player. Am J Sports Med 2005;33(5):693–8.
23. Reagan KM, Meister K, Horodyski MB, et al. Humeral retroversion and its relationship to glenohumeral rotation in the shoulder of college baseball players. Am J Sports Med 2002;30(3):354–60.
24. Sethi PM, Tibone JE, Lee TQ. Quantitative assessment of glenohumeral translation in baseball players: a comparison of pitchers versus nonpitching athletes. Am J Sports Med 2004;32(7):1711–5.
25. Crockett HC, Gross LB, Wilk KE, et al. Osseous adaptation and range of motion at the glenohumeral joint in professional baseball pitchers. Am J Sports Med 2002;30(1):20–6.
26. Dempster WT. Mechanisms of shoulder movement. Arch Phys Med Rehabil 1965;46:49–70.
27. Edelson G. The development of humeral head retroversion. J Shoulder Elbow Surg 2000;9(4):316–8.
28. Edelson G. Variations in the retroversion of the humeral head. J Shoulder Elbow Surg 1999;8(2):142–5.
29. Yamamoto N, Itoi E, Minagawa H, et al. Why is the humeral retroversion of throwing athletes greater in dominant shoulders than in nondominant shoulders? J Shoulder Elbow Surg 2006;15(5):571–5.

30. Andrews JR, Broussard TS, Carson WG. Arthroscopy of the shoulder in the management of partial tears of the rotator cuff: a preliminary report. Arthroscopy 1985;1(2):117–22.

31. Davidson PA, Elattrache NS, Jobe CM, et al. Rotator cuff and posterior-superior glenoid labrum injury associated with increased glenohumeral motion: a new site of impingement. J Shoulder Elbow Surg 1995;4(5):384–90.

32. Burkhart SS, Morgan CD, Kibler WB. The disabled throwing shoulder: spectrum of pathology. Part II: evaluation and treatment of SLAP lesions in throwers. Arthroscopy 2003;19(5):531–9.

33. Walch G, Boileau J, Noel E, et al. Impingement of the deep surface of the supraspinatus tendon on the posterior superior glenoid rim: an arthroscopic study. J Shoulder Elbow Surg 1992;1:238–43.

34. Jobe CM. Superior glenoid impingement. Orthop Clin North Am 1997;28(2):137–43.

35. Jobe CM. Superior glenoid impingement. Current concepts. Clin Orthop Relat Res 1996;330:98–107.

36. Burkhart SS, Morgan CD, Kibler WB. The disabled throwing shoulder: spectrum of pathology part I: pathoanatomy and biomechanics. Arthroscopy 2003;19(4):404–20.

37. Grossman MG, Tibone JE, McGarry MH, et al. A cadaveric model of the throwing shoulder: a possible etiology of superior labrum anterior-to-posterior lesions. J Bone Joint Surg Am 2005; 87(4):824–31.

38. Burkhart SS, Morgan CD. The peel-back mechanism: its role in producing and extending posterior type II SLAP lesions and its effect on SLAP repair rehabilitation. Arthroscopy 1998;14(6):637–40.

39. Kibler WB. The role of the scapula in athletic shoulder function. Am J Sports Med 1998;26(2):325–37.

40. Kibler WB, McMullen J. Scapular dyskinesis and its relation to shoulder pain. J Am Acad Orthop Surg 2003;11(2):142–51.

41. Lukasiewicz AC, McClure P, Michener L, et al. Comparison of 3-dimensional scapular position and orientation between subjects with and without shoulder impingement. J Orthop Sports Phys Ther 1999;29(10):574–83 [discussion: 584–6].

42. Myers JB, Laudner KG, Pasquale MR, et al. Scapular position and orientation in throwing athletes. Am J Sports Med 2005;33(2):263–71.

43. Kibler WB, Livingston B. Closed-chain rehabilitation for upper and lower extremities. J Am Acad Orthop Surg 2001;9(6):412–21.

44. Burkhart SS, Morgan CD, Kibler WB. The disabled throwing shoulder: spectrum of pathology part III: the SICK scapula, scapular dyskinesis, the kinetic chain, and rehabilitation. Arthroscopy 2003;19(6): 641–61.

45. Gerber C, Krushell RJ. Isolated rupture of the tendon of the subscapularis muscle. Clinical features in 16 cases. J Bone Joint Surg Br 1991; 73(3):389–94.

46. Hertel R, Ballmer FT, Lombert SM, et al. Lag signs in the diagnosis of rotator cuff rupture. J Shoulder Elbow Surg 1996;5(4):307–13.

47. O'Brien SJ, Pagnani MJ, Fealy S, et al. The active compression test: a new and effective test for diagnosing labral tears and acromioclavicular joint abnormality. Am J Sports Med 1998;26(5):610–3.

48. Stetson WB, Templin K. The crank test, the O'Brien test, and routine magnetic resonance imaging scans in the diagnosis of labral tears. Am J Sports Med 2002;30(6):806–9.

49. Field LD, Savoie FH III. Arthroscopic suture repair of superior labral detachment lesions of the shoulder. Am J Sports Med 1993;21(6):783–90 [discussion: 790].

50. Snyder SJ, Banas MP, Karzel RP. An analysis of 140 injuries to the superior glenoid labrum. J Shoulder Elbow Surg 1995;4(4):243–8.

51. Kibler WB. Specificity and sensitivity of the anterior slide test in throwing athletes with superior glenoid labral tears. Arthroscopy 1995;11(3):296–300.

52. Kim SH, Ha KI, Ahn JH, et al. Biceps load test II: a clinical test for SLAP lesions of the shoulder. Arthroscopy 2001;17(2):160–4.

53. Mimori K, Muneta T, Nakagawa T, et al. A new pain provocation test for superior labral tears of the shoulder. Am J Sports Med 1999;27(2):137–42.

54. Bencardino JT, Beltran J, Rosenberg ZS, et al. Superior labrum anterior-posterior lesions: diagnosis with MR arthrography of the shoulder. Radiology 2000; 214(1):267–71.

55. Tirman PF, Smith ED, Stoller DW, et al. Shoulder imaging in athletes. Semin Musculoskelet Radiol 2004;8(1):29–40.

56. Conway JE. Arthroscopic repair of partial-thickness rotator cuff tears and SLAP lesions in professional baseball players. Orthop Clin North Am 2001; 32(3):443–56.

57. Connor PM, Banks DM, Tyson AB, et al. Magnetic resonance imaging of the asymptomatic shoulder of overhead athletes: a 5-year follow-up study. Am J Sports Med 2003;31(5):724–7.

58. Wilk KE, Obma P, Simpson CD, et al. Shoulder injuries in the overhead athlete. J Orthop Sports Phys Ther 2009;39(2):38–54.

59. Burkhart SS, Morgan CD, Kibler WB. The disabled throwing shoulder: spectrum of pathology Part I: pathoanatomy and biomechanics. Arthroscopy 2003;19(4):404–20.

60. McClure P, Balaicuis J, Heiland D, et al. A randomized controlled comparison of stretching procedures for posterior shoulder tightness. J Orthop Sports Phys Ther 2007;37(3):108–14.

61. Kibler WB, Chandler TJ. Range of motion in junior tennis players participating in an injury risk modification program. J Sci Med Sport 2003;6(1):51–62.

62. Kibler WB, McMullen J, Uhl T. Shoulder rehabilitation strategies, guidelines, and practice. Orthop Clin North Am 2001;32(3):527–38.

63. Morgan CD. The thrower's shoulder. In: McGinty JB, editor. Operative arthroscopy. 3rd edition. Charleston (SC): Lippincott, Williams & Wilkins; 2002. p. 570–84.

64. Mileski RA, Snyder SJ. Superior labral lesions in the shoulder: pathoanatomy and surgical management. J Am Acad Orthop Surg 1998;6(2):121–31.

65. Enad JG, ElAttrache NS, Tibone JE, et al. Isolated electrothermal capsulorrhaphy in overhand athletes. J Shoulder Elbow Surg 2004;13(2):133–7.

66. Levitz CL, Dugas J, Andrews JR. The use of arthroscopic thermal capsulorrhaphy to treat internal impingement in baseball players. Arthroscopy 2001;17(6):573–7.

67. Yoneda M, Nakagawa S, Mizuno N, et al. Arthroscopic capsular release for painful throwing shoulder with posterior capsular tightness. Arthroscopy 2006;22(7):801 e1-e5.

68. Snyder SJ, Karzel RP, Del Pizzo W, et al. SLAP lesions of the shoulder. Arthroscopy 1990;6(4): 274–9.

69. Maffet MW, Gartsman GM, Moseley B. Superior labrum-biceps tendon complex lesions of the shoulder. Am J Sports Med 1995;23(1):93–8.

70. Cordasco FA, Steinmann S, Flatow EL, et al. Arthroscopic treatment of glenoid labral tears. Am J Sports Med 1993;21(3):425–30 [discussion: 430–1].

71. Yoneda M, Hirooka A, Saito S, et al. Arthroscopic stapling for detached superior glenoid labrum. J Bone Joint Surg Br 1991;73(5):746–50.

72. Pagnani MJ, Speer KP, Altchek DW, et al. Arthroscopic fixation of superior labral lesions using a biodegradable implant: a preliminary report. Arthroscopy 1995;11(2):194–8.

73. Samani JE, Marston SB, Buss DD. Arthroscopic stabilization of type II SLAP lesions using an absorbable tack. Arthroscopy 2001;17(1):19–24.

74. Segmuller HE, Hayes MG, Saies AD. Arthroscopic repair of glenolabral injuries with an absorbable fixation device. J Shoulder Elbow Surg 1997;6(4): 383–92.

75. Burkart A, Imhoff AB, Roscher E. Foreign-body reaction to the bioabsorbable suretac device. Arthroscopy 2000;16(1):91–5.

76. Wilkerson JP, Zvijac JE, Uribe JW, et al. Failure of polymerized lactic acid tacks in shoulder surgery. J Shoulder Elbow Surg 2003;12(2):117–21.

77. Kartus J, Kartus C, Brownlow H, et al. Repair of type-2 SLAP lesions using Corkscrew anchors. A preliminary report of the clinical results. Knee Surg Sports Traumatol Arthrosc 2004;12(3):229–34.

78. Kim SH, Ha KI, Kim YM. Arthroscopic revision Bankart repair: a prospective outcome study. Arthroscopy 2002;18(5):469–82.

79. Morgan CD, Burkhart SS, Palmeri M, et al. Type II SLAP lesions: three subtypes and their relationships to superior instability and rotator cuff tears. Arthroscopy 1998;14(6):553–65.

80. Yian E, Wang C, Millett PJ, et al. Arthroscopic repair of SLAP lesions with a bioknotless suture anchor. Arthroscopy 2004;20(5):547–51.

81. Ide J, Maeda S, Takagi K. Sports activity after arthroscopic superior labral repair using suture anchors in overhead-throwing athletes. Am J Sports Med 2005; 33(4):507–14.

82. Brockmeier SF, Voos JE, Williams RJ III, et al. Outcomes after arthroscopic repair of type-II SLAP lesions. J Bone Joint Surg Am 2009;91(7): 1595–603.

83. Snyder SJ. Arthroscopic treatment of partial articular surface tendon avulsions. Presented at: AAOS/ AOSSM Comprehensive Sports Medicine: The Athletic Perspective to Treatment, Controversies and Problem Solving. Lake Tahoe (NV), February 28 to March 4, 2001.

84. Weber SC. Arthroscopic debridement and acromioplasty versus mini-open repair in the treatment of significant partial-thickness rotator cuff tears. Arthroscopy 1999;15(2):126–31.

85. Mazzocca AD, Rincon LM, O'Connor RW, et al. Intra-articular partial thickness rotator cuff tears: analysis of injured and repaired strain behavior. Presented at: AOSSM Annual Meeting. Hershey (PA), June 29 to July 2, 2006.

86. Reynolds SB, Dugas JR, Cain EL, et al. Debridement of small partial-thickness rotator cuff tears in elite overhead throwers. Clin Orthop Relat Res 2008; 466(3):614–21.

87. Ide J, Maeda S, Takagi K. Arthroscopic transtendon repair of partial-thickness articular-side tears of the rotator cuff: anatomical and clinical study. Am J Sports Med 2005;33(11):1672–9.

88. Park MC, Elattrache NS, Ahmad CS, et al. "Transosseous-equivalent" rotator cuff repair technique. Arthroscopy 2006;22(12):1360, e1–5.

89. Apreleva M, Ozbaydar M, Fitzgibbons PG, et al. Rotator cuff tears: the effect of the reconstruction method on three-dimensional repair site area. Arthroscopy 2002;18(5):519–26.

90. Mc P, Cadet ER, Levine WN, et al. Tendon-to-bone pressure distributions at a repaired rotator cuff footprint using transosseous suture and suture anchor fixation techniques. Am J Sports Med 2005;33(8): 1154–9.

91. Ahmad CS, Stewart AM, Izquierdo R, et al. Tendon-bone interface motion in transosseous suture and suture anchor rotator cuff repair techniques. Am J Sports Med 2005;33(11):1667–71.

92. Mazoue CG, Andrews JR. Repair of full-thickness rotator cuff tears in professional baseball players. Am J Sports Med 2006;34(2):182–9.

Arthroscopic Management of Anterior Instability: Pearls, Pitfalls, and Lessons Learned

Matthew T. Provencher, MD[a,b,]*, Neil Ghodadra, MD[c], Anthony A. Romeo, MD[d,e]

KEYWORDS

- Anterior shoulder instability • Arthroscopy
- Bankart lesion • Arthroscopic management
- Revision • Glenoid bone loss

The diagnosis and treatment of recurrent anterior shoulder instability continue to evolve. Although open capsular plication with Bankart repair has long been considered the optimal method for surgical management of shoulder instability, advancements in arthroscopic techniques have led to a recent shift to arthroscopic Bankart repair. Advances in instrumentation and implants coupled with the ability to produce more of an open type of arthroscopic repair have all led to improved results with the arthroscopic technique.[1–4]

To obtain a successful outcome for patients with anterior instability, it is imperative that the surgeon be aware of preoperative, intraoperative, and postoperative factors associated with the recognition and proper treatment of instability pathology. In this article, the authors present several important pearls and pitfalls of how to effectively diagnose and treat patients with recurrent anterior instability using arthroscopic techniques. In addition, the authors highlight the importance of the recognition of anterior instability pathology and provide the important principles for successful arthroscopic management.

ANATOMY

Improvements in our understanding of the biomechanical and pathoanatomical features of anterior shoulder instability have led to advances in clinical diagnosis and recognition of associated pathology. The stability of the glenohumeral joint is conferred by three major mechanisms: (1) concavity-compression, (2) coordinated contraction of the rotator cuff to permit fluid and complete range of motion of the humeral head onto the glenoid surface, and (3) contribution of the glenohumeral ligaments.[5] When considering instability, the most pertinent anatomy includes the dynamic and static stabilizers of the shoulder joint. The

The views expressed in this article are those of the authors and do not reflect the official policy or position of the Department of the Navy, Department of Defense, or the United States Government.

[a] Division of Shoulder and Sports Surgery, Department of Orthopedics Surgery, Naval Medical Center San Diego, 34800 Bob Wilson Drive, Suite 112, San Diego, CA 92134-1112, USA

[b] Department of Surgery, Orthopedics, USUHS, USA

[c] Department of Orthopedics Surgery, Rush University, Chicago, IL, USA

[d] Section of Shoulder and Elbow, Division of Sports Medicine, Department of Orthopedics Surgery, Rush University Medical Center, 1611 West Harrison Avenue, Suite 300, Chicago, IL 60612, USA

[e] Division of Sports Medicine, Department of Orthopedic Surgery, Rush University Medical Center, 1611 West Harrison Avenue, Suite 300, Chicago, IL 60612, USA

* Corresponding author. Division of Shoulder and Sports Surgery, Department of Orthopedics Surgery, Naval Medical Center San Diego, 34800 Bob Wilson Drive, Suite 112, San Diego, CA 92134-1112.

E-mail address: matthew.provencher@med.navy.mil

Orthop Clin N Am 41 (2010) 325–337

doi:10.1016/j.ocl.2010.02.007

static stabilizers include the bony anatomy, capsular ligaments, and the rotator interval, whereas the dynamic stabilizers include the rotator cuff and scapular rotator musculature (**Fig. 1**).

→ Pearl: Understand the pathoanatomy of anterior shoulder instability.

The glenohumeral capsuloligamentous complex serves to statically restrain the glenohumeral joint against excessive translation in varying positions of arm rotation. The anterior band of the inferior glenohumeral ligament (AIGHL) attaches to the glenoid at the anteroinferior labrum and is the primary static restraint to anterior translation in the abducted externally rotated shoulder.

The bony anatomy of the glenohumeral joint plays a major role in anterior shoulder stability. Because of the small size of the glenoid compared with the humeral head, even a small loss of bone, such as a glenoid rim fracture, can compromise stability by decreasing the bony surface area for glenohumeral articulation.[6–8] Several clinical studies have shown that bone loss of either the humeral head or glenoid surface is the most common cause of failed arthroscopic stabilization procedures[8–11] and that recurrence of

glenohumeral instability is increased when there is 15% to 20% glenoid bone loss.[8,10,11]

The labrum is the portion of fibrocartilage that is circumferentially attached to the rim of the glenoid. It is critical for the orthopedic surgeon to recognize the normal anatomy and anatomic variants of the labrum to prevent misdiagnoses and inadvertent treatment. The anteroinferior attachment of the labrum to the glenoid rim is normally tight, and injury to this structure is typically referred to as the essential lesion, or the Bankart lesion (**Fig. 2**). The normal superior attachment of the labrum to the glenoid is loose, has tremendous anatomic variation,[12–14] and is complicated by the attachment of the long head of the biceps tendon as it originates from the supraglenoid tubercle. The function of the labrum as it relates to stability of the shoulder joint is threefold. First, the labrum deepens the concavity of the glenoid up to 9 mm in the superior-inferior direction and also doubles the anteroposterior depth to 5 mm.[15] Second, the labrum increases glenohumeral stability by increasing the surface area through which the glenoid contacts the humeral head through an arc of motion. Finally, the labrum is the site of attachment for the various glenohumeral ligaments that confer static stability to the joint.[5]

→ Pearl: A comprehensive evaluation of the scapular and rotator cuff musculature is important because dynamic stability is critical to glenohumeral function.

The rotator cuff musculature and parascapular muscles are critical to the overall function of the glenohumeral joint and confer important dynamic stability to the shoulder. A careful evaluation of the rotator cuff (especially in patients who present with an initial dislocation more than 40 years old) and scapular function is paramount to ensure that the dynamic stability of the glenohumeral joint is optimized.

There are several other intra-articular lesions associated with anterior instability and include a superior labral anterior posterior[16] lesion, which is a detachment of the glenoid labrum at the insertion of the long head of the biceps tendon; a medial displacement of the labrum and periosteal sleeve of the anterior glenoid labrum and capsule (Anterior Labral Periosteal Sleeve Avulsion [ALPSA]); and the humeral avulsion of the glenohumeral ligament or detachment of the capsuloligamentous structures off the humeral head (HAGL lesion). See the article by Boselli and colleagues elsewhere in this issue for a thorough review of these lesions. The presence of these lesions can lead to recurrent instability and future subluxation events if not properly addressed.

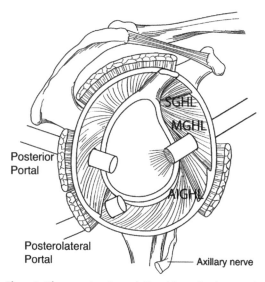

Fig. 1. The anatomic relationship of the static restraints for glenohumeral stability. The coracohumeral ligament, anterior band of the inferior glenohumeral ligament, and posterior band of the inferior glenohumeral ligament are highlighted. AIGHL, anterior band of the inferior glenohumeral ligament; CHL, coracohumeral ligament ;MGHL, middle glenohumeral ligament; PIGHL, band of the inferior glenohumeral ligament; SGHL, superior glenohumeral ligament. (Copyright Anthony A. Romeo, MD; with permission.)

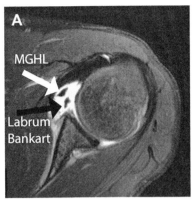
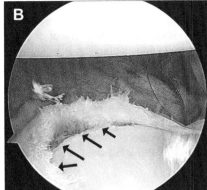

Fig. 2. (*A*) MR arthrogram axial image of a soft-tissue Bankart tear anteriorly. Arrow points to anteroinferior labrum. (*B*) Corresponding arthroscopic image of the anterior Bankart soft-tissue only tear. Posterior view of glenohumeral joint with probe on anteroinferior labrum.

PATIENT HISTORY

Understanding the source and type of instability that patients are experiencing is critical to the ultimate success of surgical treatment. A thorough history should always include type of instability (dislocation, subluxation); direction of instability (anterior, posterior, multidirectional); requirement for medically assisted reduction versus self-reduction; age and amount of time that had elapsed from the first dislocation; activity level, including contact versus non-contact sports; and any treatment that has been rendered to date.

→ Pearl: if patients experience an initial dislocation at more than 40 years of age, it is imperative to rule out an associated rotator cuff tear.

In addition, the provocative anterior instability position (almost always the abducted externally rotated position) and the amount of trauma necessary for the instability episode to occur has implications in management. Patients whose shoulders slip out during sleep or with simple activities, such as reaching overhead, may have an entirely different diagnosis (ie, multidirectional instability, glenoid hypoplasia, and so forth) and may require a different surgical plan compared with those who experience instability only with more significant trauma. If patients demonstrate the ability to easily dislocate the shoulder they should be closely evaluated for a volitional component, especially in the absence of glenoid bone loss, glenoid dysplasia, connective tissue disorders, or prior surgery.

Patients with anterior shoulder instability most often present with feelings of impending instability or pain in extremes of motion, and may experience subluxation or even frank dislocation during certain shoulder positions (namely abduction and external rotation and with overhead activities).

Although most patients complain of subjective feelings of instability during repetitive overhead activities, such as throwing or swimming, some patients may present with reports of transient sharp pain, numbness, or weakness that usually resolves briefly as their only symptom of instability.

PHYSICAL EXAMINATION

After obtaining the appropriate history from patients, a complete physical examination is integral to making the correct diagnosis and implementing the appropriate treatment plan. Range of motion, neurovascular examination, and overall strength (shoulder girdle and parascapular muscles) should all be normal in the majority of patients with shoulder instability. Specific provocative tests are the hallmark of assessing anterior shoulder instability, including the apprehension, relocation, and anterior release tests. Especially important to investigate is the ease with which the humerus begins to dislocate and engage on the glenoid; if this occurs at 30° of external rotation at the side, for example, it is highly likely that there is a significant engaging Hill-Sachs lesion or associated glenoid bone loss.[8] Patients with engaging Hill-Sachs lesions also usually report a history of shoulder instability in midranges of the shoulder abduction/external rotation.

It is imperative that the surgeon discerns between laxity and instability. Instability is generally regarded as symptomatic laxity and is the perception *by patients* experiencing the shoulder subluxation or dislocation event. Laxity is a normal finding of the glenohumeral joint, because the humerus needs to have a minimum obligate translation on the glenoid for normal shoulder function.[17,18] The amount of laxity and instability are both assessed with translation testing for laxity (anterior, posterior, and inferior sulcus) and symptomatic directional laxity, which is a critical diagnostic indicator of shoulder instability. A positive sulcus sign that does not decrease with external rotation at the side indicates a pathologic rotator interval (**Fig. 3**).[19,20] Increased generalized ligamentous laxity should also be assessed, including thumb to forearm, elbow recurvatum, metacarpophalangeal hyperextension, and increased external rotation in the abducted position.

RADIOGRAPHIC EVALUATION

Upon initial evaluation of patients with a traumatic shoulder dislocation, routine radiographs should be obtained, including true anteroposterior, axillary lateral, and scapular-Y views. In patients with a history of recurrent anterior instability, or if a bone defect is suspected, further radiographic imaging is warranted, including the apical oblique,[16,21] West Point view,[22] or Didiee[23] views. For humeral head defects, such as a Hill-Sachs injury, the Stryker Notch view[23] and a true anteroposterior in internal rotation should be obtained. Hill-Sachs injuries may be well demonstrated on anteroposterior internal rotation views (**Fig. 4**).

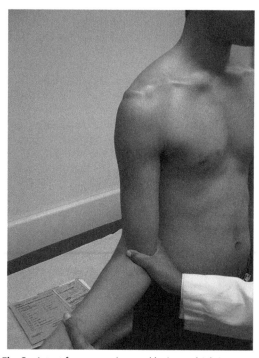

Fig. 3. A test for rotator interval lesion, which is a positive sulcus sign that does not decrease with external rotation at the side.

EVALUATION OF GLENOID AND HUMERAL HEAD BONE LOSS

In evaluating patients with glenohumeral instability, it essential that the surgeon assess for patient demographic and examination factors associated with glenoid and humeral head bone loss. Patients with high energy trauma to the shoulder leading to dislocation should be evaluated for glenoid bone loss. The position when instability of the shoulder is first experienced should be carefully assessed on examination to determine if the instability is present in midranges of motion (suggestive of bone loss).

→ Pearl: Patients that present with numerous instability episodes, a long history of instability, or progressive ease of instability symptoms suggests a larger anatomic problem, namely glenoid or humeral head bone loss.

→ Pearl: Patients who demonstrate instability in midranges of motion (45° abduction with external rotation), have a progressive ease of instability symptoms, or have a long, documented history of recurrence, should be evaluated closely for glenoid or humeral head bone loss.

For a comprehensive evaluation of glenoid bone loss, advanced imaging is necessary. An MRI and MR Arthrogram, although helpful in diagnosis of soft-tissue pathology, may also be used to assess the degree of bone loss by evaluating the most lateral glenoid cut on sagittal oblique images (**Fig. 5**). However, the most accurate method to measure glenoid bone loss is a three-dimensional CT scan with digital subtraction of the humeral head on sagittal oblique imaging. The humeral head may also be isolated in three-dimensional reconstruction to assess the size, depth, and orientation of the Hill-Sachs defect.

→ Pearl: Nearly all patients with recurrent anterior instability have some amount of glenoid bone loss (either of glenoid, humeral head, or both) and the surgeon should seek to determine the extent of bone loss to make informed decisions regarding optimal treatment.

Huysmans and colleagues[24] have described the inferior two thirds of the glenoid as a well-conserved circle, and deficiencies within this circle are used to quantify the amount of glenoid bone loss. (**Fig. 6**) A best-fit circle is drawn on the inferior two thirds of the en face sagittal image, and is well conserved for normal glenoid geometry.[24] The amount of bone missing is determined by assessing surface area losses from the anteroinferior part of the circle. The reason for the precision of bone loss measurement is that the glenoid bone stock from anterior to posterior is only about 24 to 28 mm[25] and varies from patient to patient. In

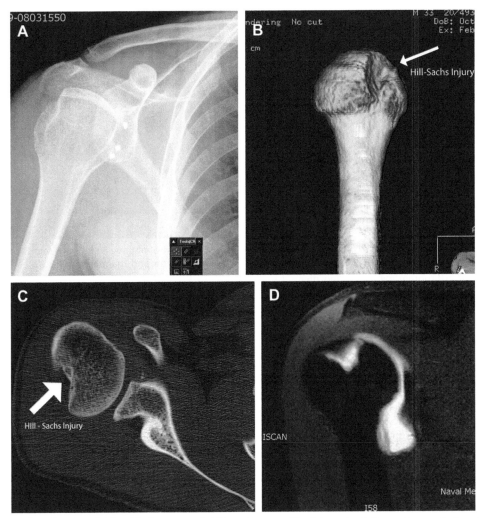

Fig. 4. A Hill-Sachs injury is identified on several different images. The internal rotation anteroposterior view (*A*); a three-dimensional CT scan with the glenoid and scapula digitally subtracted that demonstrates the hatchet-type injury of the humerus (*B*); the same image on the axial CT scan (*C*); and a coronal MR arthrogram demonstrating the injury adjacent to the rotator cuff posterolaterally (*D*).

addition, for approximately each 1.5 to 1.7 mm of glenoid bone loss, this corresponds to a 5% increase in loss of glenoid bone stock.[26] Glenoid bone loss occurs along a line parallel to the long axis of the glenoid (parallel to the 12- to 6-o'clock line).[27,28] (**Fig. 7**) Glenoid bone loss greater than 20% to 25% can lead to the glenoid taking on the shape of an inverted pear when viewed arthroscopically from the anterosuperior portal (**Fig. 8**).[25,29] Although a Hill-Sachs lesion is present in up to 80% to 100% of patients with anterior instability, it is usually insignificant.[8] However, in patients with glenoid bone loss, it is now well appreciated that a Hill-Sachs lesion can become more significant and engage the glenoid with much less force and anterior translation than those without glenoid bone loss.[30,31] Thus, one should

look at glenoid and humeral head bone loss as a bipolar problem, and make informed decisions regarding treatment based upon the amount of bone loss, patient expectations, and associated recurrent instability risk factors.

→ Pearl: Glenoid bone loss of between 6 to 8 mm indicates an approximately 20% to 25% bone stock loss of the glenoid from anterior to posterior and may necessitate a change in surgical strategy (ie, soft-tissue procedure to bone augmentation).

Ideally, the amount of glenoid and humeral head bone loss is determined preoperatively in order to have an informed discussion with patients regarding treatment options and expected outcomes of arthroscopic versus bone augmentation repair. However, if the presence of bone loss is not evaluated preoperatively, the glenoid bone

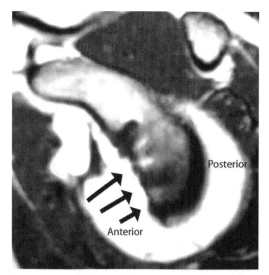

Fig. 5. MR arthrogram demonstrating glenoid bone loss on the sagittal oblique image. Arrow points to bone defect.

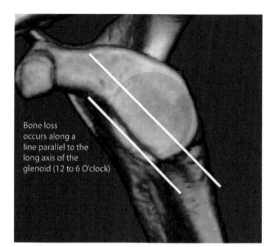

Fig. 7. A sagittal oblique CT image demonstrating the typical location and manner in which glenoid bone loss occurs; along a line parallel with the long axis of the glenoid (12 o'clock–6 o'clock).

stock may be assessed arthroscopically. The bare spot of the glenoid is a well-described landmark for assessing glenoid bone loss via a calibrated probe inserted from the posterior shoulder while the arthroscope is in the anterosuperior portal. Lo and colleagues[25] have described a method of quantifying glenoid bone loss by measuring the anterior-posterior width of the defect at the level of the bare spot. A calibrated probe is inserted from the posterior portal to measure the distance from the anterior and posterior rims to the bare spot. The difference between the anterior and posterior radii can be determined and referenced

as a percentage of the diameter of the normal inferior glenoid using the following equation:

Distance from the bare spot to the posterior rim percent bone loss = distance from the bare spot to the anterior rim)/2x distance from the bare spot to the posterior rim × 100

The arthroscopic determination of glenoid bone loss remains a well-accepted technique and has been validated clinically[25,32] and in the laboratory setting.[27] In addition, the amount of glenoid bone loss may be measured intraoperatively to confirm the surgical plan and preoperative findings.

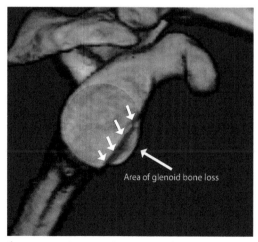

Fig. 6. CT evaluation of a sagittal oblique glenoid en face view demonstrating the best-fit circle as a gold standard to determine the amount of glenoid bone loss.

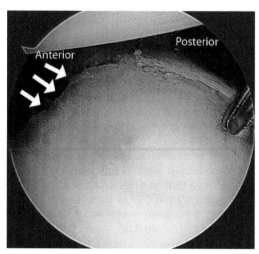

Fig. 8. Arthroscopic image from the anterosuperior portal demonstrating an inverted pear glenoid with significant (>20%–25%) glenoid bone loss.

Historically, arthroscopic treatment of glenoid bone defects have had a high recurrence rate (from 61%–67%).[8] Mologne and colleagues[29] demonstrated a 14% recurrence rate in patients with a mean loss of 25% glenoid bone loss treated arthroscopically, and noted that all of their failures (three total) were in patients deemed to have attritional bone loss and no glenoid bone fragment to incorporate into the repair. In another study, Sugaya and colleagues[33] demonstrated only an 8% recurrence rate in patients with a mean 25% bone loss treated arthroscopically when the bony fragment was incorporated into the repair. These studies illustrate the importance of glenoid bone stock for the success of arthroscopic instability repair.

The management of patients with humeral bone loss is less well quantified, owing to the difficulty in determining when a Hill-Sachs lesion is clinically important. Burkhart and De Beer[8] defined a Hill-Sachs lesion as "engaging" when the posterolateral humeral head engages the anterior glenoid with the arm in abduction and externally rotation. Yamamoto and colleagues[34] demonstrated in a cadaveric model that the engagement phenomenon is potentiated in the setting of glenoid bone loss (ie, the humeral head engages the glenoid easier if the anterior glenoid has a bone deficiency present). However, in the presence of humeral head engagement, or for sizable Hill-Sachs defects (usually >5–7 mm in depth), the typical solution is glenoid bone augmentation. In rare circumstances, there are a variety of surgical management options for a Hill-Sachs injury that range from soft-tissue augmentation (Remplissage), glenoid-based bone augmentation, humeral-head options, and occasionally both (See the article by Boselli and colleagues elsewhere in this issue for further exploration of this topic).

→ Pearl: Based upon preoperative evaluation, including age; sports participation (risky contact sports); and amount of glenoid bone loss, an informed consent regarding expected treatment outcomes will allow patients to decide upon soft-tissue versus bony stabilization. The key is to recognize that not all patients are candidates for soft-tissue instability repair (either arthroscopic or open), as many in high-risk groups (bone loss, contact athletics) may not fare as well with a soft-tissue instability repair.

ASSOCIATED PATHOLOGY WITH INSTABILITY

→ Pearl: Understand the pathology that is commonly associated with anterior instability and how to treat if encountered.

- HAGL: the capsuloligamentous structures have avulsed and torn off the humeral head instead of at the glenoid. See the article by Boselli and colleagues elsewhere in this issue for further exploration of this topic.
- ALPSA: a soft-tissue or bony Bankart injury (see later discussion) has occurred and healed in a medially displaced position on the glenoid neck. See the article by Boselli and colleagues elsewhere in this issue for further exploration of this topic.
- Glenoid labrum articular disruption: an articular cartilage injury of the anteroinferior glenoid. See the article by Boselli and colleagues elsewhere in this issue for further exploration of this topic.
- Bony Bankart: injury at the bony glenoid, instead of at the bone-labral junction. Usually includes component of capsular stretch and injury. See the article by Boselli and colleagues elsewhere in this issue for further exploration of this topic.
- Soft-tissue Bankart: tear of the anteroinferior labrum off the glenoid. Usually includes component of capsular stretch and injury.
- Capsular stretch and injury: almost always present in anterior instability. Some level of anterior capsular stretch and injury is required to have an instability event.

→ Pearl: The pathology of capsular stretch and the Bankart injury (soft tissue or bony) need to be corrected for successful outcomes.

TREATMENT PEARLS AND PITFALLS
Nonoperative

The natural history of acute anterior instability events has been evaluated through numerous prospective studies with age at the time of initial dislocation being the most significant prognostic factor for future instability events. Active patients less than 30 years of age treated with a supervised physical therapy program instead of surgically have had reported recurrence rates of 17% to 96%, whereas those treated with arthroscopic repair had failure rates ranging from 4% to 22%.[35,36] This data indicates early arthroscopic repair following first-time dislocation is applicable for young, highly active patients or those engaged in activities involving overhead use of their arms.

Nonoperative treatment for anterior shoulder instability consists of physical therapy tailored toward the acuity and mechanism of instability. Immobilization is only necessary until pain control is achieved, which is typically 1 to 3 weeks. Although controversial, immobilization in external rotation after an initial instability event decreases recurrence rates in some populations.[37–39]

Operative

Indications

Although open repair of anterior shoulder instability has been considered the gold standard, arthroscopic shoulder instability repair has become a key component in the diagnosis and management of shoulder instability. Given that there are a multitude of factors associated with successful anterior shoulder instability repair, it is critical that the surgeon identify and address each of these operative pearls during arthroscopic repair.

Operative pearls

1. Appropriate preoperative evaluation: Evaluate for glenoid/humeral head bone loss.
2. Evaluation under anesthesia: This evaluation should confirm the preoperative plan and assist with amount of capsular shift to perform.
3. Patient positioning: Although it is surgeon preference, the lateral decubitus provides for ease of access to the superior, posterior, inferior, and anterior labrum and capsule (**Fig. 9**).
4. Anterosuperior portal: *Always* view the pathology from the anterosuperior portal to avoid missing ALPSA lesions, it is better to evaluate anteroinferior glenoid bone loss and to assess extent of tear posteriorly.
5. Glenoid preparation: Make sure that the soft tissue is removed from the intended repair site and that there is a bleeding bed of bone to enhance healing. Visualization of the posterior subscapularis muscle fibers indicates an adequate preparation of the labrum and capsular attachments to the glenoid and allows for sufficient mobilization for repair (**Fig. 10**). The axillary nerve is closest at the 6-o'clock position, between 12.5 to 15 mm, and should be avoided.
6. Labral preparation: Use an elevator device and ensure labrum is visible, release subperiosteally to prepare the glenoid and allow the capsulolabral tissue to easily float up to the glenoid face.
7. Suture anchor placement: Make sure anchors are placed at the articular cartilage margin to avoid non-anatomic medial scapular neck placement.
8. Suture anchor quantity: For most anteroinferior labral tears a minimum of three suture anchors should be used (3–6 o'clock on a right shoulder; 6–9 o'clock on a left shoulder). A standard repair is three anchors below 3 o'clock (the equator).
9. Capsular plication: Abrasion of the capsule should be performed to enhance healing to the labrum. The plication can be performed to an intact labrum if there is robust labral tissue.

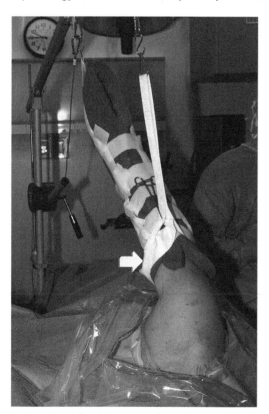

Fig. 9. Lateral decubitus setup for arthroscopic instability procedure. Arrow points to lateral arm traction.

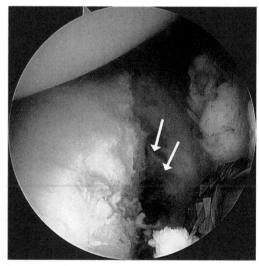

Fig. 10. Arthroscopic image of an adequately prepared anterior glenoid labrum. The posterior subscapularis fibers (*arrows*) are just visualized and the labrum and capsule easily float up to the glenoid face indicating adequate preparation.

If there is any question, a suture anchor is preferred.

Pearls for patient setup in the operating room

Based on the preference of the surgical team and patient, shoulder arthroscopy can be performed with general anesthesia, inter-scalene block or a combination of the two. The authors prefer regional anesthesia supplemented with a light general anesthetic to facilitate lateral decubitus positioning in the outpatient setting.

With regard to setup for patients undergoing arthroscopic anterior shoulder instability repair, patients can be placed in either the lateral decubitus or beach-chair position. The beach-chair position affords several advantages, including ease of access, ability to see the anterosuperior, inferior and anterior aspect of the glenohumeral joint, and ability to easily convert to an open procedure if indicated.

For cases of shoulder instability, however, the authors prefer to place patients in a lateral decubitus position because it allows ease of access and visualization of the entire capsulolabral complex. With the ability to provide longitudinal and direct lateral suspension, the lateral position affords greater distension of the glenohumeral joint and better ability to make the necessary passes with instrumentation for optimal repair. One of the pitfalls of lateral decubitus positioning is the difficulty in achieving rotational control during instability repair. For instance, proper tensioning of the capsule and inferior glenohumeral ligament is particularly challenging in the lateral decubitus position and can lead to postoperative stiffness and decreased external rotation. In addition, subscapularis repair in athletes with shoulder instability and rotator interval closure are ideally done in 30° to 45° of external rotation, which can be difficult to achieve in patients in the lateral position.

Examination under anesthesia and arthroscopic evaluation

→ Pearl: The examination under anesthesia (EUA) is usually used to confirm what is known preoperatively about patients, including direction of instability, symptoms, and associated findings.

→ Pearl: The EUA can offer information about the amount of translation in the anterior, posterior, and inferior directions, and can serve to tailor specific operative planning, such as how much capsular plication to perform.

Pearls for portals

Proper portal placement is pivotal in performing an accurate diagnostic arthroscopy and complete Bankart repair while providing facile soft-tissue mobilization and accurate anchor placement. After patient positioning, the standard posterior and anterior-superior portals (high in the rotator interval) are made and a full diagnostic arthroscopy is performed. Once a Bankart lesion has been identified, an anterior mid-glenoid portal can be established in line with the 3-o'clock position on the glenoid using an 18-gauge needle for localization just superior to the subscapularis tendon. Although accurate portal placement is essential for labral preparation and anchor placement for anteroinferior labral defects, the 4- to 6-o'clock labral pathology can prove to be increasingly difficult to appropriately repair through these standard portals. A 7-o'clock portal can be established approximately 2 to 3 cm lateral and 1 cm inferior to the posterior portal (or 3 to 4 cm lateral to the posterolateral edge of the acromion) and provides excellent access to the inferior glenoid and may be used to percutaneously place suture anchors in the most inferior aspect of the glenoid (**Fig. 11**).

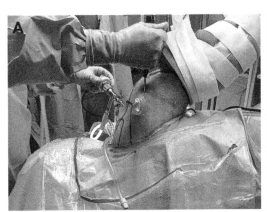
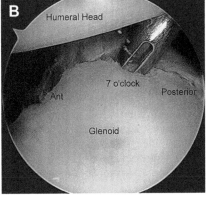

Fig. 11. The posterolateral 7-o'clock portal as viewed from outside (*A*) and inside (*B*) the shoulder demonstrating ease of access and anchor placement in the inferior aspects of the glenoid.

Pearl/pitfalls of portal placement

- The initial posterior portal in the lateral decubitus position is made in line with the lateral edge of the acromion and 1 cm inferior to the posterior tip. This position allows the posterior portal to have a slightly downward trajectory on the glenoid surface to facilitate ease of instrumentation during the case.
- The anterosuperior portal is made high in the rotator interval. After initial diagnostic arthroscopy, the arthroscope is transferred to the anterosuperior portal for excellent visualization of the anterior glenoid.
- The mid-glenoid portal is also made in the rotator interval, just superior to the subscapularis tendon. The mid-glenoid and anterosuperior portals should have enough skin bridge separation (2–3 cm) to avoid intraarticular crowding for performing the case.
- Although not always used, a 7-o'clock (posterolateral) portal may be made for percutaneous anchor placement, or a small cannula may be inserted to facilitate glenoid anchor placement and repair inferiorly.
- The axillary nerve is closest at the 6-o'clock position on the glenoid (12.5 mm –15 mm), which increases with abduction.

Pearls for labrum preparation

Proper labral preparation is a critical portion of anterior shoulder instability repair as inadequate labral preparation can lead to insufficient capsulolabral plication and symptoms of recurrent instability. It is imperative that the surgeon spend time preparing and mobilizing the labrum-bone interface before anchor insertion and fixation. The authors prefer to use an elevator device to peel the labrum from the glenoid neck while viewing the labral pathology from the anterosuperior portal.

→ Pearl: A small bone-cutting type of shaver (3.0 to 3.5 mm) is useful to prepare the anterior glenoid neck on a high-speed reverse setting, keeping in mind that this is a glenoid bone preserving procedure.

Labral preparation should be completed before preparing the glenoid for anchor placement and special care should be taken to preserve the remaining labrum for plication. With either the shaver or small bone-cutting shaver on forward or the burr on reverse, the glenoid can be prepared, allowing for adequate bone preservation during glenoid preparation.

Besides bone loss, the most frequent reasons for failure after instability repair include unaddressed capsular laxity, improper anchor positioning, and recurrent trauma in an otherwise well-done reconstruction. Accurate positioning of suture anchors on the glenoid with penetration at the margin of the articular surface allows recreation of the glenoid concavity during repair and avoids repairing the labrum complex too medially down the glenoid neck. Boileau and colleagues[10] recommend at least four suture anchors, because less than three suture anchors in their study was associated with failure after instability repair. Their study finding speaks to well-placed suture anchors that correctly address the pathology of instability. Lastly, asymmetric tensioning during open or arthroscopic capsulorrhaphy can also create instability in the opposite direction.

Anchors

The standard arthroscopic Bankart repair typically uses three anchors placed below 3 o'clock with ideal anchor placement on the glenoid rim at a 45° angle relative to the glenoid surface 2 to 3 mm inside the anterior glenoid rim (**Fig. 12**). Additional anchors are placed approximately 7 mm apart depending on the size and extent of the labral defect. Some have advocated a balanced repair, which includes repair of the anterior tear and posterior plication sutures to the intact posterior labrum.[40] The posterior labrum may not always be intact and may present as an extension of the anterior tear posteriorly. In this case, suture anchors are used to repair the labrum and perform plication of the capsule as necessary. However, if a balanced repair is desired and the

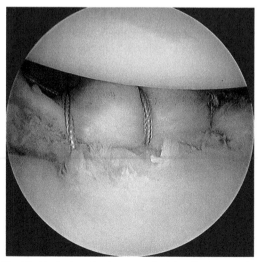

Fig. 12. Posterior viewing portal of the final anteroinferior labral repair with anatomic restoration of the labral-ligamentous complex.

posterior labrum is intact, it has been shown biomechanically that an intact labrum provides similar fixation strength to a suture anchor.[41] In performing adequate capsulolabral tensioning, the surgeon can use knots from a suture anchor or knotless anchors for fixation of the labrum to the glenoid.

Pearl and pitfalls for capsular plication

- Tension the capsulolabral structures with the arm in slight external rotation.
- Use a minimum of three suture anchors.
- The anchors should be placed 2 mm onto the glenoid rim and not medially on the glenoid neck.
- Pull on sutures before knot tying and after the capsulolabral repair stitch has been placed to visualize capsular plication and to ensure that adequate capsular tissue has been incorporated.
- A balanced repair may be performed if there is significant posterior laxity and capsular volume with either plication stitches (if labrum intact) or suture anchor repair after an anterior instability repair.[40]

Choosing the right rehabilitation

Proper postoperative rehabilitation begins with thorough *preoperative* patient counseling combined with the intraoperative findings. Factors to consider are type of pathology (traumatic vs atraumatic); direction of instability (anterior, posterior, multidirectional); integrity of tissue at time of repair; comfort level with quality of repair; and possible associated findings and treatment (ie, biceps tendon tear, rotator cuff tear). Routine postoperative immobilization varies based on the procedures performed. The authors recommend an abduction sling for most anterior instability repairs (this type of sling keeps the shoulder in a neutral position).

Physical therapy typically starts 7 to 10 days following most routine instability repairs. Unidirectional instability repair will progress with passive and active-assisted range of motion for the first 4 weeks (forward elevation [FE] to 130°; external rotation [ER] to 30°). From 4 to 6 weeks these ranges will be increased to FE 130° to180° and ER 30° to 60°. Active range of motion exercises progress thereafter with resistive strengthening from 8 to 12 weeks and the return to full sports and activities at 4 to 6 months in most cases.

SUMMARY

The successful management of patients with anterior shoulder instability can be a significant challenge and is predicated on the accurate assessment and treatment of the offending pathologies. It is essential that the surgeon have an understanding of the pathoanatomy of recurrent anterior shoulder instability and to recognize the associated conditions. With a thorough understanding of the principles of arthroscopic instability repair, the pearls provided should allow a comprehensive approach to patients with shoulder instability with the hope of continued improvement in patient outcomes.

REFERENCES

1. Kim SH, Ha KI. Bankart repair in traumatic anterior shoulder instability: open versus arthroscopic technique. Arthroscopy 2002;18(7):755–63.
2. Bottoni CR, Smith EL, Berkowits MJ, et al. Arthroscopic versus open shoulder stabilization for recurrent anterior instability: a prospective randomized clinical trial. Am J Sports Med 2006;34(11):1730–7.
3. Kim SH, Ha KI, Park JH, et al. Arthroscopic posterior labral repair and capsular shift for traumatic unidirectional recurrent posterior subluxation of the shoulder. J Bone Joint Surg Am 2003;85(8): 1479–87.
4. Freedman KB, Smith AP, Romeo AA, et al. Open Bankart repair versus arthroscopic repair with transglenoid sutures or bioabsorbable tacks for Recurrent Anterior instability of the shoulder: a meta-analysis. Am J Sports Med 2004;32(6): 1520–7.
5. Levine WN, Flatow EL. The pathophysiology of shoulder instability. Am J Sports Med 2000;28(6): 910–7.
6. Ferrari DA. Capsular ligaments of the shoulder. Anatomical and functional study of the anterior superior capsule. Am J Sports Med 1990;18(1):20–4.
7. Bigliani LU, Newton PM, Steinmann SP, et al. Glenoid rim lesions associated with recurrent anterior dislocation of the shoulder. Am J Sports Med 1998;26(1):41–5.
8. Burkhart SS, De Beer JF. Traumatic glenohumeral bone defects and their relationship to failure of arthroscopic Bankart repairs: significance of the inverted-pear glenoid and the humeral engaging Hill-Sachs lesion. Arthroscopy 2000; 16(7):677–94.
9. Bushnell BD, Creighton RA, Herring MM. Bony instability of the shoulder. Arthroscopy 2008;24(9):1061–73.
10. Boileau P, Villalba M, Héry JY, et al. Risk factors for recurrence of shoulder instability after arthroscopic Bankart repair. J Bone Joint Surg Am 2006;88(8): 1755–63.
11. Tauber M, Resch H, Forstner R, et al. Reasons for failure after surgical repair of anterior shoulder instability. J Shoulder Elbow Surg 2004;13(3):279–85.

12. Snyder SJ, Karzel RP, Del Pizzo W, et al. SLAP lesions of the shoulder. Arthroscopy 1990;6(4): 274–9.

13. Williams MM, Snyder SJ. A sublabral foramen must not be confused with a Bankart lesion. Arthroscopy 1994;10(5):586.

14. Williams MM, Snyder SJ, Buford D Jr. The Buford complex–the "cord-like" middle glenohumeral ligament and absent anterosuperior labrum complex: a normal anatomic capsulolabral variant. Arthroscopy 1994;10(3):241–7.

15. Howell SM, Galinat BJ, Renzi A, et al. Normal and abnormal mechanics of the glenohumeral joint in the horizontal plane. J Bone Joint Surg Am 1988; 70(2):227–32.

16. Garth WP, Slappey CE, Ochs CW. Roentgenographic demonstration of instability of the shoulder: the apical oblique projection. J Bone Joint Surg Am 1984;66:1450–3.

17. Arciero RA, Taylor DC. Primary anterior dislocation of the shoulder in young patients. A ten-year prospective study. J Bone Joint Surg Am 1998; 80(2):299–300.

18. Bigliani LU, Kelkar R, Flatow EL, et al. Glenohumeral stability. Biomechanical properties of passive and active stabilizers. Clin Orthop Relat Res 1996;330: 13–30.

19. Ikeda H. ["Rotator interval" lesion. Part 1: clinical study]. Nippon Seikeigeka Gakkai Zasshi 1986; 60(12):1261–73 [in Japanese].

20. Ovesen J, Nielsen S. Stability of the shoulder joint. Cadaver study of stabilizing structures. Acta Orthop Scand 1985;56(2):149–51.

21. Kornguth PJ, Salazar AM. The apical oblique view of the shoulder: its usefulness in acute trauma. AJR Am J Roentgenol 1987;149(1):113–6.

22. Roukos JR, Feagin JA. Modified axillary roentgenogram: a useful adjunct in the diagnosis of recurrent instability of the shoulder. Clin Orthop Relat Res 1972;82:84–6.

23. Pavlov H, Warren RF, Weiss CB Jr, et al. The roentgenographic evaluation of anterior shoulder instability. Clin Orthop Relat Res 1985;194:153–8.

24. Huysmans PE, Haen PS, Kidd M, et al. The shape of the inferior part of the glenoid: a cadaveric study. J Shoulder Elbow Surg 2006;15(6):759–63.

25. Lo IK, Parten PM, Burkhart SS. The inverted pear glenoid: an indicator of significant glenoid bone loss. Arthroscopy 2004;20(2):169–74.

26. Detterline AJ, Provencher MT, Ghodadra N, et al. A new arthroscopic technique to determine anterior-inferior glenoid bone loss: validation of the secant chord theory in a cadaveric model. Arthroscopy 2009;25(11):1249–56.

27. Provencher MT, Detterline AJ, Ghodadra N, et al. Measurement of glenoid bone loss: a comparison of measurement error between 45 degrees and

0 degrees bone loss models and with different posterior arthroscopy portal locations. Am J Sports Med 2008;36(6):1132–8.

28. Saito H, Itoi E, Sugaya H, et al. Location of the glenoid defect in shoulders with recurrent anterior dislocation. Am J Sports Med 2005;33(6): 889–93.

29. Mologne TS, Provencher MT, Menzel KA, et al. Arthroscopic stabilization in patients with an inverted pear glenoid: results in patients with bone loss of the anterior glenoid. Am J Sports Med 2007;35(8):1276–83.

30. Ito H, Takayama A, Shirai Y. Radiographic evaluation of the Hill-Sachs lesion in patients with recurrent anterior shoulder instability. J Shoulder Elbow Surg 2000;9(6):495–7.

31. Saito H, Itoi E, Minagawa H, et al. Location of the Hill-Sachs lesion in shoulders with recurrent anterior dislocation. Arch Orthop Trauma Surg 2009;129(10): 1327–34.

32. Burkhart SS, Debeer JF, Tehrany AM, et al. Quantifying glenoid bone loss arthroscopically in shoulder instability. Arthroscopy 2002;18(5): 488–91.

33. Sugaya H, Kon Y, Tsuchiya A, et al. Arthroscopic osseous Bankart repair for chronic recurrent traumatic anterior glenohumeral instability. Surgical technique. J Bone Joint Surg Am 2006;88 (Suppl 1 Pt 2):159–69.

34. Yamamoto N, Itoi E, Abe H, et al. Contact between the glenoid and the humeral head in abduction, external rotation, and horizontal extension: a new concept of glenoid track. J Shoulder Elbow Surg 2007;16(5):649–56.

35. DeBerardino TM, Arciero RA, Taylor DC, et al. Prospective evaluation of arthroscopic stabilization of acute, initial anterior shoulder dislocations in young athletes. Two- to five-year follow-up. Am J Sports Med 2001;29(5):586–92.

36. Bottoni CR, Wilckens JH, DeBerardino TM, et al. A prospective, randomized evaluation of arthroscopic stabilization versus nonoperative treatment in patients with acute, traumatic, first-time shoulder dislocations. Am J Sports Med 2002; 30(4):576–80.

37. Itoi E, Hatakeyama Y, Sato T, et al. Immobilization in external rotation after shoulder dislocation reduces the risk of recurrence. A randomized controlled trial. J Bone Joint Surg Am 2007; 89(10):2124–31.

38. Hovelius L, Olofsson A, Sandström B, et al. Nonoperative treatment of primary anterior shoulder dislocation in patients forty years of age and younger. A prospective twenty-five-year follow-up. J Bone Joint Surg Am 2008;90(5):945–52.

39. Miller BS, Sonnabend DH, Hatrick C, et al. Should acute anterior dislocations of the shoulder be

immobilized in external rotation? A cadaveric study. J Shoulder Elbow Surg 2004;13(6):589–92.

40. Snyder SJ, Strafford BB. Arthroscopic management of instability of the shoulder. Orthopedics 1993; 16(9):993–1002.

41. Provencher MT, Verma N, Obopilwe E, et al. A biomechanical analysis of capsular plication versus anchor repair of the shoulder: can the labrum be used as a suture anchor? Arthroscopy 2008;24(2):210–6.

.

Arthroscopic Management of Posterior Instability

James P. Bradley, MD[a,b,c], Sam G. Tejwani, MD[d,e,*]

KEYWORDS

- Shoulder dislocation • Posterior instability
- Arthroscopy • Posterior stabilization

In comparison with anterior shoulder instability, posterior instability is uncommon, occurring in 2% to 10% of cases.[1–5] A posteriorly directed blow to an adducted, internally rotated, and forward-flexed upper extremity is classically described as the sentinel traumatic event.[6] However, recurrent or locked posterior shoulder dislocations from macrotrauma are exceedingly rare in the athletic population.[2,7] Instead, athletes typically present with posterior shoulder instability secondary to repetitive microtrauma, which can occur in multiple arm positions and under a variety of loading conditions. In 1952, McLaughlin[2] first acknowledged the existence of a wide clinical spectrum of posterior shoulder instability, ranging from locked posterior dislocation to the often subclinical recurrent posterior subluxation (RPS).

In athletics, RPS has been observed in weight-lifters, football linemen, golfers, tennis players, butterfly and freestyle swimmers, overhead throwers, and baseball hitters, among others.[8–10] The origin of RPS is repetitive microtrauma, most commonly leading to posterior capsular attenuation and labral tearing. Regardless of the sport, athletes with RPS typically present with ambiguous complaints of diffuse pain and shoulder fatigue, without distinct injury, often making it challenging to elucidate the underlying pathology and diagnosis.

A thorough history and physical examination, coupled with specific imaging studies, are required to determine the exact pathogenesis of and appropriate treatment options for RPS. With increased clinical awareness, imaging advances such as magnetic resonance arthrography (MRA), and the development of specific provocative physical examination tests, the identification of RPS in the athletic population is improving. Several variables that must be considered during the workup include mechanism of injury (true posterior traumatic dislocation vs repetitive microtrauma vs an acute on chronic subluxation), specific direction of instability (posterior vs posteroinferior or posterosuperior), and the pattern of instability (unidirectional or multidirectional), as these factors will ultimately affect treatment and outcome.[11]

Successful treatment of RPS begins with thorough identification of all of the structural abnormalities present in the affected shoulder, which can include any combination of the labrum, capsule, supporting ligaments, and rotator cuff. Over time, posterior glenohumeral stabilization has evolved from various open procedures to an anatomic-based arthroscopic approach, which allows for enhanced identification and repair of intra-articular pathology including posterior capsular laxity, complete or incomplete

Financial disclosure: J.P.B.: Research support from Arthrex Inc; S.G.T.: None.
[a] Pittsburgh Steelers, Pittsburgh, PA, USA
[b] Department of Orthopaedic Surgery, University of Pittsburgh Medical Center, Pittsburgh, PA, USA
[c] Burke and Bradley Orthopaedics, 200 Delafield Road, Suite 4010, Pittsburgh, PA 15215, USA
[d] Department of Orthopaedic Surgery, Division of Sports Medicine, Southern California Permanente Medical Group, Kaiser Permanente Hospital, Fontana, CA, USA
[e] 9985 Sierra Avenue, Medical Office Building 3, Fontana, CA 92335, USA
* Corresponding author. 9985 Sierra Avenue, Medical Office Building 3, Fontana, CA 92335.
E-mail address: samtejwani@yahoo.com

doi:10.1016/j.ocl.2010.02.002

detachment of the posterior capsulolabral complex, and inferior capsular tears.[12] While postoperative results are generally good to excellent after stabilization for RPS, there is room for improvement. Accordingly, research continues on both the biomechanical and clinical fronts to further refine diagnostic and treatment approaches to RPS.

PATHOANATOMY

The pathogenesis of RPS varies among athletes, in direct relationship to the particular repetitive stresses placed on the posterior structures of the glenohumeral joint during competition and training. For example, activities like push-ups, bench-press weight lifting, and blocking in football linemen all place direct stress on the posterior capsulolabral complex of the shoulder, potentially resulting in RPS. Similarly, the follow-through phase of throwing, pull-through phase in swimming, tennis backhand stroke, and golf backswing can all lead to RPS.

The posterior labrum, capsule, and posterior band of the inferior glenohumeral ligament (IGHL) are the primary stabilizers to posterior translation of the humeral head, particularly between 45° and 90° of glenohumeral abduction.[13] The posterior capsule is delineated by the area between the intra-articular portion of the biceps tendon and the posterior band of the IGHL. The posterior capsule is the thinnest segment of the shoulder capsule, devoid of any supporting ligamentous structures, thus making it prone to attenuation from applied stress.[14] It has been postulated that overhead throwers, tennis players, and swimmers develop shoulder pain associated with progressive laxity of the posterior capsule and fatigue of the static and dynamic stabilizers.[15] Recurrent posterior subluxation can lead to plastic deformation of the posterior capsule, and a patulous posteroinferior capsular pouch with an associated increased joint volume.[16] After a traumatic posterior subluxation or dislocation, athletes may sustain a capsulolabral detachment known as a reverse Bankart tear, further contributing to recurrent instability and symptoms (**Figs. 1** and **2**).

Many investigators have reported an elaborate role of the anterior IGHL and shoulder capsule in preventing posterior instability, which varies with shoulder position and applied forces.[14,17–19] Warren and colleagues[19] studied the static restraints to posterior translation with the arm in the vulnerable position of shoulder flexion and internal rotation.[14] Transection of the infraspinatus, teres minor, and entire posterior capsule was insufficient to produce posterior dislocation;

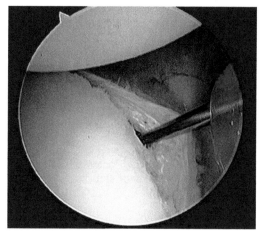

Fig. 1. Posterior labral tear from the glenoid (right shoulder, viewed from the anterior portal).

however, when the anterosuperior capsule and superior glenohumeral ligament (SGHL) were transected, a posterior dislocation would develop. This finding led to the development of the "circle concept," which proposed that dislocation in one direction requires capsular damage on both the same side and the opposite side of the joint. A biomechanical study by Cole and colleagues[20] demonstrated that the rotator interval and SGHL provide static glenohumeral stability by limiting inferior and posterior joint translations with the arm adducted. However, recent work by Provencher and colleagues[21] has demonstrated that rotator interval closure, though associated with a predictable loss of external rotation, has no

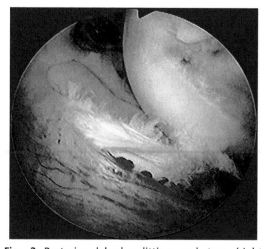

Fig. 2. Posterior labral splitting and tear (right shoulder, viewed from the posterior portal). Placing the patient in the lateral decubitus position facilitates posterior labral visualization and repair.

effect on reducing posterior instability of the glenohumeral joint. Thus, it appears that rotator interval closure is not clinically indicated in the athlete with unidirectional posterior instability, and may actually have a deleterious effect on overhead throwers who rely on functioning in the abduction-external rotation (ABER) position.

Muscular forces from the deltoid and rotator cuff also contribute to the dynamic concavity-compression effect on the humeral head within the glenoid.[22] Of the rotator cuff muscles, the subscapularis provides the most resistance to posterior translation of the shoulder, acting as a dynamic supporter of the action of the posterior band of the IGHL.[23,24] In one cadaveric study examining the effect of rotator cuff imbalance on the development of labral tear, it was concluded that decreased subscapularis muscle strength in the position simulating the late cocking phase of throwing motion results in increased maximum glenohumeral external rotation and increased glenohumeral contact pressure.[25] It was inferred from these findings that throwers who develop subscapularis fatigue from repetitive throwing may be more susceptible to these forces and a resultant Type II superior labral anterior posterior (SLAP) tear. In their clinical experience with both throwers and nonthrowers, the authors have found that Type II SLAP tears can propagate posteroinferiorly around the glenoid rim, resulting in the Type VIII SLAP tear and symptomatic RPS.[25,26]

While a full understanding of the pathology contributing to decreased performance in the elite throwing athlete has yet to be established, an evidence-based biomechanical model regarding RPS is taking shape. The humeral head possesses an oblong, or cam, shape due to the presence of the greater and lesser tuberosities. In the ABER position, the anterior band of the IGHL becomes taut as it is draped over the anteroinferior aspect of the eccentrically positioned humeral head, providing a check-rein against excessive external rotation in that position.[27,28] In pitchers, increased glenohumeral external rotation is favored at the expense of internal rotation in an effort to prime the late cocking phase of throwing, primarily because an enhanced late cocking phase leads to more rapid internal humeral rotation in follow-through and increased pitch velocity. Chronic use of the shoulder in this manner, with external rotation priming, ultimately results in a glenohumeral internal rotation deficit (GIRD), which manifests structurally as a posterior capsular contracture.

Burkhart and colleagues[27,28] have postulated that the cam effect of the humerus is overcome by the thrower, who by developing a posterior capsular contracture shifts the rotational fulcrum posterosuperiorly; this shift of the rotational fulcrum allows the humeral head to clear the anteroinferior labroligamentous restraints and achieve more external rotation in abduction. With this adaptation, it is felt that the posterior and posterosuperior glenohumeral restraints in overhead throwers are susceptible to repetitive microtrauma events during the follow-through phase with the shoulder in the adducted, flexed, and internally rotated position.[4,15,29] Throwers who have GIRD are thought to experience repetitive microtrauma after ball release, resulting in progressive tearing of the superior, and potentially posterior labrum (**Fig. 3**).[26]

The resultant posteroinferior capsular thickening from contracture associated with GIRD has been visualized on magnetic resonance (MR) examinations of the throwing athlete.[30] In addition, throwing athletes who have painful posterior shoulder instability and commonly perform with the shoulder in the ABER position have been found on dynamic MRA to undergo a phenomenon described as posterosuperior labral "peel back."[31] During the "peel back" event, when the arm is placed in the ABER position during MRA, the detached posterosuperior labral tissue is seen separating from and moving medially to the glenoid rim. This dynamic phenomenon can also be visualized arthroscopically with the arm in the ABER position.

Not all throwing athletes demonstrate concurrent findings of GIRD and posterior labral tear, highlighting the complexity of the pathogenesis of RPS in this population. It has been observed

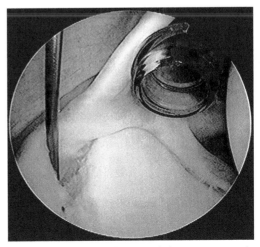

Fig. 3. Complete detachment of the posterosuperior labrum from the glenoid in an overhead thrower, as localized by the spinal needle (right shoulder, viewed from the posterior portal).

that some adaptive changes can occur in the throwing shoulder without negative consequence, while other athletes reach a tipping point that may lead to symptoms. After approximately 25° of GIRD, the posterosuperior shift in the glenohumeral center of rotation ceases to be adaptive and instead leads to pathologic shearing forces on the posterosuperior labrum and rotator cuff.[32] In effect, the excessive external rotation in the ABER position exposes the posterosuperior labrum, long head of the biceps tendon, and undersurface rotator cuff tendons to large rotatory lever arm forces, resulting in the "peel back" phenomenon.[33] In addition, the posterosuperior shift of the humeral head in the ABER position has been found to result in a relative redundancy of the anteroinferior capsuloligamentous complex. This redundancy in the anteroinferior shoulder capsule is caused by a decrease in the cam effect of the proximal humerus, and may have clinical implications in the pathophysiology of the disabled throwing shoulder.

The clinical presentation of a posterosuperior labral tear in combination with posteroinferior capsular contracture in throwing athletes differs from the spectrum of pathology seen in offensive linemen, weightlifters, and those athletes who are frequently subjected to repetitive high loads with the arm in the forward flexed and adducted position.[9] In the latter, these high shearing forces on the posterior labrum result in labral tearing, posterior capsular laxity, and capsular redundancy. This condition is best treated with arthroscopic posterior labral repair and additional posterior capsular plication as indicated. On the contrary, when GIRD and RPS are present in the overhead thrower, stretching of the posteroinferior capsular contracture by way of "sleeper stretches" is a more appropriate initial treatment.[28,34] In addition, subscapularis muscle strengthening may play a role. Ultimately, arthroscopic posterior labral repair with optional posterior capsular release can be performed to treat recalcitrant symptoms in the thrower with GIRD and RPS. In these cases, the GIRD is typically successfully treated preoperatively with stretching, and the associated capsulolabral avulsion is treated with arthroscopic repair; in rare cases of recalcitrant GIRD a limited capsular release is concomitantly performed during surgery.

Of additional importance is the identification and treatment of scapular dyskinesia, which has variable clinical implications. Scapular winging can act as a compensatory mechanism to prevent posterior subluxation of the humeral head in some patients, although in other patients scapular winging is thought to be the primary cause of

subluxation.[4] In a recent study of 8 elite golfers with posterior shoulder instability, fatigue developed in the serratus anterior muscle during competitive play, possibly contributing to scapulothoracic asynchrony and the combination of posterior shoulder instability and subacromial impingement.[35] Further study of the relationship between scapular mechanics and shoulder stability is warranted. Typically a periscapular muscle strengthening program is incorporated into the physical therapy protocol for RPS to account for the possible contribution of scapular dyskinesia.

Finally, in baseball hitters "batter's shoulder" has recently been described by Dines and colleagues[36] as a cause of RPS. This syndrome affects the lead shoulder during a baseball swing, as dynamic posterior pulling forces approach 500 N, resulting in posterior labral tearing. Typically the nondominant arm is affected, resulting in pain with batting. It has been inferred that golfers may suffer from a similar mechanism of injury. Of note, arthroscopic posterior labral repair (n = 9) or labral debridement (n = 2) was reported to allow return to previous level of batting in 10 of 11 patients with this condition.

HISTORY AND PHYSICAL EXAMINATION

Thorough knowledge of an athlete's sport, position, and training regimen is critical in deducing the pathogenesis and specific pathology associated with RPS. Pollock and Bigliani noted that two-thirds of athletes who ultimately required surgery presented with complaints of difficulty using the shoulder outside of sports, particularly with the arm above the horizontal.[37] An inquiry should also be made regarding mechanical symptoms, as one study found that 90% of patients with symptomatic RPS noted clicking or crepitation with motion.[38] Often this crepitus can be reproduced during examination, and is caused by discrete posterior capsulolabral pathology.

Physical examination of a shoulder suspected of RPS begins with inspection, focusing on asymmetry, scapular dysrhythmia, and muscular atrophy. A skin dimple over the posteromedial deltoid of both shoulders has been found to be 62% sensitive and 92% specific in correlating with posterior instability.[39] Tenderness to palpation as a result of inflammation is next assessed at the posterior glenohumeral joint line, greater tuberosity, and biceps tendon. Patients with posterior instability have been found to have posterior joint line tenderness, likely caused by posterior synovitis or posterior rotator cuff tendinosis secondary to multiple episodes of instability.[37]

Range of motion (ROM) of both shoulders is assessed in forward elevation, abduction in the scapular plane, external rotation with the arm at the side, and internal rotation behind the back to the highest vertebral level. With the patient supine, the arm is abducted 90°, the scapula stabilized, and internal and external glenohumeral rotation measured. These supine measurements are compared with the contralateral shoulder and are used to calculate total arc of rotation (total external rotation plus total internal rotation) and GIRD (side-to-side difference in internal rotation).

Strength testing is performed bilaterally, with a focus on the rotator cuff musculature, and graded on a typical 5-point scale. The majority of athletes with RPS who are tested have Grade 4 or Grade 5 strength. Supraspinatus strength is tested with a downward force while the arm is abducted 90° in the scapular plane. Infraspinatus and teres minor strength are assessed with resisted external rotation, with the arm adducted and elbow flexed 90°. Subtle weakness can be detected in side-to-side comparison if the posterior rotator cuff has damage. Lastly, subscapularis strength is tested with the lumbar lift-off and belly press tests.

Glenohumeral stability is assessed on both shoulders with the patient supine. The load and shift maneuver is performed with the arm held in 60° of abduction and neutral rotation.[23] In this position, a moderate axial load is applied to the glenohumeral joint in combination first with an anterior force in an attempt to translate the humeral head over the anterior glenoid rim. The test is repeated with a posterior directed force (**Fig. 4**). Anterior and posterior laxity is quantified as 0 for a humeral head that does not translate to the glenoid rim, 1+ for a humeral head that translates to but does not translate over the glenoid rim, 2+ for a humeral head that translates over the glenoid rim but spontaneously reduces, and 3+ for a humeral head that translates over the glenoid rim and does not spontaneously reduce.

To assess for excessive IGHL and SGHL laxity, a "sulcus" test is performed by applying longitudinal traction with the arm adducted and in neutral rotation, with the patient seated. The test is repeated in 30° of external rotation. Laxity is quantified as 1+ for an acromiohumeral distance less than 1 cm, 2+ for an acromiohumeral distance between 1 and 2 cm, or 3+ for an acromiohumeral distance greater than 2 cm. A 3+ "sulcus sign" that remains 2+ or greater in 30° of external rotation is considered pathognomonic for an incompetent rotator interval.

Generalized ligamentous laxity may also contribute to multidirectional instability (MDI) and thus should be graded on the 9-point Beighton Scale with the following tests: (1) ability to hyperextend the elbows (1 point for each extremity), (2) ability to passively touch the thumb to the adjacent forearm with the wrist in flexion (1 point for each extremity), (3) ability to passively hyperextend the small finger metacarpophalangeal joint more than 90° (1 point for each extremity), (4) ability to hyperextend the knees (1 point for each extremity), and (5) ability to touch the palms to the floor with feet together (1 point).[40] Patients who score 5 points or greater on the Beighton Scale are considered ligamentously lax.

Several specialized tests have been devised to further elucidate capsulolabral pathology in the shoulder. The Jerk Test is used to assess to assess posterior stability in the seated position. The medial border of the scapula is stabilized with one hand, and the other hand applies a posteriorly directed force to the 90° forward flexed, adducted, and internally rotated arm. The test is positive if posterior subluxation or dislocation of the humeral head occurs while simultaneously reproducing the symptoms of pain and apprehension.[7,41,42]

The Kim Test can also aid in the diagnosis of posterior and posteroinferior shoulder instability. The patient is seated and the arm is placed in 90° of abduction in the scapular plane, and an axial load is applied. The arm is subsequently forward elevated an additional 45°, and a posteroinferior vector is placed on the glenohumeral joint. Kim and colleagues[43] concluded that the test is positive with a sudden onset of posterior subluxation with pain. This test, in combination with the Jerk Test, was found to be 97% sensitive in detecting a posteroinferior labral lesion. The investigators also found that patients who experienced pain

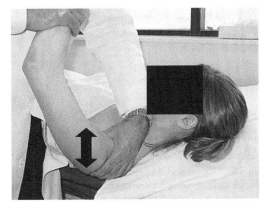

Fig. 4. The "load and shift" test is performed to assess anterior and posterior glenohumeral stability.

with the Kim Test were more likely to require operative intervention to alleviate their symptoms than those who did not experience pain.

The Circumduction Test is particularly useful in higher grades of chronic posterior instability, and is performed with the patient seated. With the elbow in full extension, the arm is brought into 90° of forward elevation and slight adduction. Similar to the Jerk Test, a posteriorly directed load is applied, which subluxates, or possibly dislocates, the humeral head posteriorly. The arm is then circumducted with a combination of abduction and extension until the head reduces into the glenoid. A positive test is a palpable, and typically audible, clunk as the posteriorly subluxated head reduces into the glenoid. In patients with chronic posterior instability, this test can often be performed without pain or muscle guarding.

In some cases of RPS, particularly involving overhead throwers, a posterior labral tear is associated with a superior labral tear, resulting in the Type VIII SLAP tear.[26] Accordingly, when examining a shoulder suspected of RPS, the Active-Compression Test for superior labral pathology should also be performed. For this test, the patient is seated and the arm is forward elevated 90°, adducted 10°, and internally rotated with the elbow in full extension. A downward force is placed on the arm. A positive test is confirmed when pain is described as "deep," and the pain is eliminated or decreased when the maneuver is repeated with the arm in external rotation.

Impingement signs may also be positive in patients with RPS, and should be sought during physical examination. It is believed that the stress-related changes that can occur in the posterior rotator cuff can manifest as a secondary impingement syndrome in some cases.

IMAGING

Three radiographs of the shoulder are routinely obtained for the workup of RPS: (1) an anteroposterior view in the plane of the scapula, (2) an axillary view, and (3) a scapular Y lateral view. In most patients with RPS radiographic images are normal, although in some cases a posterior glenoid lesion or impaction of anterior humeral head (Reverse Hill-Sachs lesion) can be visualized. In rare instances, a fracture of the lesser tuberosity will give evidence of a previous posterior dislocation.[44] In addition, the West Point radiographic view can be useful for detecting fractures of the glenoid rim or subtle ectopic bone formation around the glenoid.[45,46]

MRA is the most sensitive diagnostic test for identifying lesions of the posterior labrum and capsule.[47] Specific MRA findings indicative of posterior shoulder instability include posterior translation of the humeral head relative to the glenoid, posterior labrocapsular avulsion, posterior labral tear or splitting, discrete posterior capsular tears or rents, reverse humeral avulsion of the glenohumeral ligaments (HAGL), posterior labrum periosteal sleeve avulsion (POLPSA), and subscapularis tendon avulsion (**Fig. 5**).[48,49] The Kim classification is used to specifically describe posterior labral tear morphology: Type I, incomplete detachment; Type II (the "Kim lesion"), a concealed complete detachment; Type III, chondrolabral erosion; and Type IV, flap tear of the posteroinferior labrum (**Figs. 6–8**).[50] The Kim lesion appears arthroscopically as a crack at the junction of the posteroinferior glenoid articular cartilage and labrum, through which a complete detachment of the deeper labrum from the glenoid rim can be identified (see **Fig. 7**).

In further work by Kim and colleagues,[51] 33 shoulders with atraumatic posterior instability were studied with MRA to examine chondrolabral changes. In comparison with age-matched normal shoulders, the affected shoulders had a glenoid that was shallower, with more osseous and chondrolabral retroversion present in the middle and inferior glenoid (**Fig. 9**). The study was not able to determine whether these changes were etiologic or pathologic, but nonetheless they should be sought when diagnosing posterior instability of the shoulder. Similar findings were presented in a 2006 study by Bradley and colleagues,[8] in

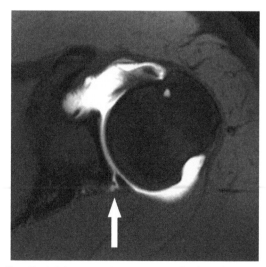

Fig. 5. Axial magnetic resonance (MR) arthrogram image (left shoulder) demonstrating a posterior capsulolabral avulsion from the glenoid with associated posterior translation of the humeral head relative to the glenoid (*arrow*).

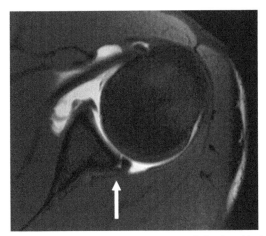

Fig. 6. Axial MR arthrogram image (left shoulder) demonstrating a Type I Kim lesion: posterior chondrolabral fissure without displacement (*arrow*).

which MRA of 48 shoulders with RPS revealed increased chondrolabral retroversion (10.7° vs 5.5°) and increased glenoid bony retroversion (7.1° vs 3.5°) in comparison with controls. More recent data by Bradley and colleagues[52] has revealed that 16 baseball pitchers with RPS examined with MRA had even higher chondrolabral retroversion (11.5°) and glenoid bony retroversion (8.4°). In addition, Tung and Hou[47] found that in 24 patients with RPS, MRA revealed more posterior humeral head translation, posterior labral tears, and posterior labrocapsular avulsions when compared with normal controls.

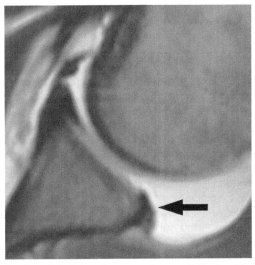

Fig. 8. Axial MR arthrogram image (left shoulder) demonstrating a Type III Kim lesion: posterior chondrolabral erosion with loss of contour (*arrow*).

As a supplementary test, dynamic MRA can be performed, as discussed earlier, to demonstrate labral "peel back" in the ABER position, which is consistent with posterosuperior labral tear.[31] This finding has been most commonly seen in the overhead thrower, who often presents with concomitant posterior and superior labral tears. Lastly, in the authors' practice the use of computed tomography is limited to cases in which a significant amount of bony glenoid retroversion is suspected,

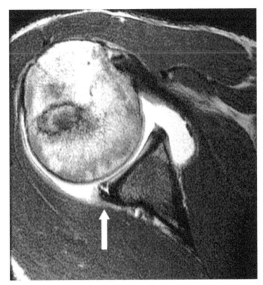

Fig. 7. Axial MR arthrogram image (right shoulder) demonstrating a Type II Kim lesion: a concealed complete detachment of the posterior labrum from the glenoid (*arrow*).

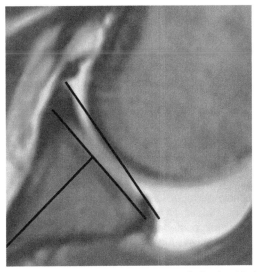

Fig. 9. Axial MR arthrogram image (left shoulder) demonstrating the technique used to measure the degree of chondrolabral retroversion, which can be increased in patients with recurrent posterior subluxation of the shoulder.

and an accurate measurement is desired when considering operative intervention.

NONOPERATIVE TREATMENT

A variety of operative and nonoperative treatment methods for posterior shoulder instability have been described. Rehabilitation with an emphasis on strengthening the rotator cuff, posterior deltoid, and periscapular muscles is frequently the first line of treatment and may allow an athlete to return to the preinjury level of sport.[7,29,37,53–56] It is recommended to maintain this physical therapy protocol for a minimum of 6 months to decrease an athlete's functional disability. Previous studies have reported subjective improvement in up to 70% of athletes with this protocol. Objectively the RPS is typically not completely eliminated, but the functional disability during athletics is improved sufficiently to allow participation in sport without significant problems. If an athlete is unable to return to the preinjury level of competition, operative treatment is a reasonable option.[15,57] Therapy has traditionally been more effective in those patients who have an atraumatic cause of RPS, as opposed to those with generalized ligamentous laxity or who have suffered a discrete traumatic event.[29,54]

SURGICAL TREATMENT

Many operative procedures have been described for the treatment of posterior instability. Overall, the results of surgical treatment of posterior instability have been less consistent compared with those for anterior instability, particularly in the overhead thrower.[15,58,59] Although in general there is a relative paucity of clinical data on posterior shoulder stabilization, the last decade has produced multiple noteworthy studies. Overall, there has been a trend from open to arthroscopic repair, and from nonanatomic to anatomic reconstruction. However, there are multiple confounding variables that make the literature difficult to analyze, including differing causes of instability (RPS vs traumatic dislocation), patterns of instability (unidirectional posterior vs MDI), surgical techniques (open vs arthroscopic), patient populations (athletic vs nonathletic, throwers vs nonthrowers), postoperative rehabilitation protocols, postoperative functional demands (return to work, sport, or neither) and definitions of clinical success and failure.

Multiple open procedures for posterior shoulder stabilization have historically been performed involving patients of wide demographics, variable patterns of instability, and differing levels of athletic competition. These techniques have included the reverse Putti-Platt procedure, biceps tendon transfer, subscapularis transfer, infraspinatus advancement, posterior opening glenoid wedge osteotomy, proximal humeral rotational osteotomy, bone block augmentation of the posterior glenoid or acromion, posterior staple capsulorrhaphy, allograft reconstruction, capsulolabral reconstruction, and open capsular shift.[2,3,7,15,29,56,59–71] Scapinelli[68] found that 10 shoulders that underwent an inverted scapular spine bone graft to the posterior border of the acromion to treat recurrent posterior shoulder instability resulted in 100% success at 9.5-year follow-up.

Notable soft tissue tightening procedures have included the reverse Putti-Platt procedure and the Boyd and Sisk procedure of rerouting the long head of the biceps tendon to the posterior glenoid.[3,69] In 1980, Neer and Foster[70] reported good results in their description of a laterally based posterior capsular shift to tighten a patulous posteroinferior capsule. Similarly, numerous investigators have attempted a medially based posterior capsular shift for posterior capsular tightening.[15,29,56] Misamore and Facibene[56] reported on 14 patients with traumatic unidirectional posterior instability treated with an open posterior capsulorrhaphy, and evaluated at mean 45-month follow-up. Based on Rowe grading criteria, 13 of 14 patients were found to have excellent results and 12 of 14 returned to their preinjury level of athletic competition.

In further pursuit of anatomic-based repair, Rhee and colleagues[63] presented a review of 33 shoulders that underwent an open, deltoid-saving posterior capsulolabral reconstruction for recurrent posterior instability. At 25-month follow-up, 4 patients (13.3%) had recurrent instability. Wolf and colleagues[62] presented similar findings in a retrospective review on 44 shoulders after open posterior glenohumeral stabilization; recurrence rate was 19%, with patients older than 37 years and those with chondral damage having poor results.

Due to interest in minimizing iatrogenic surgical trauma, arthroscopic techniques have been implemented with increasing popularity for the treatment of shoulder instability. Arthroscopic thermal capsulorrhaphy has been used in the treatment of shoulder instability with mixed results. Bisson[72] presented results of 14 shoulders with unidirectional posterior instability without labral detachment, which were treated with thermal capsulorrhaphy; 3 patients (21%) were found to have failure at 2-year follow-up. D'Alessandro and colleagues[73] found that 37% of patients who underwent thermal capsulorrhaphy for anterior, anteroinferior, or multidirectional shoulder instability had unsatisfactory results based on American Shoulder and Elbow Surgeons (ASES) scores, at 2- to 5-year follow-up, lending additional skepticism to the reliability of this surgical technique. Miniaci and McBirnie[74] presented similar disappointing results in another study of 19 shoulders with MDI treated with thermal capsulorrhaphy, in which 9 patients (47%) had recurrent instability at an average of 9 months postoperatively, 5 patients (26%) had stiffness, and 4 patients (21%) had neurologic complications. Therefore, the authors presently do not advocate thermal capsulorrhaphy for the treatment of RPS, due to the variable response patients have demonstrated to thermal energy.

Over time there has been an evolution toward arthroscopic capsulolabral repair for RPS, which is an anatomic and minimally invasive procedure, and the authors' preferred method of treatment. Indications for surgery include failure of 6 or more months of physical therapy, large labral tear on MRA, chondrolabral retroversion of greater than 10°, reverse HAGL or discrete posterior capsular tear, or an inability to return to sport or activity at preinjury level.

ARTHROSCOPIC POSTERIOR SHOULDER STABILIZATION: SURGICAL TECHNIQUE
Setup and Examination Under Anesthesia

Arthroscopic posterior shoulder stabilization is performed under general anesthesia, with an optional interscalene block performed perioperatively to optimize postoperative pain control. After intubation, examination under anesthesia (EUA) is performed on the affected and contralateral shoulder with the patient in the supine position on the operating table. Particular attention is paid to measurements of anterior, posterior, and inferior glenohumeral translation using the "load and shift" and "sulcus" tests, as described earlier.

The authors' preference is then to place the patient on a beanbag in the lateral decubitus position, with the affected shoulder oriented superior. Arthroscopic posterior shoulder stabilization can also be performed with the patient in the beach chair position. However, this requires manual adjustments of arm position intraoperatively by an assistant or arm holder, and also may provide suboptimal visualization of the posteroinferior labrum and capsule in some cases.

The upper extremity is prepped from the fingers to the level of the sternum anteriorly and the medial border of the scapula posteriorly. The operative shoulder is placed in 10 pounds of longitudinal traction with a commercially available arm holder and positioned in 45° of abduction and 20° of forward flexion. This position displaces the humeral head anteriorly and inferiorly, bringing the posterior labrum into clear, unobstructed view (see **Fig. 2**). A prefabricated bump or additional traction in a tangential vector can be applied to create more distraction between the humeral head and glenoid if desired, thus facilitating visualization and access to the labrum and capsule circumferentially.

Portal Creation and Diagnostic Arthroscopy

Arthroscopic posterior labral repair is performed using a 2-portal technique. An 18-gauge spinal needle is directed into the glenohumeral joint from a posterior approach and the glenohumeral joint is injected with 50 mL of sterile saline for distention. This distention facilitates safe insertion of the arthroscope cannula and blunt trochar, thereby minimizing potential damage to the articular cartilage of the humeral head and glenoid.

Location of the posterior portal for posterior stabilization is critical to properly establish access to the posterior glenoid rim for labral preparation and repair. The posterior portal is created in a "modified" location, approximately 1 cm distal and 1 cm lateral to a standard posterior portal; this allows an advantageous trajectory of instruments toward the posterior glenoid rim. Difficulty in the placement of suture anchors and the use of suture passers can be encountered if the posterior portal is located too far superior or medial in the posterior capsule. The conventional posterior portal is located near the 10-o'clock position on the right glenoid, which makes approach to the posteroinferior glenoid difficult for the placement of suture anchors. A spinal needle is used to localize the modified posterior portal at the 7-o'clock position on the glenoid rim in a right shoulder, approximately 1 to 2 cm lateral to the glenoid rim. Cadaveric study has shown the 7-o'clock portal to be located a safe distance from the axillary nerve and posterior humeral circumflex artery (39 ± 4 mm), and the suprascapular nerve and artery (29 ± 3 mm).[75] If the posterior portal has been made too far superior or medial, a supplementary posterior portal is made further inferior and lateral to the existing posterior portal.

A 30° arthroscope is introduced into the glenohumeral joint via the posterior portal, and systematic diagnostic arthroscopy is performed. The anterior portal is created in the rotator interval, approximately 1 cm lateral to the coracoid process, using either an outside-in technique with spinal needle localization or an inside-out technique with a switching stick.

To best visualize and address the posterior structures, the arthroscope is switched to the anterior portal. Typical pathology associated with posterior instability includes posterior labral fraying and splitting, posterior labral detachment from the glenoid rim, a patulous posterior capsule, discrete posterior capsular tear, undersurface partial-thickness rotator cuff tears, and widening of the rotator interval (**Fig. 10**). The surgeon must also be cognizant of the subtle "Kim lesion"— a concealed incomplete detachment of the posterior labrum.[50]

An 8.25-mm threaded clear plastic cannula is placed (Arthrex Inc, Naples, FL, USA), in either 7-cm or 9-cm lengths, depending on the musculature girth of the patient. This cannula allows unobstructed passage of the required arthroscopic drill guide and 45° angled or curved suture passers for work on the labrum and capsule.

Labral Preparation

The posterior labrum is visualized from both the posterior and anterior portals to appreciate the full extent of the tear. The arthroscope then remains in the anterior portal, and the posterior portal serves as the working portal for the repair. An arthroscopic chisel is first used to elevate the torn labrum, which is often scarred medially, away from the glenoid rim, throughout the entire extent of the tear (**Fig. 11**). An angled rasp or motorized shaver is then used to decorticate the glenoid rim and abrade the labral undersurface to remove scar tissue and achieve a vascularized surface for healing (**Fig. 12**). Debridement of the labrum with an arthroscopic shaver is limited to

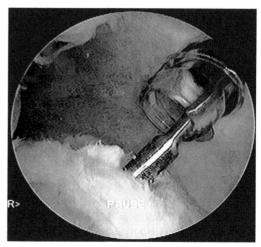

Fig. 11. An arthroscopic chisel is used to elevate the torn labrum, which is scarred medially, away from the glenoid rim. In this case, a split in the labrum is used to access the scarred tissue (right shoulder, viewed from the anterior portal).

only those portions involving free flaps of tissue or extensive fraying, as the goal is to preserve as much tissue as possible for incorporation into the repair.

Labral Repair

The posterior labrum is repaired to the glenoid rim with suture anchors. The authors typically use the 2.4-mm Biocomposite Suture-Tak anchor (Arthrex Inc, Naples, FL, USA), which is single-loaded with

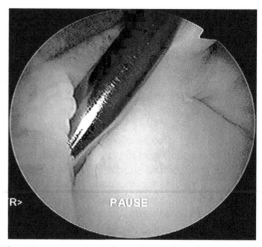

Fig. 12. A motorized shaver is used at the posterosuperior extent of the labral tear to decorticate the glenoid rim and abrade the labral undersurface (right shoulder, viewed from the posterior portal). To complete the abrasion posteroinferiorly, the shaver is switched to the posterior portal and the arthroscope is placed in the anterior portal.

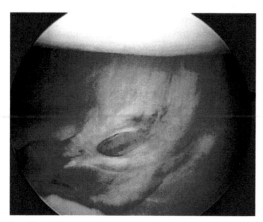

Fig. 10. A discrete posterior capsular tear in an athlete with recurrent posterior subluxation of the shoulder (right shoulder, viewed from the anterior portal).

a #2 FiberWire suture and has been found to have equivalent pull-out strength to the 3.0-mm and 3.7-mm anchors with the same design. Multiple similar anchors are commercially available. The anchors should be placed on the chondral rim of the glenoid, as opposed to on the glenoid neck, thereby enabling labral tissue to be repaired in an anatomic position on the glenoid face. An offset drill guide for this specific purpose is commercially available (Arthrex Inc, Naples, FL, USA), and allows the guide to be securely positioned on the rim of the glenoid while simultaneously directing the drill onto the chondral surface (**Fig. 13**). During placement of the suture anchor, care must be taken to avoid inadvertent injury to the articular cartilage; this typically occurs with a low, tangential drilling angle (<30°) and can be avoided by a properly placed posterior portal that allows a higher angle (>30°) of approach to the glenoid rim. Suture anchors are placed along the posterior glenoid rim in an inferior to superior direction, and the labrum is secured to the articular margin to restore the length tension relationship of the posterior band of the IGHL.

The number of suture anchors used is dependent on the size of the labral tear. The o'clock nomenclature is used describe the location and extent of labral tear. For example, a posterior labral tear extending from the 6-o'clock to 9-o'clock position in a right shoulder is typically repaired with suture anchors at the 6:30, 7:30, 8:30, and 9:30 positions. The first anchor is typically placed more superiorly than the inferior extent of the tear, in order to perform a superior shift of the capsulolabral complex concomitantly. For example, in this scenario the first anchor would be placed at the 6:30 position to advance the labral tissue from the 6-o'clock position. Advancing the suture passer in this fashion restores tension in the posterior band of the IGHL, which is necessary to restore posterior stability.

On insertion, the suture anchor is rotated to orient the sutures perpendicular to the glenoid rim to facilitate passage of the most posterior suture through the torn labrum; this suture will be used as the post for arthroscopic knot tying, thus allowing the knot to be positioned away from the chondral surfaces of the glenoid and humeral head (**Fig. 14**). This knot position is selected in an attempt to minimize postoperative iatrogenic chondral injury from knot abrasion.

Following placement of the first suture anchor, one of several commercially available suture passers can be used to shuttle one limb of the #2 FiberWire suture around the labrum to be repaired (**Fig. 15**). The authors prefer either the 45° Spectrum suture hook (Linvatec Corp, Largo, FL, USA), which is loaded with a number-0 polydiaxanone (PDS) suture (Ethicon, Somerville, NJ, USA), or the Suture Lasso (Arthrex, Naples, FL, USA). The suture passer is passed through the labral tissue beginning posteriorly, and exits at the edge of the glenoid articular surface at the level of the suture anchor.

When using the Spectrum, the PDS is then fed into the glenohumeral joint and the suture passer

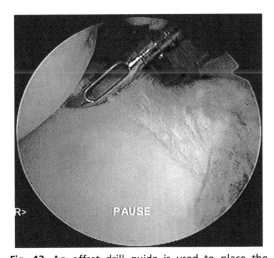

Fig. 13. An offset drill guide is used to place the suture anchor directly on the border of glenoid face (right shoulder, viewed from the anterior portal). The most inferior anchor is placed first. The advantageous position of the 7-o'clock portal and working cannula is appreciated in relation to the location of the posterior labral tear and the required approach to the repair.

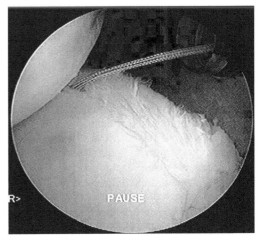

Fig. 14. The first suture anchor is placed on the glenoid face. The two suture limbs are visualized exiting the anchor (right shoulder, viewed from the anterior portal).

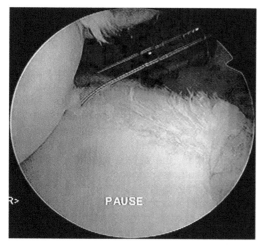

Fig. 15. Using a suture passing technique, one limb of the suture from the suture anchor is shuttled around the posterior labrum (right shoulder, viewed from the anterior portal).

is withdrawn through the posterior cannula. While withdrawing the suture passer from the posterior cannula, additional suture is advanced into the joint to prevent inadvertently pulling the PDS back through the torn edge of the labrum. An arthroscopic suture grasper is used to withdraw both the most posterior #2 FiberWire suture from the suture anchor and the end of the PDS suture that has been advanced through the torn labrum. The PDS is then fashioned into a single loop and tightly tied over the FiberWire, approximately 5 cm from the end. By pulling on the other end of the PDS suture, the more posterior FiberWire suture from the suture anchor is shuttled behind the labral tear. At this point, with one suture limb on either side of the torn labrum, the authors' preference is to tie a sliding-locking arthroscopic Weston knot to begin the repair; multiple alternative knots can be used. Of utmost importance is the surgeon's familiarity and proficiency with the knot technique, whichever is selected. The posterior suture limb serves as the post, which in effect will advance the labrum to the glenoid rim when the knot is tightened. An emphasis should be made to secure the knot posteriorly and not on the rim of the glenoid to prevent humeral head abrasion from the knot. Regardless of the knot-tying technique used, each half-hitch must be completely seated before the next half-hitch is thrown. Placing tension on the nonpost suture and advancing the knot-pusher "past point" will lock the Weston knot. A total of 3 half-hitches are placed to secure the Weston knot.

Additional suture anchors are then placed in similar fashion to complete the labral repair. The labral tear at the 7-o'clock position is advanced

to the 7:30 suture anchor, the 8-o'clock labral tear position is advanced to the 8:30 suture anchor, and the labral tear at 9-o'clock labral tear position is advanced to the 9:30 suture anchor (**Fig. 16**). In the case of the Type VIII SLAP tear, additional anchors are incrementally placed superiorly, up to the 12-o'clock or 1-o'clock position as indicated, to repair the associated superior labral tear.[26]

On completion of the capsulolabral repair, an arthroscopic awl is used to penetrate the bare area of the humeral head, under the infraspinatus tendon, in an effort to allow egress of stem cells and marrow elements into the intra-articular space to augment the healing response.[26] Finally, the posterior capsular portal incision is closed by partially withdrawing the arthroscopic cannula, then passing a PDS suture through one side of the portal site with a crescent Spectrum suture passer and retrieving the suture through the other side of the portal with an arthroscopic penetrating suture grasper. Varying the distance that the penetrator is passed from the border of the portal incision allows titration of the capsulorrhaphy performed with the closure. The PDS is then tied over the capsule, with care to taken to avoid incorporating the overlying musculature into the knot.

Labral Repair with Capsular Plication

The clinical history, EUA, MRA images, and arthroscopic findings regarding posterior capsular pathology dictate the specific type of capsular procedure performed in addition to the labral repair. Patients with acute injuries and minimal evidence of capsular stretching do not require the same degree of capsular advancement as

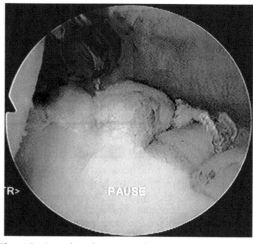

Fig. 16. Completed repair of the posterior labrum (right shoulder, viewed from the anterior portal).

those with more chronic instability or MDI. Based on these factors, the surgeon may consider capsular plication at the time of labral repair or immediately after the labrum has been repaired.

When a patulous posterior capsule is observed at the onset of the procedure, this tissue is also abraded in preparation for a concomitant capsular plication using the sutures from the suture anchors. The authors have found this technique to have superior clinical results in comparison with the placement of independent plication sutures in the posterior capsule without suture anchors.[8] Care should be taken in the use of the motorized shaver when abrading the posterior capsule, which is thin and can be easily penetrated with an overly aggressive technique; the authors typically favor the rasp for this purpose. In the setting of a labral tear with excessive posterior capsular laxity, the suture passer is advanced through the posterior capsule approximately 1 cm lateral to the edge of the labral tear and then is advanced as described previously, underneath the labral tear, to the edge of the articular cartilage, creating a "pleat stitch." Placing as many of these pleat stitches as necessary in the face of a patulous shoulder capsule will reduce the associated capsular redundancy while simultaneously repairing the torn labrum.

If the labrum has been repaired in isolated fashion initially and it is then determined that the capsule requires further tension, suture capsulorrhaphy can be performed in the intervals between the suture anchors directly to the newly secured labrum. Knots are tied following passage of each suture approximately 1 cm lateral to the edge of the labral border, allowing continued assessment of the repair and the degree of the capsular shift achieved by each suture. Care must be taken with the sharp Spectrum suture passer tip to avoid cutting or placing undue tension on previously tied sutures from the suture anchors.

Isolated Capsular Plication

In some instances, patients with unidirectional posterior instability or primary posterior MDI do not have a posterior labral tear, but rather display only significant capsular laxity at arthroscopy. In this setting, an isolated posterior capsulorrhaphy is performed with suture anchors in a similar fashion to that described above. For example, in a right shoulder, suture anchors are typically placed beginning inferior (6:30), and progressing superior (9:30) incrementally, as indicated. Depending on the degree of capsular laxity present, the 1-cm 6-o'clock capsular pleat suture is typically advanced to the 6:30 position on the

glenoid. This suture is tied, as described previously, and the reduction in capsular volume is assessed. Restoring adequate tension in the posterior band of the IGHL and capsule is critical to the success of the reconstruction. If necessary, a second 1-cm capsulorrhaphy pleat suture is placed at the 7-o'clock position on the capsule and advanced to the 7:30 position on the glenoid. Likewise, if indicated, additional sutures are then placed at the 8-o'clock and 9-o'clock positions on the capsule, advancing to the 8:30 and 9:30 positions on the glenoid, respectively.[8]

Labral Repair with Posterior Capsular Release

It has been observed, as previously discussed, that some overhead throwers such as baseball pitchers develop GIRD, which is associated with a posterior capsular contracture, in conjunction with a posterosuperior, or isolated posterior, labral tear. Accordingly, both elements of this pathology need to be addressed for alleviation of symptoms. Initially, the authors treat the GIRD with preoperative "sleeper stretches." In a majority of throwers this is successful; however, in rare cases the GIRD is recalcitrant to stretching. In these scenarios, an arthroscopic posterior labral repair is first performed, as described previously. Next, to treat the posterior capsular contracture and associated GIRD, a limited arthroscopic posterior capsular release is performed with a thermal device, which is used to create a full-thickness incision in the posterior capsular tissue. The posterior capsular release is performed while viewing from the anterior portal, beginning approximately 5 mm away from the glenoid rim, at the 7-o'clock position (right shoulder), and progressing superiorly with the thermal device to the 8-o'clock position, thereby incising the contracted posterior band of the IGHL. On rare occasions, the authors extend this release slightly more superiorly, as indicated, based on the extent of the contracture.

Rotator Interval Closure

Biomechanical study has demonstrated that in the setting of unidirectional posterior shoulder instability, the rotator interval need not be addressed with closure to restore glenohumeral stability.[21] However, in the setting of MDI with a primary posterior component, the rotator interval requires closure to restore stability. These patients are defined preoperatively by having a 2+ or greater sulcus sign that does not decrease in 30° of external rotation. The goal is to plicate the tissue between the supraspinatus and subscapularis tendons. Specifically, this requires suturing the anterior capsule, superior tissue of the rotator interval, and SGHL to the anterior capsule and middle glenohumeral ligament (MGHL). The closure begins medially and is performed with a number-0 PDS suture, which is passed through the superior tissue with a Spectrum suture passer and retrieved with an arthroscopic penetrating grasper passed through the inferior tissue. A Weston knot is tied through the anterior cannula. Additional interrupted plication sutures are placed in a similar fashion progressing laterally, as needed, to complete the closure.

POSTOPERATIVE REHABILITATION

At the conclusion of surgery the shoulder is placed in an Ultrasling (DonJoy, Carlsbad, CA) with an abduction pillow, which immobilizes the shoulder in 30° of abduction and prevents internal rotation. A cryotherapy device is used for the first 3 postoperative days to minimize swelling and pain. The day after surgery, patients begin active ROM of the elbow, wrist, and fingers. At 1 week after the operation formal physical therapy for the shoulder is initiated, beginning with passive forward flexion and abduction in the scapular plane to 90°. Over the subsequent 5 weeks, full passive ROM is achieved. At 6 weeks postoperatively, the sling is discontinued and active-assisted ROM begins, progressing to full active ROM as able. Full active ROM should be achieved by 3 months postoperatively. Strengthening of the rotator cuff, deltoid, and periscapular muscles begins at 2 to 3 months after surgery.

Once patients are able to achieve 80% of the strength of their contralateral shoulders, as measured by isokinetic testing, a sport-specific rehabilitation protocol is initiated. This protocol typically takes place between 4 and 6 months postoperatively. Athletes are cleared to return to sport when they demonstrate full ROM and strength, along with restoration of glenohumeral stability, typically between 6 and 9 months postoperatively.

Throwing athletes require special consideration, and follow a specific protocol designed to monitor their throwing distance and speed, which is slowly advanced over 2 to 3 months. Initially, at 6 months postoperatively, an easy tossing program is commenced at a distance of 20 ft, without a windup. Before each session, stretching and heat application is performed to increase circulation and improve ROM. At 7 months, light throwing with an easy windup at a distance of 30 ft is allowed for 2 to 3 days per week, for 10 minutes per session. Easy throws from 150 to 200 ft are permitted at 9 months postoperatively and stronger throws from the same distance are allowed at 10 months. Pitchers can throw half to three-quarters speed from the mound, with an emphasis on accuracy and technique, at 11 months. At 12 months, pitchers can throw at three-quarters to full speed. Throwers are released to full competition when they are able to throw at full speed without discomfort for 2 weeks, typically between 9 and 12 months after surgery.

CLINICAL RESULTS

Several clinical series were reported in the 1990s documenting successful accounts of arthroscopic posterior glenohumeral stabilization.[16,76,77] In 1998, Wolf and Eakin[16] reported on 14 patients who had arthroscopic posterior capsular plication for unidirectional posterior instability; at 33-month follow-up 86% had good or excellent results and 93% had restoration of stability. With improvement in arthroscopic techniques and surgical implants, research has led to the evolution of suture-anchor–based arthroscopic posterior glenohumeral stabilization. Multiple recent studies have revealed a majority of good or excellent results, fueling interest in these methods.

Williams and colleagues[12] retrospectively reported on 27 shoulders with symptomatic posterior capsulolabral complex detachment from the posterior glenoid rim, with minimal posterior capsular laxity, after a distinct traumatic event. Isolated arthroscopic posterior capsulolabral repair was performed with bioabsorbable tack fixation in all patients. Subjective instability and pain were eliminated in 92% of patients, with all of these patients returning to unlimited athletic activity by 6 months. Kim and colleagues[50] prospectively reported on 27 athletes with traumatic unidirectional RPS treated with arthroscopic posterior labral repair and capsular shift; all patients had a labral lesion, and 81% also had stretching of the posterior band of the IGHL. The posterior capsule was shifted superiorly in all cases. All complete labral lesions were repaired directly, and incomplete labral lesions were converted to complete tears and then repaired. The mean ASES scores improved from 51.2 to 96.5. All but one patient had restoration of stability and were able to return to previous athletic activities with little or no limitations. Multiple additional studies on between 13 and 33 shoulders have presented similar successful results for arthroscopic posterior stabilization, with recurrence rates between 0% and 12% at a minimum mean follow-up of 3 years.[6,8,78–80]

In 2006, Bradley and colleagues[8] presented a prospective study on 91 athletes (100 shoulders) treated with arthroscopic capsulolabral reconstruction for posterior instability. At 27-month mean follow-up the mean ASES scores improved from 50.4 to 85.7, with 89% returning to sport and 67% returning to their same level as preoperatively. Several potential reasons elucidated for the 11 failures included undiagnosed MDI, inadequate capsular shift due to unappreciated capsular laxity, inadequate recognition of poor capsular tissue quality in those patients referred after thermal capsulorrhaphy, and capsular plication performed in an isolated fashion without suture anchors. These conclusions led to further refinement of the surgical approach to posterior instability.

In 2008, Radkowski and colleagues[78] reported on arthroscopic capsulolabral repair for posterior shoulder instability in throwing athletes as compared with nonthrowing athletes. At mean 27-month follow-up, there were no differences in the ASES score or scores for stability, ROM, strength, pain, and function between the 27 throwing shoulders and the 80 nonthrowing shoulders, with both groups showing significant improvement in all categories. Excellent or good results were achieved in 89% of throwers and 93% of nonthrowers. However, throwing athletes were less likely to return to the preinjury level of sport (55%) compared with nonthrowing athletes (71%). Due to the relatively small patient population in this study, the investigators had difficulty elucidating the reasoning for the lower rate of return to sport in throwers, although it was found that all of the 3 throwers who failed underwent capsulolabral repair without suture anchors. Based on the findings of this study, the investigators presently advocate repair with suture anchors. Also, within the thrower group there were more athletes unable to return to their previous levels of sport than there were failures based on the subjective instability scale, suggesting it is possible that some of these athletes had lower levels of subjective instability but enough to keep them from returning the same high level of competition and the unique demands required from the shoulder during throwing activities.

Recent prospective data have been presented by Bradley and colleagues[52] on 161 shoulders in athletes treated with arthroscopic capsulolabral reconstruction for posterior instability. All patients had unidirectional posterior instability and failed a course of nonoperative management. At mean follow-up of 32 months (minimum 27 months), mean ASES scores increased from 46.9 to 86.0, with no difference between contact and noncontact athletes. Good or excellent results were reported in 90% of the 161 patients in the study and in 93% of the 90 contact athletes. Overall return to sport was 89%, with return at the preinjury level successful in 67% of all patients and 69% of contact athletes. Return to sport rates at limited level were 22% of all patients and 24% of contact athletes. Among throwers in the study, 97% returned to sport, with 67% at the preinjury level and 30% reporting some limitation. For the future, with enhanced understanding of the pathogenesis of shoulder instability in the throwing athlete, the goal exists to return a higher percentage of throwing athletes to sport at their preinjury level postoperatively. Further biomechanical and larger prospective clinical studies on throwers are warranted to gain enhanced understanding of this complex athletic population.

SUMMARY

Posterior shoulder instability poses a significant challenge, both diagnostically and therapeutically. Posterior shoulder instability is a broad clinical entity, ranging from RPS to locked posterior dislocations. The pathogenesis varies tremendously, based on the stressed placed on the involved shoulder. As opposed to a singular traumatic event, athletes with RPS typically suffer from chronic, repetitive microtrauma that leads to posterior labral tearing, posterior capsular laxity, and symptoms. Overhead throwers are a unique patient population, often with a varied presentation that can include posterior capsular contracture and the Type VIII SLAP tear. Extensive basic science and clinical research is ongoing to elucidate a biomechanical explanation of the pathogenesis of RPS in throwers. Increased clinical awareness as well as advances in imaging and physical examination techniques has improved diagnosis in athletes and patients from wide demographic presentations. Multiple distinct pathologic lesions can be identified on MRA in patients with RPS; these should be sought carefully during the workup of symptomatic patients. Likewise, specific provocative physical examination tests have been found to be useful in making the diagnosis of posterior shoulder instability.

Successful outcomes can be achieved with physical therapy, although many patients still require surgical intervention to alleviate symptoms and return to sport at their preinjury level. The transition from open to arthroscopic surgical techniques has facilitated more comprehensive identification and treatment of coexisting structural pathologies in RPS. For patients with unidirectional posterior instability, an arthroscopic repair of the capsulolabral complex is recommended. When a patulous posterior capsule or a posteroinferior component of instability is also present, an arthroscopic superiorly directed capsular shift and capsular plication is added. In throwers with RPS and a posterior labral tear, the authors advocate repairing the posterior labrum only, while treating excessive GIRD, if present, initially with preoperative "sleeper stretches" and, if recalcitrant, with a limited posterior capsular release at the time of surgery. Regarding addressing capsular pathology, the authors generally tend toward over-tightening contact athletes and those with significant capsular laxity, and under-tightening overhead throwers.

At mid-term follow-up, promising success rates between 80% and 100% have been achieved with arthroscopic repair techniques, with generally lower results in throwers. Longer-term studies are necessary to evaluate the durability of arthroscopic techniques in the treatment of posterior glenohumeral instability. Further work is also needed to elucidate the complex mechanics of the elite thrower's shoulder, and the best path to alleviating the symptoms of RPS while simultaneously allowing return to sport at a preinjury level.

REFERENCES

1. Antoniou J, Duckworth DT, Harryman DT II. Capsulolabral augmentation for the management of posteroinferior instability of the shoulder. J Bone Joint Surg Am 2000;82(9):1220–30.
2. McLaughlin H. Posterior dislocation of the shoulder. J Bone Joint Surg Am 1952;24-A-3:584–90.
3. Boyd HB, Sisk TD. Recurrent posterior dislocation of the shoulder. J Bone Joint Surg Am 1972;54(4): 779–86.
4. Robinson CM, Aderinto J. Recurrent posterior shoulder instability. J Bone Joint Surg Am 2005; 87(4):883–92.
5. Arciero RA, Mazzocca AD. Traumatic posterior shoulder subluxation with labral injury: suture anchor-technique. Tech Shoulder Elbow Surg 2004; 5:13–24.
6. Bottoni CR, Franks BR, Moore JH, et al. Operative stabilization of posterior shoulder instability. Am J Sports Med 2005;33(7):996–1002.
7. Hawkins RJ, Koppert G, Johnston G. Recurrent posterior instability (subluxation) of the shoulder. J Bone Joint Surg Am 1984;66(2):169–74.
8. Bradley JP, Baker CL III, Kline AJ, et al. Arthroscopic capsulolabral reconstruction for posterior instability of the shoulder: a prospective study of 100 shoulders. Am J Sports Med 2006;34(7):1061–71.
9. Kaplan LD, Flanigan DC, Norwig J, et al. Prevalence and variance of shoulder injuries in elite collegiate football players. Am J Sports Med 2005;33(8): 1142–6.
10. Mair SD, Zarzour RH, Speer KP. Posterior labral injury in contact athletes. Am J Sports Med 1998; 26(6):753–8.
11. Fuchs B, Jost B, Gerber C. Posterior-inferior capsular shift for the treatment of recurrent voluntary posterior subluxation of the shoulder. J Bone Joint Surg Am 2000;82(1):16–25.
12. Williams RJ III, Strickland S, Cohen M, et al. Arthroscopic repair for traumatic posterior shoulder instability. Am J Sports Med 2003;31(2):203–9.
13. O'Brien SJ, Schwartz RE, Warren RF, et al. Capsular restraints to anterior-posterior motion of the abducted shoulder: a biomechanical study. J Shoulder Elbow Surg 1995;4(4):298–308.
14. Pagnani MJ, Warren RF. Stabilizers of the glenohumeral joint. J Shoulder Elbow Surg 1994;3:173–90.
15. Tibone JE, Bradley JP. The treatment of posterior subluxation in athletes. Clin Orthop Relat Res 1993;291:124–37.
16. Wolf EM, Eakin CL. Arthroscopic capsular plication for posterior shoulder instability. Arthroscopy 1998; 14(2):153–63.
17. Bigliani LU, Kelkar R, Flatow EL, et al. Glenohumeral stability. Biomechanical properties of passive and active stabilizers. Clin Orthop Relat Res 1996;330: 13–30.
18. O'Brien SJ, Schwartz RE, Warren RF. Capsular restraints to anterior-posterior motion of the shoulder. Orthop Trans 1988;12:143.
19. Warren RF, Kornblatt IB, Marchland R. Static factors affecting shoulder stability. Orthop Trans 1984;8:89.
20. Cole BJ, Rodeo SA, O'Brien SJ, et al. The anatomy and histology of the rotator interval capsule of the shoulder. Clin Orthop Relat Res 2001;390:129–37.
21. Provencher MT, Mologne TS, Hongo M, et al. Arthroscopic rotator interval closure: effect on glenohumeral translation and range of motion in an anterior and posterior stabilization model. Presented at the American Orthopaedic Society for Sports Medicine annual meeting. Calgary (AB), July 11–15, 2007.
22. Lee SB, An KN. Dynamic glenohumeral stability provided by three heads of the deltoid muscle. Clin Orthop Relat Res 2002;400:40–7.
23. Murrell GA, Warren RF. The surgical treatment of posterior shoulder instability. Clin Sports Med 1995;14(4):903–15.
24. Blasier RB, Soslowsky LJ, Mallicky DM, et al. Posterior glenohumeral subluxation: active and passive stabilization in a biomechanical model. J Bone Joint Surg Am 1997;79(3):433–40.
25. Mihata T, Gates J, McGarry MH, et al. Effect of rotator cuff musculature imbalance on forceful internal impingement and peel-back of the superior labrum: a cadaveric study. Am J Sports Med 2009; 37(9):2222–7.
26. Seroyer S, Tejwani SG, Bradley JP. Arthroscopic capsulolabral reconstruction of the type VIII superior

labrum anterior posterior lesion: mean 2-year follow-up on 13 shoulders. Am J Sports Med 2007;35(9): 1477–83.

27. Burkhart SS, Morgan CD, Kibler WB. The disabled throwing shoulder: spectrum of pathology. Part I: pathoanatomy and biomechanics. Arthroscopy 2003;19(4):404–20.

28. Burkhart SS, Lo IK. The cam effect of the proximal humerus: its role in the production of relative capsular redundancy of the shoulder. Arthroscopy 2007;23(3):241–6.

29. Fronek J, Warren RF, Bowen M. Posterior subluxation of the glenohumeral joint. J Bone Joint Surg Am 1989;71(2):205–16.

30. Tuite MJ, Petersen BD, Wise SM, et al. Shoulder MR arthrography of the posterior labrocapsular complex in overhead throwers with pathologic internal impingement and internal rotation deficit. Skeletal Radiol 2007;36(6):495–502.

31. Borrero CG, Casagranda BU, Towers JD, et al. Magnetic resonance appearance of posterosuperior labral peel back during humeral abduction and external rotation. Skeletal Radiol 2010;39(1): 19–26.

32. Myers JB, Laudner KG, Pasquale MR, et al. Glenohumeral range of motion deficits and posterior shoulder tightness in throwers with pathologic internal impingement. Am J Sports Med 2006; 34(3):385–91.

33. Burkhart SS, Morgan CD, Kibler WB. The disabled throwing shoulder: spectrum of pathology. Part II: evaluation and treatment of SLAP lesions in throwers. Arthroscopy 2003;19(5):531–9.

34. Kibler WB. The relationship of glenohumeral internal rotation deficit to shoulder and elbow injuries in tennis players: a prospective evaluation of posterior capsular stretching. Presented at the Annual Closed Meeting of American Shoulder and Elbow Surgeons. New York (NY), October 1998.

35. Hovis WD, Dean MT, Mallon WJ, et al. Posterior instability of the shoulder with secondary impingement in elite golfers. Am J Sports Med 2002;20(6): 886–90.

36. Dines JS, Wanich T, Gambardella RA, et al. "Batter's Shoulder" as a cause of posterior instability. Accepted for Presentation at the American Orthopaedic Society for Sports Medicine annual meeting. Providence (RI), July 15–18, 2010.

37. Pollock RG, Bigliani LU. Recurrent posterior shoulder instability. Diagnosis and treatment. Clin Orthop Relat Res 1993;291:85–96.

38. Cyprien JM, Vasey HM, Burdet A, et al. Humeral retrotorsion and glenohumeral relationship in the normal shoulder and in recurrent anterior dislocation (scapulometry). Clin Orthop Relat Res 1983;175:8–17.

39. Von Raebrox A, Campbell B, Ramesh R, et al. The association of subacromial dimples with recurrent posterior dislocation of the shoulder. J Shoulder Elbow Surg 2006;15(5):591–3.

40. Beighton P, Solomon L, Soskolne CL. Articular mobility in an African population. Ann Rheum Dis 1973;32(5):413–8.

41. Bigliani LU, Endrizzi DP, McIlveon SJ. Operative management of posterior shoulder instability. Orthop Trans 1989;13:232.

42. Hernandez A, Drez D. Operative treatment of posterior shoulder dislocations by posterior glenoidplasty, capsulorrhaphy and infraspinatus advancement. Am J Sports Med 1986;14(3):187–91.

43. Kim SH, Park JS, Jeong WK, et al. The Kim test: a novel test for posteroinferior labral lesion of the shoulder—a comparison to the jerk test. Am J Sports Med 2005;33(8):1188–92.

44. Pagnani MJ, Warren RF. Instability of the shoulder. In: Nicholas JA, Hershman EB, editors. The upper extremity and spine in sports medicine. Philadelphia: J.B. Lippincott; 1994. p. 173.

45. Engebretsen L, Craig EV. Radiologic features of shoulder instability. Clin Orthop Relat Res 1993; 291:29–44.

46. Pavlov H, Warren RF, Weiss CB Jr, et al. The roentgenographic evaluation of anterior shoulder instability. Clin Orthop Relat Res 1985;194:153–8.

47. Tung GA, Hou DD. MR arthrography of the posterior labrocapsular complex: relationship with glenohumeral joint alignment and clinical posterior instability. Am J Roentgenol 2003;180(2):369–75.

48. Safran O, Defranco MJ, Hatem S, et al. Posterior humeral avulsion of the glenohumeral ligament as a case of posterior shoulder instability. A case report. J Bone Joint Surg Am 2004;86(12): 2732–6.

49. Yu JS, Ashman CJ, Jones G. The POLPSA lesion: MR imaging findings with arthroscopic correlation in patients with posterior instability. Skeletal Radiol 2002;31(7):396–9.

50. Kim SH, Ha KI, Park JH, et al. Arthroscopic posterior labral repair and capsular shift for traumatic unidirectional recurrent posterior subluxation of the shoulder. J Bone Joint Surg Am 2003;85(8): 1479–87.

51. Kim SH, Noh KC, Park JS, et al. Loss of chondrolabral containment of the glenohumeral joint in atraumatic posteroinferior multidirectional instability. J Bone Joint Surg Am 2005;87(1):92–8.

52. Bradley JP, Lesniak BP, McClincy M. Arthroscopic capsulolabral reconstruction for posterior shoulder instability in athletes: a prospective study of 161 shoulders. Presented at the Annual Closed Meeting of the American Shoulder and Elbow Society. New York (NY), October 24–27, 2009.

53. Bell RH, Noble JS. An appreciation of posterior instability of the shoulder. Clin Sports Med 1991; 10(4):887–99.

54. Burkhead WZ Jr, Rockwood CA Jr. Treatment of instability of the shoulder with an exercise program. J Bone Joint Surg Am 1992;74:890–6.

55. Hawkins RJ, Janda DH. Posterior instability of the glenohumeral joint: a technique of repair. Am J Sports Med 1996;24(3):275–8.

56. Misamore GW, Facibene WA. Posterior capsulorrhaphy for the treatment of traumatic recurrent posterior subluxations of the shoulder in athletes. J Shoulder Elbow Surg 2000;9(5):403–8.

57. Hurley JA, Anderson TE, Dear W, et al. Posterior shoulder instability. Surgical versus conservative results with evaluation of glenoid version. Am J Sports Med 1992;20(4):396–400.

58. Tibone JE, Preitto C, Jobe FW, et al. Staple capsulorrhaphy for recurrent posterior shoulder dislocation. Am J Sports Med 1981;9(3):135–9.

59. Schwartz E, Warren RF, O'Brien SJ, et al. Posterior shoulder instability. Orthop Clin North Am 1987;18(3):409–19.

60. Bigliani LU, Pollock RG, McIlveen SJ, et al. Shift of the posteroinferior aspect of the capsule for recurrent posterior glenohumeral instability. J Bone Joint Surg Am 1995;77(7):1011–20.

61. Hawkins RJ, Belle RM. Posterior instability of the shoulder. Instr Course Lect 1989;38:211–5.

62. Wolf BR, Strickland S, Williams RJ, et al. Open posterior shoulder stabilization for recurrent posterior glenohumeral instability. J Shoulder Elbow Surg 2005;14(2):157–64.

63. Rhee YG, Lee DH, Lim CT. Posterior capsulolabral reconstruction in posterior shoulder instability: deltoid saving. J Shoulder Elbow Surg 2005;14(4):355–60.

64. Chaudhuri GK, Sengupta A, Saha AK. Rotation osteotomy of the shaft of the humerus for recurrent dislocation of the shoulder: anterior and posterior. Acta Orthop Scand 1974;45(2):193–8.

65. Surin V, Blåder S, Markhede G, et al. Rotational osteotomy of the humerus for posterior instability of the shoulder. J Bone Joint Surg Am 1990;72(2):181–6.

66. Scott DJ Jr. Treatment of recurrent posterior dislocations of the shoulder by glenoidplasty. Report of three cases. J Bone Joint Surg Am 1967;49(3):471–6.

67. Jones V. Recurrent posterior dislocation of the shoulder: report of a case treated by posterior bone block. J Bone Joint Surg Br 1958;40(2):203–7.

68. Scapinelli R. Posterior addition acromioplasty in the treatment of recurrent posterior instability of the shoulder. J Shoulder Elbow Surg 2006;15(4):424–31.

69. Severin A. Anterior and posterior recurrent dislocation of the shoulder: the Putti-Platt operation. Acta Orthop Scand 1953;23:14–22.

70. Neer CS II, Foster CR. Inferior capsular shift for involuntary inferior and multidirectional instability of the shoulder. A preliminary report. J Bone Joint Surg Am 1980;62(6):897–908.

71. Gerber C, Lambert SM. Allograft reconstruction of segmental defects of the humeral head for treatment of chronic locked posterior dislocation of the shoulder. J Bone Joint Surg Am 1996;78(3):376–82.

72. Bisson LJ. Thermal capsulorrhaphy for isolated posterior instability of the glenohumeral joint without labral detachment. Am J Sports Med 2005;33:1898–904.

73. D'Alessandro DF, Bradley JP, Fleischli JE, et al. Prospective evaluation of thermal capsulorrhaphy for shoulder instability: indications and results, two- to five-year follow-up. Am J Sports Med 2004;32(1):21–33.

74. Miniaci A, McBirnie J. Thermal capsular shrinkage for treatment of multidirectional instability of the shoulder. J Bone Joint Surg Am 2003;85(12):2283–7.

75. Davidson PA, Rivenburgh DW. The 7-o'clock posteroinferior portal for shoulder arthroscopy. Am J Sports Med 2002;30(5):693–6.

76. Papendick LW, Savoie FH III. Anatomy-specific repair techniques for posterior shoulder instability. J South Orthop Assoc 1995;4:169–76.

77. McIntyre LF, Caspari RB, Savoie FH III. The arthroscopic treatment of posterior shoulder instability: two-year results of a multiple suture technique. Arthroscopy 1997;13(4):426–32.

78. Radkowski CA, Chhabra A, Baker CL III, et al. Arthroscopic capsulolabral repair for posterior shoulder instability in throwing athletes compared with nonthrowing athletes. Am J Sports Med 2008;36(4):693–9.

79. Goubier JN, Iserin A, Duranthon LD, et al. A 4-portal arthroscopic stabilization in posterior shoulder instability. J Shoulder Elbow Surg 2003;12(4):337–41.

80. Provencher MT, Bell SJ, Menzel KA, et al. Arthroscopic treatment of posterior shoulder instability: results in 33 patients. Am J Sports Med 2005;33(10):1463–71.

Arthroscopic Management of Multidirectional Instability

John-Erik Bell, MD

KEYWORDS

- Multidirectional instability • Arthroscopy
- Capsular plication • Shoulder • Sports medicine

In 1980, Charles S. Neer provided the first description of multidirectional instability (MDI) and the operation, the open inferior capsular shift, which was established as the gold standard.[1] He described it as "involuntary inferior and multidirectional subluxation and dislocation." This original article outlined the basis for much of our modern thinking about this condition. Although it is surprising how little has changed during the past 30 years, one aspect of MDI that has altered our thinking significantly is the advent of arthroscopic surgery and the innovation of arthroscopic techniques to restore stability and minimize morbidity.

Shoulder instability is best understood as a spectrum of disease. The most common type of instability, traumatic unidirectional instability, lies at one end of the spectrum, while multidirectional instability lies at the other extreme. Many cases fall somewhere in between these two classic examples. The most critical step in successful treatment of shoulder instability does not lie in surgical technique, but in accurate assessment of factors contributing to instability. Diagnostic precision is confounded further by variations in the definition of multidirectional instability.[2] In general, MDI consists of symptomatic, involuntary instability of the glenohumeral joint in more than one direction. It is often bilateral and usually atraumatic. One of the frequent findings in MDI compared with traumatic unidirectional instability is pathologically increased capsular volume.[3] MDI should not be confused with asymptomatic hyperlaxity or voluntary instability.

MDI is initially treated with rehabilitation, which requires patience and an extended period of time and effort on the part of the patient. The primary goal of rehabilitation is strengthening of the dynamic stabilizers, including the rotator cuff and scapular stabilizers. Proprioceptive training is also important. Nonoperative management is successful in approximately 80% of compliant patients with MDI.[4] In the recalcitrant case in which nonoperative treatment fails, surgical management is appropriate. There are several surgical techniques described to manage MDI, ranging from the classic Neer inferior capsular shift to a multitude of arthroscopic procedures. This article focuses on the arthroscopic management of MDI.

ANATOMIC CONSIDERATIONS

Shoulder stability is imparted by a combination of static and dynamic stabilizers. The most important static stabilizers include the glenohumeral ligaments, which are thickenings in the glenohumeral joint capsule that tighten and relax depending on the position of the shoulder. As a group, they render the shoulder stable through the full range of motion. The inferior glenohumeral ligaments (anterior and posterior) form a sling beneath the glenohumeral joint that stabilizes the joint in positions of abduction, preventing anterior, posterior, and inferior translation.[5,6] The middle glenohumeral ligament provides anterior stability in the midrange of abduction, limiting external rotation and

Department of Orthopaedic Surgery, Dartmouth-Hitchcock Medical Center, One Medical Center Drive, Lebanon, NH 03756, USA
E-mail address: John.E.Bell@hitchcock.org

Orthop Clin N Am 41 (2010) 357–365
doi:10.1016/j.ocl.2010.02.006

orthopedic.theclinics.com

inferior translation.[7] The superior glenohumeral ligament and coracohumeral ligament stabilize the shoulder in the adducted position, primarily limiting inferior translation and external rotation. These ligaments also comprise the structural portion of the rotator interval, the area of capsule between the superior edge of the subscapularis tendon, and the anterior edge of the supraspinatus tendon. Incompetence of the rotator interval has been shown to result in a 50% increase in posterior translation and a 100% increase in inferior translation.[8]

The most important dynamic stabilizers include the rotator cuff muscles, scapular stabilizers, and the long head of the biceps. The rotator cuff is able to resist humeral head translation through the mechanism of concavity-compression, in which the humeral head is centered into the glenoid and the rotator cuff imparts a balanced contact pressure to the articulation.[9] The labrum increases the concavity of the socket by up to 50%, but only provides 20% of the concavity-compression stability of the glenohumeral joint.[9,10] Depth of the socket (including sufficient glenoid bone stock and labral integrity) and adequate compressive force (including intact rotator cuff and sufficient rotator cuff strength) are important for shoulder stability.

Scapular stabilizers are shown to be important for shoulder stability, and abnormal scapular kinematics and periscapular muscle function have been identified in patients with MDI.[11–13] Decreased upward rotation and increased internal rotation in scapular plane abduction were found in patients with MDI in comparison with asymptomatic control patients.[11] Stabilizing the scapula results in stabilization of the glenoid, the platform on which the humeral head must function.

MAKING THE DIAGNOSIS

There are several potential causes of MDI. Genetic disorders such as Ehlers-Danlos syndrome can result in abnormal connective tissue properties that are present from birth and cannot be changed. Repetitive microtrauma such as can occur with swimming, throwing, or gymnastics can cause capsular damage that builds up over time. Patients with generalized ligamentous laxity are especially prone to develop MDI.[1] Signs of laxity include elbow or knee hyperextension beyond 10°, small finger metacarpophalangeal hyperextension more than 90°, or the ability to abduct the thumb to the forearm with the wrist fully flexed.[14,15] If the patient has 3 out of 4 of these signs, he or she is believed to have generalized ligamentous laxity (**Fig. 1**). Skin hyperelasticity

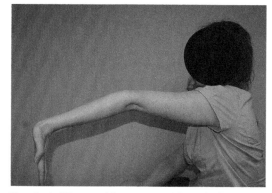

Fig. 1. A 23-year-old woman with multidirectional shoulder instability. Physical examination demonstrates extreme elbow hyperextension (recurvatum). (*Courtesy of* Center for Shoulder, Elbow and Sports Medicine, Columbia University.)

should also be noted. If severe generalized ligamentous laxity is found, a genetic workup for Ehlers-Danlos syndrome or other connective tissue disorders may be warranted. Patients who voluntarily dislocate their shoulders for reasons of psychiatric pathology or for secondary gain must be identified.[16] These patients typically have poor results after surgery.

Patients may present with frank instability or with nebulous descriptions of pain exacerbated by positions that provoke instability such as throwing (anterior instability), carrying heavy loads (inferior instability), or pushing (posterior instability). Physical examination maneuvers for anterior instability include the apprehension, relocation, and anterior release tests, the load and shift test, and the anterior drawer test. Tests for posterior instability include the posterior stress test, the jerk test, the load and shift test, and the posterior drawer test. The most important maneuver in the MDI examination, however, is the sulcus test, initially described by Neer and Foster.[1] Inferior traction is placed on the affected limb with the arm adducted at the side in neutral rotation. A positive finding is the presence of a dimple in the lateral subacromial aspect of the shoulder (**Fig. 2**). This maneuver is repeated with the arm in 30° external rotation to determine whether the rotator interval is intact. If the sulcus decreases, the rotator interval is competent. The sulcus test has good interobserver reliability and high positive predictive value for MDI when it is 2 cm or more.[17,18] Because the diagnosis of MDI is so dependent on accurate physical examination, surgery should not be planned unless the diagnosis is clear. If confusion remains after a thorough physical examination, an examination under anesthesia (EUA) may be warranted.[19] EUA is highly

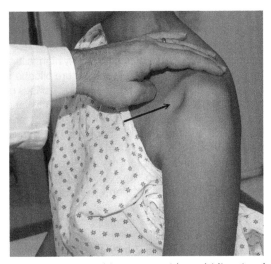

Fig. 2. A 20-year-old woman with multidirectional instability. Physical examination demonstrates a pathologic sulcus that does not decrease with external rotation at the side (*arrow* pointing to dimple caused by inferior humeral subluxation). (*Courtesy of* Center for Shoulder, Elbow and Sports Medicine, Columbia University.)

sensitive and specific, and despite the risks of anesthesia, EUA is preferable to failure of a well-done surgery on a misdiagnosed patient.

Advanced imaging plays a limited role in confirming the diagnosis of MDI. It does, however, often need to be used to rule out other causes of shoulder pain and dysfunction. Plain radiographs and computed tomography may be necessary to evaluate glenoid bone stock and the presence of a Hill-Sachs lesion. Location of glenoid and humeral head lesions can offer clues regarding the direction of instability. Magnetic resonance imaging can be used to rule out labral injury, rotator cuff injury, or humeral avulsion of the glenohumeral ligaments lesions, but the most common finding in MDI patients is capsular redundancy.

TREATMENT
Nonoperative Management

The standard of care for initial treatment of MDI is rehabilitation, with a focus on rotator cuff strengthening to maximize the concavity-compression mechanism and scapular stabilization to stabilize the glenoid platform. A dynamic stabilization protocol should also focus on proprioception once the rotator cuff and scapular stabilizers are adequately conditioned. Patient education, medical pain management with nonsteroidal anti-inflammatory medications, and avoidance of high-risk activities are also necessary components of successful nonoperative treatment.

Nonoperative treatment is effective in approximately 80% of patients compliant with their exercise program.[4] If a long-term physical therapy program is not effective, surgical options can be considered. If severe generalized ligamentous laxity or skin hyperelasticity is found, a workup for Ehlers-Danlos or other connective tissue disorder is advisable before deciding on surgical intervention.

Open Inferior Shift

The open inferior shift emerged as a successful method of treatment of MDI following its introduction by Neer and Foster in 1980.[1] In this technique, the subscapularis is tenotomized and the capsule is released from the humerus from anterior to posterior. A T-shaped capsulotomy is then performed and the inferior leaflet is shifted superiorly while the superior leaflet is shifted inferiorly. The net effect is to decrease capsular volume.[20] Overall, this procedure is highly effective. Neer and Foster reported elimination of instability in 39 out of 40 shoulders.[1] Since then, multiple other studies have shown satisfactory outcomes.[21–26] The major drawback to this procedure is the obligate damage to the subscapularis. Postoperative subscapularis insufficiency can have a negative impact on outcomes.[27]

Arthroscopic Techniques

Advantages of arthroscopic treatment include preservation of the subscapularis and the ability to visualize the entire capsulolabral anatomy. In most cases, the technique focuses on retensioning and volume reduction of the patulous capsule, with special focus on the anterior and posterior inferior glenohumeral ligaments. In some cases, this may also require closure of an incompetent rotator interval or attention to labral pathology. Arthroscopic treatment of MDI has advanced significantly since it was first described in 1993 by Duncan and Savoie,[28] who based their arthroscopic capsular shift on a modification of the inferior shift described by Altchek and colleagues.[29] Ten patients were treated and followed up for 1 to 3 years. All patients had satisfactory results according to the Neer criteria, but 2 out of 10 patients required a second operation to remove symptomatic knots.

Results of transglenoid technique
Treacy and colleagues[30] treated 25 patients with a transglenoid suture technique with a minimum 2-year follow-up, and reported 88% satisfactory results but recurrence of instability in 3 patients (12%). These patients were athletes, and return

to previous level of competition was low for football players, at 2 out of 5. All other players were able to return to their sport. McIntyre and colleagues[31] described 19 patients with mean 34-month follow-up, reporting 95% good and excellent results and 1 episode of recurrent instability (5%). In this study, 89% were able to return to previous level of competition.

Results of capsular plication technique

Capsular plication uses sutures to reduce capsular volume. This procedure can be done with or without suture anchors and can use either permanent or resorbable suture material. It has been shown that suture plication alone can restore normal range of motion and reduce volume, but rotator interval closure may be necessary to reduce translation.[32,33] Wichman and Snyder[34] reported on this in 1997, using a technique in which the capsule is abraded with a rasp and a 1-cm infolding was created at the capsulolabral junction using a horizontal mattress suture configuration. Gartsman and colleagues[35] described a pancapsular plication technique used in 47 MDI patients with an average follow-up of 35 months. Suture anchors were used in 27 of the patients because of labral deficiency. Good or excellent results were obtained in 94% of patients, 85% of patients returned to previous level of competition, and there was 1 case of recurrent instability (2%). Baker and colleagues[36] recently reported on 40 patients with MDI who underwent arthroscopic capsular plication with or without suture anchors and were followed for 2 to 5 years postoperatively; 86% were able to return to sport. These investigators reported 4 failures (2 because of instability), but all patients reported feeling that the surgery was worthwhile and said they would have it again. Joshua and colleagues[37] reported on 13 patients with MDI and a labral tear of 270° or greater, who underwent arthroscopic repair with mean follow-up of 56 months, with a minimum 2-year follow-up. The investigators reported 84% completely or mostly satisfied, with a recurrent instability rate of 15%.

Results of thermal capsulorrhaphy

Thermal capsulorrhaphy has been used alone or in conjunction with suture plication in the treatment of MDI. In this technique, radiofrequency or laser is applied to the capsule, heating it and damaging the ultrastructure, resulting in cell necrosis and destruction of collagen cross-links with the net effect of shrinking the capsule. At 2 weeks, this tissue is weaker and vulnerable to injury, but over time it is repaired and regains its mechanical properties by 12 weeks.[38] Unfortunately, if the temperature limits are exceeded the matrix is destroyed, which can result in capsular necrosis.[39] This technique is no longer recommended even as an adjunct because of unacceptably high failure rates compared with arthroscopic suture plication. Hawkins and colleagues[40] reported on 17 cases of MDI treated with thermal capsulorrhaphy and found a 57% failure rate. D'Alessandro and colleagues[41] described 53 shoulders with MDI treated with thermal capsulorrhaphy and reported a 41% rate of unsatisfactory results. Fitzgerald and colleagues[42] reported on experience with 30 shoulders treated with thermal capsulorrhaphy and found a 30% failure rate at mean follow-up of 33 months. Noonan and colleagues[44] described 11 patients with MDI treated with thermal capsulorrhaphy and found 7 failures (64%).[43] Miniaci and McBirnie[44] also reported on 19 patients with MDI treated with thermal capsulorrhaphy, with a 47% recurrence rate at minimum 2-year follow-up.

In addition to these unacceptably high failure rates, there is also a small risk of catastrophic complications, including capsular necrosis, glenohumeral chondrolysis, and axillary nerve injury.[39,45–48] The high rate of failure and the possibility of these catastrophic complications considerably outweigh the technical ease of the procedure.

The Author's Preferred Technique

The author uses a technique described in detail by Bahu and colleagues.[49] The procedure is performed in the lateral decubitus position, which improves access to the posterior and inferior aspects of the glenohumeral joint. A comprehensive EUA is performed to grade the amount and direction of instability and to document the range of motion. The EUA includes a sulcus test in neutral forearm rotation and in external rotation, then anterior and posterior load and shift testing. Approximately 10 lb (4.53 kg) of in-line traction is used through a sterile arm holder to allow repositioning, and repeat EUA is performed if necessary during the case. The joint is initially accessed through the posterior portal about 2 cm beneath the posterior-inferior corner of the acromion but not the typical 1 to 2 cm medial, because this allows better access to the posterior labrum if necessary. Anterior portal placement is made using an outside-in technique and depends on the presence of anterior pathology. If anterior plication or labral repair is necessary, 2 anterior portals are created with a skin bridge of approximately 3 to 4 cm, one entering in the superiormost aspect of the rotator interval immediately behind the long head of the biceps tendon and the second at the inferior and lateral aspect of the rotator interval just adjacent to the superior border of the subscapularis tendon. Cannulae placement through the subscapularis is avoided. Diagnostic arthroscopy usually reveals a capacious capsule and obvious drive-through sign (**Fig. 3**). Occasionally, the rotator interval is widened. Concomitant pathology such as labral or rotator cuff tears is rarely found. It is also important to assess the posterior aspect of the joint accurately, and this requires visualization with the arthroscope in the anterior portal.

The first capsular plication stitch is placed in the posterior band of the inferior glenohumeral ligament. While viewing from the anterosuperior portal, a rasp is brought in through the posterior cannula and the posteroinferior capsule is abraded to promote healing (**Fig. 4**). If the labrum is substantial and firmly attached, it can be used to anchor the plication stitch. If attenuated or torn, then a suture anchor is placed at the edge of the glenoid face at the inner edge of the labrum after abrading it with a rasp or shaver. The anchor (or plication stitch) is placed percutaneously, which minimizes rotator cuff damage and allows for greater accuracy of anchor placement, because direction is not limited by location of the cannula. A spinal needle is placed approximately 2 cm inferior and slightly lateral to the posterior cannula, and is used to identify the perfect angle for anchor insertion. Then a 2-mm nick is made in the skin, through which the drill guide and trocar

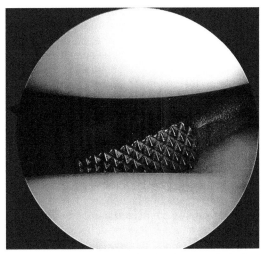

Fig. 4. A rasp is used to abrade the capsule before plication, stimulating a healing response. (*Courtesy of* Center for Shoulder, Elbow and Sports Medicine, Columbia University.)

assembly are introduced into the joint at the same angle as the spinal needle. The glenoid is drilled and the anchor is inserted through the same drill guide (**Fig. 5**). Then the suture limb on the labral side is brought out through the posterior cannula. A 90° suture lasso (Arthrex, Naples, FL, USA) is then passed through the same percutaneous skin nick into the joint. The author usually captures about 5 mm of the capsule starting approximately 1 cm from the edge of the labrum, depending on

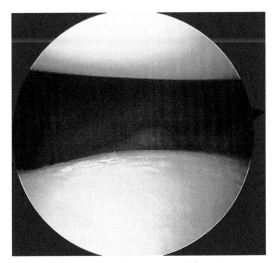

Fig. 3. Anterosuperior viewing portal showing a capacious posterior capsule in a patient with MDI (LEFT shoulder, lateral decubitus position). (*Courtesy of* Center for Shoulder, Elbow and Sports Medicine, Columbia University.)

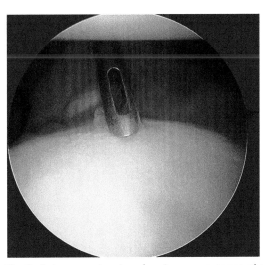

Fig. 5. Anterosuperior view showing a percutaneously placed drill guide. Note how inferior on the glenoid the drill guide can be placed when not constrained by a cannula (LEFT shoulder, lateral decubitus position). (*Courtesy of* Center for Shoulder, Elbow and Sports Medicine, Columbia University.)

the degree of pathology present. The suture lasso is then passed through the labrum and the nitinol wire is retrieved through the same posterior cannula as the previously retrieved suture limb, allowing the suture to be shuttled through the capsule as the suture lasso is removed from the joint (**Fig. 6**). Both limbs are the brought out through the posterior cannula and tied. If the labrum is substantial, the suture lasso is passed under the labrum, the nitinol wire is retrieved, and a #2 FiberWire suture (Arthrex, Naples, FL, USA) is shuttled back through the capsule as the lasso is removed from the joint. A similar technique is repeated posteriorly as needed; typically 2 to 3 posterior sutures are placed and tied sequentially (**Fig. 7**). The scope is then switched to the posterior portal from the anterior portal. The same procedure is performed, beginning inferiorly with the anterior band of the inferior glenohumeral ligament and proceeding superiorly as pathology dictates, but usually 2 to 3 anterior plication stitches are placed. The goal is to balance the plication so that there is no relative laxity or over-tightening anteriorly or posteriorly (**Fig. 8**). The author typically uses a second anterior cannula to simplify the procedure, because there is less morbidity to a second rotator interval cannula. The percutaneous technique is preferred posteriorly to minimize trauma to the posterior rotator cuff.

Finally, a decision regarding rotator interval closure must be made. If the sulcus diminishes

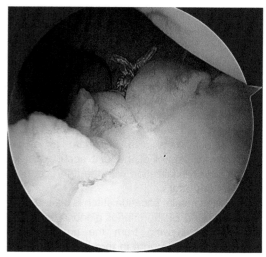

Fig. 7. Anterosuperior view showing completed capsular plication. The knots are kept as far from the joint surface as possible (LEFT shoulder, lateral decubitus position). (*Courtesy of* Center for Shoulder, Elbow and Sports Medicine, Columbia University.)

with external rotation on examination under anesthesia, the interval is typically competent. However, in cases where the rotator interval is incompetent, closure should be performed. Closure is achieved by placing the anterosuperior cannula in an extracapsular position and introducing a #2 nonabsorbable, high-strength suture through the superior aspect of the middle glenohumeral ligament laterally with a penetrating

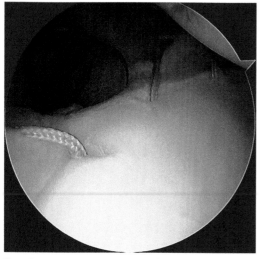

Fig. 6. Anterosuperior view showing 2 plication sutures (4 and 5 o'clock). The sutures go through the posteroinferior capsule, then through the labrum (LEFT shoulder, lateral decubitus position). (*Courtesy of* Center for Shoulder, Elbow and Sports Medicine, Columbia University.)

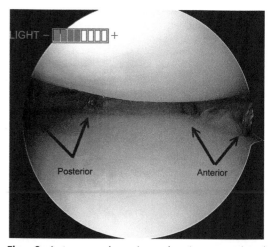

Fig. 8. Anterosuperior view showing completed capsular plication with 2 anterior and 2 posterior plication sutures. Note that the humeral head is perfectly centered on the glenoid (LEFT shoulder, lateral decubitus position). (*Courtesy of* Center for Shoulder, Elbow and Sports Medicine, Columbia University.)

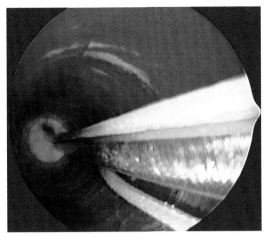

Fig. 9. Rotator interval closure. View down the anterosuperior cannula showing the sutures being tied in the cannula (but outside the joint). (*Courtesy of* Center for Shoulder, Elbow and Sports Medicine, Columbia University.)

grasper. The end is the brought out of the joint through the anteroinferior portal.

The penetrating grasper is then reintroduced through the extracapsular anterosuperior cannula and through the superior glenohumeral ligament laterally. The end of the suture is retrieved such that both free suture ends are within the anterosuperior cannula that rests just on the outside of the capsule, and the knot is tied on the external aspect of the capsule (**Figs. 9** and **10**). One or 2 sutures are used dependent on the amount of relative patholaxity in this part of the capsule.

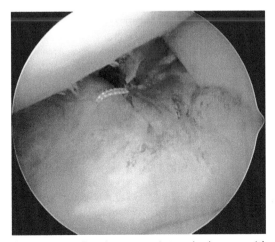

Fig. 10. Completed rotator interval closure with a single suture (LEFT shoulder, lateral decubitus position—posterior viewing portal). (*Courtesy of* Center for Shoulder, Elbow and Sports Medicine, Columbia University.)

Postoperative Management

The patient is placed in slight external rotation and immobilized for 6 weeks postoperatively before formal physical therapy is initiated. Despite this long period of immobilization, the author has not encountered long-term postoperative stiffness in this patient population. Beginning at 6 weeks, range of motion and strengthening exercises are progressively initiated. Return to sport is allowed at 6 months.

SUMMARY

Since Neer's initial work, there has been remarkably little change in the understanding of the anatomy and pathophysiology of MDI.[1] Although rehabilitation remains the initial recommended treatment and is typically successful, the indications for surgery continue to be refined. Although thermal capsulorrhaphy is no longer recommended for the treatment of MDI, capsular plication with or without anchors has been shown to be successful. The technology available for treatment has advanced significantly, and arthroscopic techniques now yield results comparable to Neer's classic open capsular shift.

REFERENCES

1. Neer CS 2nd, Foster CR. Inferior capsular shift for involuntary inferior and multidirectional instability of the shoulder. A preliminary report. J Bone Joint Surg Am 1980;62:897.
2. McFarland EG, Kim TK, Park HB, et al. The effect of variation in definition on the diagnosis of multidirectional instability of the shoulder. J Bone Joint Surg Am 2003;85:2138.
3. Dewing CB, McCormick F, Bell SJ, et al. An analysis of capsular area in patients with anterior, posterior, and multidirectional shoulder instability. Am J Sports Med 2008;36:515.
4. Burkhead WZ Jr, Rockwood CA Jr. Treatment of instability of the shoulder with an exercise program. J Bone Joint Surg Am 1992;74:890.
5. O'Brien SJ, Neves MC, Arnoczky SP, et al. The anatomy and histology of the inferior glenohumeral ligament complex of the shoulder. Am J Sports Med 1990;18:449.
6. Warner JJ, Deng XH, Warren RF, et al. Static capsuloligamentous restraints to superior-inferior translation of the glenohumeral joint. Am J Sports Med 1992;20:675.
7. Ferrari DA. Capsular ligaments of the shoulder. Anatomical and functional study of the anterior superior capsule. Am J Sports Med 1990;18:20.
8. Harryman DT 2nd, Sidles JA, Harris SL, et al. The role of the rotator interval capsule in passive motion

and stability of the shoulder. J Bone Joint Surg Am 1992;74:53.

9. Lippitt S, Matsen F. Mechanisms of glenohumeral joint stability. Clin Orthop Relat Res 1993;291:20.

10. Howell SM, Galinat BJ. The glenoid-labral socket. A constrained articular surface. Clin Orthop Relat Res 1989;243:122.

11. Ogston JB, Ludewig PM. Differences in 3-dimensional shoulder kinematics between persons with multidirectional instability and asymptomatic controls. Am J Sports Med 2007;35:1361.

12. Ozaki J. Glenohumeral movements of the involuntary inferior and multidirectional instability. Clin Orthop Relat Res 1989;238:107.

13. Warner JJ, Micheli LJ, Arslanian LE, et al. Scapulothoracic motion in normal shoulders and shoulders with glenohumeral instability and impingement syndrome. A study using Moire topographic analysis. Clin Orthop Relat Res 1992;285:191.

14. Beighton PH, Horan FT. Dominant inheritance in familial generalised articular hypermobility. J Bone Joint Surg Br 1970;52:145.

15. Schwartz E, Warren RF, O'Brien SJ, et al. Posterior shoulder instability. Orthop Clin North Am 1987; 18:409.

16. Rowe CR, Pierce DS, Clark JG. Voluntary dislocation of the shoulder. A preliminary report on a clinical, electromyographic, and psychiatric study of twenty-six patients. J Bone Joint Surg Am 1973; 55:445.

17. Tzannes A, Murrell GA. Clinical examination of the unstable shoulder. Sports Med 2002;32:447.

18. Tzannes A, Paxinos A, Callanan M, et al. An assessment of the interexaminer reliability of tests for shoulder instability. J Shoulder Elbow Surg 2004; 13:18.

19. Cofield RH, Nessler JP, Weinstabl R. Diagnosis of shoulder instability by examination under anesthesia. Clin Orthop Relat Res 1993;291:45.

20. Wiater JM, Brady TV. Glenohumeral joint volume reduction with progressive release and shifting of the inferior shoulder capsule. J Shoulder Elbow Surg 2007;16:810.

21. Bak K, Spring BJ, Henderson JP. Inferior capsular shift procedure in athletes with multidirectional instability based on isolated capsular and ligamentous redundancy. Am J Sports Med 2000; 28:466.

22. Bigliani LU, Kurzweil PR, Schwartzbach CC, et al. Inferior capsular shift procedure for anterior-inferior shoulder instability in athletes. Am J Sports Med 1994;22:578.

23. Cooper RA, Brems JJ. The inferior capsular-shift procedure for multidirectional instability of the shoulder. J Bone Joint Surg Am 1992;74:1516.

24. Hamada K, Fukuda H, Nakajima T, et al. The inferior capsular shift operation for instability of the shoulder. Long-term results in 34 shoulders. J Bone Joint Surg Br 1999;81:218.

25. Lebar RD, Alexander AH. Multidirectional shoulder instability. Clinical results of inferior capsular shift in an active-duty population. Am J Sports Med 1992;20:193.

26. Pollock RG, Owens JM, Flatow EL, et al. Operative results of the inferior capsular shift procedure for multidirectional instability of the shoulder. J Bone Joint Surg Am 2000;82:919.

27. Sachs RA, Williams B, Stone ML, et al. Open Bankart repair: correlation of results with postoperative subscapularis function. Am J Sports Med 2005;33:1458.

28. Duncan R, Savoie FH 3rd. Arthroscopic inferior capsular shift for multidirectional instability of the shoulder: a preliminary report. Arthroscopy 1993;9:24.

29. Altchek DW, Warren RF, Skyhar MJ, et al. T-plasty modification of the Bankart procedure for multidirectional instability of the anterior and inferior types. J Bone Joint Surg Am 1991;73:105.

30. Treacy SH, Savoie FH 3rd, Field LD. Arthroscopic treatment of multidirectional instability. J Shoulder Elbow Surg 1999;8:345.

31. McIntyre LF, Caspari RB, Savoie FH 3rd. The arthroscopic treatment of multidirectional shoulder instability: two-year results of a multiple suture technique. Arthroscopy 1997;13:418.

32. Jon KS, James AW, Mark DM, et al. Arthroscopic multi-pleated capsular plication compared with open inferior capsular shift for reduction of shoulder volume in a cadaveric model. Arthroscopy 2007;23:1145.

33. Shafer BL, Mihata T, McGarry MH, et al. Effects of capsular plication and rotator interval closure in simulated multidirectional shoulder instability. J Bone Joint Surg Am 2008;90:136.

34. Wichman M, Snyder S. Arthroscopic capsular plication for multidirectional instability of the shoulder. Oper Tech Sports Med 1997;5:238.

35. Gartsman GM, Roddey TS, Hammerman SM. Arthroscopic treatment of multidirectional glenohumeral instability: 2- to 5-year follow-up. Arthroscopy 2001;17:236.

36. Baker CL, Mascarenhas R, Kline AJ, et al. Arthroscopic treatment of multidirectional shoulder instability in athletes. Am J Sports Med 2009;37:1712.

37. Joshua MA, Nikhil V, Robert W, et al. Arthroscopic treatment of multidirectional shoulder instability with minimum 270° labral repair: minimum 2-year follow-up. Arthroscopy 2008;24:704.

38. Hecht P, Hayashi K, Cooley AJ, et al. The thermal effect of monopolar radiofrequency energy on the properties of joint capsule. An in vivo histologic study using a sheep model. Am J Sports Med 1998;26:808.

39. Rath E, Richmond JC. Capsular disruption as a complication of thermal alteration of the glenohumeral capsule. Arthroscopy 2001;17:E10.

40. Hawkins RJ, Krishnan SG, Karas SG, et al. Electro-thermal arthroscopic shoulder capsulorrhaphy: a minimum 2-year follow-up. Am J Sports Med 2007;35:1484.

41. D'Alessandro DF, Bradley JP, Fleischli JE, et al. Prospective evaluation of thermal capsulorrhaphy for shoulder instability: indications and results, two- to five-year follow-up. Am J Sports Med 2004;32:21.

42. Fitzgerald BT, Watson BT, Lapoint JM. The use of thermal capsulorrhaphy in the treatment of multidirectional instability. J Shoulder Elbow Surg 2002;11:108.

43. Noonan TJ, Tokish JM, Briggs KK, et al. Laser-assisted thermal capsulorrhaphy. Arthroscopy 2003;19:815.

44. Miniaci A, McBirnie J. Thermal capsular shrinkage for treatment of multidirectional instability of the shoulder. J Bone Joint Surg Am 2003;85:2283.

45. Ciccone WJ 2nd, Weinstein DM, Elias JJ. Glenohumeral chondrolysis following thermal capsulorrhaphy. Orthopedics 2007;30:158.

46. Good CR, Shindle MK, Kelly BT, et al. Glenohumeral chondrolysis after shoulder arthroscopy with thermal capsulorrhaphy. Arthroscopy 2007;23:797, e1.

47. Levine WN, Clark AM Jr, D'Alessandro DF, et al. Chondrolysis following arthroscopic thermal capsulorrhaphy to treat shoulder instability. A report of two cases. J Bone Joint Surg Am 2005;87:616.

48. Wong KL, Williams GR. Complications of thermal capsulorrhaphy of the shoulder. J Bone Joint Surg Am 2001;83(Suppl 2 Pt 2):151.

49. Bahu MJ, Trentacosta N, Vorys GC, et al. Multidirectional instability: evaluation and treatment options. Clin Sports Med 2008;27:671.

Management of Failed Instability Surgery: How to Get It Right the Next Time

Julienne L. Boone, MD[a], Robert A. Arciero, MD[b],*

KEYWORDS

- Instability • Shoulder instability
- Bankart lesion • Arthroscopic Bankart repair
- Revision instability surgery • Bone defect

Traumatic anterior shoulder dislocations are the most frequent type of joint dislocation and affect approximately 1.7% of the general population.[1] The literature supports the consideration of primary stabilization in high-risk patients because of reported recurrences as high as 80% to 90% with nonoperative treatment regimens.[2–4] Successful stabilization of anterior glenohumeral instability relies on not only good surgical techniques but also careful patient selection. Failure rates after open and arthroscopic stabilization have been reported to range from 2% to 8% and 4% to 13%, respectively.[5–9] Recurrent shoulder instability leads to increased morbidity to the patient, increased pain, decreased activity level, prolonged time away from work and sports, and a general decrease in quality of life. This article reviews the potential pitfalls in anterior shoulder stabilization and discusses appropriate methods of addressing them in revision surgery.

PATHOANATOMY

The stability of the glenohumeral joint relies on the balance maintained by its static and dynamic stabilizers.[10] Dynamic components include the rotator cuff muscles,[11] and the critical static components include the glenolabral complex and capsuloligamentous structures. The labrum increases the surface area and depth of the glenoid socket by as much as 50%, thereby improving osseous conformity.[12] Detachment of the anteroinferior labrum with its attached inferior glenohumeral ligament complex denotes the classic Bankart lesion and is the most common pathologic finding associated with anterior shoulder instability.[13] With recurrent episodes of instability, elongation of the anteroinferior and inferior capsule has been shown to occur, further adding to the underlying pathology of this clinical entity.[14]

In addition to soft tissue injury, recurrent instability can facilitate progressive bony injury. Sugaya and colleagues[15] identified an osseous Bankart lesion in 50% of patients with traumatic anterior shoulder instability. Although most of these fragments were less than 10.6% of the glenoid fossa, they also noted that an additional 40% of patients showed blunting on oblique radiographs, suggestive of mild erosion. Griffith and colleagues[16] reported similar results, with a 41% incidence of glenoid bone loss in first-time anterior shoulder dislocators. This condition increased to 86% in recurrent dislocators, and the severity of the bone defect significantly correlated to the number of dislocations.

[a] Department of Orthopedic Surgery, Washington University School of Medicine, 660 South Euclid Avenue, St Louis, MO 63110, USA
[b] Department of Orthopedic Surgery, University of Connecticut Health Center, 263 Farmington Avenue, Farmington, CT 06030-4037, USA
* Corresponding author.
E-mail address: arciero@nso.uchc.edu

Orthop Clin N Am 41 (2010) 367–379
doi:10.1016/j.ocl.2010.02.009

The clinical applicability of these findings was characterized by Itoi and colleagues,[17] who elucidated the minimum sized defect that led to clinical instability after a Bankart repair. In a cadaveric study they showed that after a Bankart repair, the capsular structures maintained stability of the joint up to a 21% (6.8 mm) anteroinferior glenoid defect. With bony defects greater than 21%, the shoulder showed persistent instability with internal rotation, and experienced limited external rotation after Bankart repair (**Fig. 1**).

Increasing anteroinferior glenoid bone loss has been associated also with increased contact pressures. Greis and colleagues[18] showed in a cadaveric study that a 30% glenoid bone defect led to a 41% decreased articular contact area of the entire glenoid and a 100% increase in mean contact pressures. These findings may have implications in the development of postoperative arthritis, and potentially support the findings of Buscayret and colleagues[19] that the presence of osseous glenoid rim lesions is a risk factor in the development of arthritis, and that the development of postoperative arthritis correlates with an increased number of preoperative dislocations.

In patients with anterior shoulder instability, bony lesions are not limited to the glenoid but frequently also affect the humeral head. The classic Hill-Sachs lesion, in which the posterolateral aspect of the anteriorly dislocated head impacts the anterior glenoid rim, occurs in up to

90% of primary dislocators, 100% of patients with recurrent instability, and 40% of patients with recurrent anterior shoulder subluxations (**Fig. 2**).[20–22] Although lesions involve less than 20% of the articular surface and are considered clinically insignificant, those larger than 20% to 30% may be relevant contributors to recurrent instability.[23,24]

From a pathoanatomic standpoint, when caring for patients for whom treatment of instability failed, both soft tissue and bony issues must be addressed. The surgeon should identify and be prepared to address not only the Bankart lesion but also any excess capsular tissue and relevant bony lesions.

CLINICAL EVALUATION

In patients for whom treatment of instability failed, a careful clinical workup is essential to diagnose and appropriately address the underlying problem. The essential question remains: "Why do we have a 'failed' instability patient?" Is the patient complaining of recurrent instability or a different complication, such as pain, loss of motion, or decreased strength? A proper diagnosis is the foundation on which to direct treatment. A thorough history and physical examination, and judicious use of imaging studies, will help separate patients with posterior instability, multidirectional instability, and other labral disorders (such as

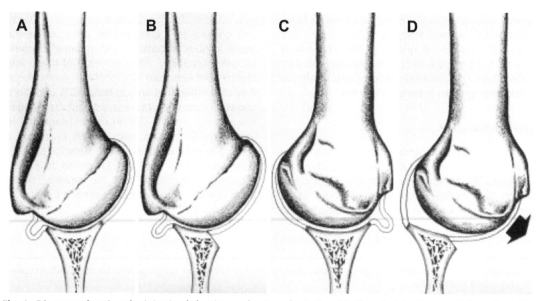

Fig. 1. Diagrams showing the joint in abduction and external rotation (*A, B*) and abduction and internal rotation (*C, D*). With external rotation, the tight anterior capsuloligamentous structures prevent anterior translation of the humeral head (*B*). With internal rotation and a glenoid rim defect, the humeral head shifts anteriorly (*D*). (*Reproduced from* Itoi E, Lee SB, Berglund LJ, et al. The effect of a glenoid defect on anteroinferior stability of the shoulder after Bankart repair: a cadaveric study. J Bone Joint Surg Am 2000;82(1):35–46; with permission.)

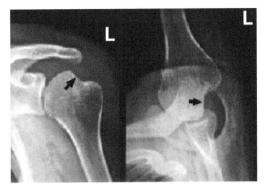

Fig. 2. Radiographs of a young active female patient with recurrent instability of the shoulder showing a large Hill-Sachs lesion (*arrows*). (*Reproduced from Flatow EL, Warner JI. Instability of the shoulder: complex problems and failed repairs: Part I. Relevant biomechanics, multidirectional instability, and severe glenoid loss. Instr Course Lect 1998;47:97–112; with permission.*)

a humeral avulsion of the glenohumeral ligament [HAGL] lesion) from those with traumatic anterior instability.

History and Physical Examination

Details of the patient's history are focused on assessing the severity of the instability, confirming the diagnosis, and identifying any associated lesions (eg, bone loss, capsular tears). Up to 89% of failed prior stabilization procedures have been shown to have some degree of glenoid bone loss.[25] Arm position during the injury should be determined, in addition to avoidance of positions that make the patient apprehensive about possible instability. These facts provide significant clues as to the type of instability the patient is experiencing.

The nature of the recurrence episode is also important to determine. A trivial event, such as one occurring during simple activities of daily living or sleeping, suggests the presence of persistent capsular laxity or an osseous defect. However, a major event, especially one requiring a reduction, suggests a disruption of the prior Bankart repair and should raise suspicion of the presence of an engaging Hill-Sachs lesion.

The physical examination should involve comparison with the contralateral shoulder and begins with observation of the shoulder's resting position. Range of motion and strength testing are important to assess. Loss of motion may be caused by chondrolysis, hardware impingement, or overtightening of the capsulolabral complex. Strength deficits may be caused by a concomitant rotator cuff deficiency or neurapraxia; in particular,

the axillary and musculocutaneous nerve functions must be examined. A thorough examination of rotator cuff function should be documented in any patient older than 40 years, because this age group has a higher incidence of rotator cuff tearing with traumatic anterior shoulder dislocations, and this may contribute to their sense of "failure."[26] Subscapularis function should be assessed by using the belly press or lift-off tests. This is especially important in patients with a previous open Bankart repair, because studies have shown that 23% of these patients will have an incompetent subscapularis with a positive lift-off test and only 27% the strength of their contralateral side.[27] In a study of patients with clinical subscapularis deficiencies, Sachs and colleagues[27] showed that only 57% reported good to excellent results and would have the surgery again.

Generalized ligamentous laxity should be tested for, because its presence may suggest increased baseline capsular redundancy. The Beighton score, which quantifies joint laxity and hypermobility, may be useful.[28] It includes assessment of elbow and knee hyperextension, metacarpophalangeal joint hyperextension, the ability to approximate the thumbs to forearm, and the ability to rest the palms resting on the floor with the knees extended.

The sulcus test should be performed to identify and quantify inferior capsular laxity. Provocative examination maneuvers, such as apprehension testing at varying degrees of abduction and external rotation followed by relocation testing, are vital to characterize the nature of the instability. These tests are greater than 72% sensitive and greater than 92% specific when apprehension is used as the end point (and not pain).[29] Patients with instability at early and midranges of motion are more likely to have a complicating bony lesion. A load-and-shift maneuver may be helpful to quantify any instability, and the examiner should pay careful attention to any crepitus at the edges, which may also suggest a bony defect.

Imaging

Adequate imaging studies are essential in the workup of a patient who underwent failed instability surgery, because they facilitate identification and quantification of bony defects. Standard radiographs, which include an anteroposterior (AP), a true AP, and an axillary view, may suggest subtle bone loss. Modified axillary views, such as the West Point view, are often helpful in visualizing anteroinferior glenoid bone defieciencies.[30] In cadaveric models, this view has been shown to accurately estimate the size of the rim defect, whereas it is significantly underestimated on the standard axillary view (**Fig. 3**).[31] Additional radiographs, such as the Stryker notch view and the AP view with the humerus in internal rotation, are often useful in defining Hill-Sachs lesions of the humerus.[32]

A

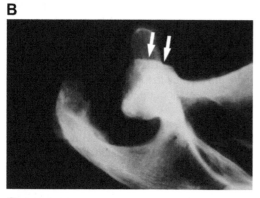

B

C

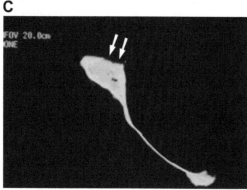

Fig. 3. Radiographs and CT scan of one specimen with a 21% defect. The defect can hardly be recognized on the axillary view (*A, arrow*), whereas it seems to be one fifth of the glenoid on the West Point view (*B, arrows; B*). The CT image (*C*) depicts the defect (*arrows*) as one half of the glenoid at the inferior one-fourth level of the glenoid. (*Reproduced from* Itoi E, Lee SB, Amrami KK, et al. Quantitative assessment of classic anteroinferior bony Bankart lesions by radiography and computed tomography. Am J Sports Med 2003;31(1):112–8; with permission.)

Further imaging studies should be performed in patients whose clinical history and examination are suspicious for glenoid bone loss or whose radiographs show any bony defect. A history of multiple dislocations, the progressive ease of dislocation and reduction, prior failed instability surgery, and marked apprehension and guarding at lower abduction angles on examination are all indications to obtain a CT scan.[33] The CT scan allows definition of both lesions of the humeral head and the glenoid fossa (**Fig. 4**). Axial and sagittal views permit precise measurement of any glenoid defects. In a review of 123 computed tomography (CT) scans in patients with anterior shoulder instability, Saito and colleagues[34] defined the common location of the glenoid defect to be centered around the 3-o'clock position, extending inferiorly. In their cadaveric study, Itoi and colleagues[17,31] showed that the critical 21% defect appears as a 50% glenoid bone loss on a single axial slice across the lower one fourth of the glenoid.

The use of three-dimensionally reconstructed CT images with the humeral head subtracted has been recommended to facilitate quantification of glenoid bone loss.[15] Because the inferior two thirds of the glenoid has been shown to consistently be a "circle," one can use the en face three-dimensional image and calculate the area of bone loss as a percentage of the circle (**Fig. 5**).[35] Three-dimensional CT imaging can also be used to measure the length of the glenoid lesion. Gerber and Nyffeler[36] found that if the length of the lesion was equal to half the widest diameter in the anteroposterior plane, then the resistance to dislocation was decreased by more than 30%.

MR arthrography can also be helpful in evaluating patients for whom instability surgery failed because it permits better delineation of associated soft-tissue pathology and may detect rotator cuff tears, HAGL, capsular tears or laxity, and posterior extension of Bankart lesions. A recent study of patients with recurrent instability showed MR arthrography to be 91.9% accurate in assessing pathologic labral conditions and other internal derangements compared with arthroscopic findings.[37] Recognition of this concomitant pathology allows for appropriate surgical planning to address these lesions and can lead to improved outcomes.

All of these imaging modalities play a role in the workup of patients for whom instability repair failed. Plain radiographs remain the baseline screening tool. Although MR arthrography excels at detecting soft-tissue injuries, it often underestimates the extent of bony lesions (**Fig. 6**). It should not substitute for CT with three-dimensional

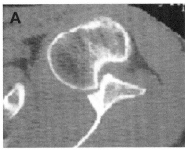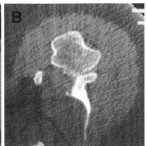

Fig. 4. Axial CT scan cuts showing a Hill-Sachs lesion (*A*) and glenoid bone loss (*B*).

imaging, which persists as the gold standard for quantification of bony defects of the glenoid fossa and humeral head.[38]

RECURRENT INSTABILITY

Recurrent instability may be caused by several potential pitfalls. Typically, the causative factors are poor patient selection (diagnostic errors), technical errors, or postsurgical trauma.[39–41] Patient selection factors include recognition of significant glenoid bone loss or a Hill-Sachs lesion, hyperlaxity, poor tissue quality, associated injuries, and potential compliance issues with postoperative rehabilitation. Technical errors may involve nonanatomic repairs with incorrect suture anchor placement, unrecognized HAGL injuries, and inadequate capsular tensioning and mobilization resulting in persistent capsular laxity. Failure to recognize and adequately

address any of these issues can result in a poor outcome and lead to failed instability.

In a recent systematic review, Brophy and Marx[42] reported that the rate of recurrent instability was roughly equal after arthroscopic suture anchor stabilization (6.4%) and open suture anchor stabilization (8.2%). Failure to address the pathologic anatomy plays a critical role in failed instability surgery. Tauber and colleagues[5] published their anatomic findings for failure after both open and arthroscopic anterior shoulder instability procedures. At revision surgery, they found 56% of patients had persistent bony Bankart lesions, 22% had a large capsule, and 5% had a laterally torn capsule. Other authors have reported similar findings, with a 46% to 50% incidence of recurrent/residual Bankart lesions and a 61% to 86% incidence of capsular redundancy.[39,40]

The importance of patient selection and surgical technique cannot be overstated, and several risk factors for recurrent instability after arthroscopic repair have been identified. In a study of 91 patients who underwent arthroscopic stabilization for recurrent anterior shoulder instability, Boileau and colleagues[43] reported that the presence of glenoid or humeral head bone loss (>25% of the articular surface), hyperlaxity, and the use of fewer than four suture anchors significantly increased the risk for recurrence. However, although their overall recurrence rate was 15.3%, patients with hyperlaxity and glenoid bone loss exhibited a 75% recurrence rate, and the authors suggested that this association of findings was a contraindication to arthroscopic repair. They advocated arthroscopic Bankart repair only in patients with minimal humeral and glenoid bone loss, with the incorporation of a technique that would permit optimal capsular tensioning.

To further help identify which patients are at increased risk for recurrent instability after arthroscopic Bankart repair, Balg and Boileau[44] introduced the instability severity index score. This 10-point score is derived risk factors identified from a prospective study of 131 patients with

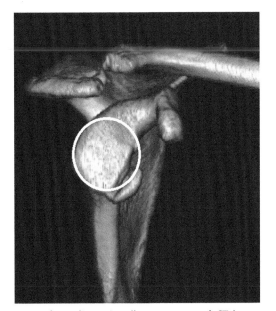

Fig. 5. Three-dimensionally reconstructed CT images showing a glenoid fragment.

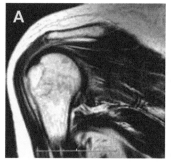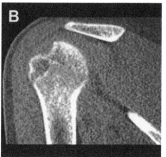

Fig. 6. MRI (*A*) and CT scan (*B*) of a Hills-Sachs lesion show that MRI can underrepresent bone defects. (*Reproduced from* Arciero RA, Spang JT. Complications in arthroscopic anterior shoulder stabilization: pearls and pitfalls. Instr Course Lect 2008;57:113–24; with permission.)

recurrent anterior instability who underwent arthroscopic Bankart repair. These investigators found that 14.5% of their population experienced recurrent instability after repair and that risk factors were age younger than 20 years; participation in competitive, contact, or overhead sports; hyperlaxity; the presence of a Hill-Sachs lesion on an AP radiograph with the humerus in external rotation; and the loss of the sclerotic inferior glenoid contour on an AP radiograph. They concluded that arthroscopic repair was contraindicated in patients with a preoperative instability severity index score greater than six because they had a 70% risk of recurrence after an arthroscopic repair.

Other authors have found similar subsets of patients to be at increased risk for recurrent instability after arthroscopic Bankart repair. Uhorchak and colleagues[45] reported a 23% rate of recurrent instability after arthroscopic stabilization in contact and collision athletes. In the presence of a bone defect, this value increases significantly to 89% recurrence in contact athletes treated arthroscopically.[25] Because Pagnani and Dome[46] noted only a 3% recurrence rate for subluxation after open stabilization in football players, many surgeons advocate initial open Bankart repair in contact athletes, especially those with bone loss.

Bone loss also plays a substantial role in the outcomes of noncontact athletes with anterior shoulder instability treated with arthroscopic stabilization. In a study of 194 athletes treated with arthroscopic Bankart repair, Burkhart and De Beer[25] noted a 4% recurrence rate in patients without a bone defect. In the 11% of patients with a significant bone defect, the recurrence rate was significantly higher at 67%. The question then becomes what defines a relevant bony defect and how the surgeon identifies this risk factor intraoperatively.

Significant glenoid bone loss is often discussed in the framework of the inverted pear glenoid, in which the normal pear-shaped glenoid has lost enough anteroinferior bone to assume the shape of an inverted pear when viewed arthroscopically from the anterosuperior portal (**Fig. 7**).[25] Yiannakopoulos and colleagues[47] reported a 15.4% incidence of the inverted pear configuration in their patients with recurrent instability. Lo and colleagues[48] quantified the amount of anterior glenoid bone loss needed to produce the inverted pear morphology as 7.5 mm or 28.8% loss of the glenoid width.

Arthroscopic quantification of glenoid bone loss has been described by Burkhart and colleagues[49] using the glenoid bare spot as a consistent reference point. Located at the center of the circle

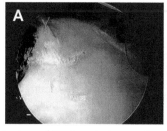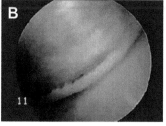

Fig. 7. (*A*) Arthroscopic view of the inverted pear glenoid as viewed from the anterosuperior portal. (*B*) Arthroscopic view of an engaging Hill-Sachs lesion.

formed by the inferior glenoid margin, the distance from the anterior and posterior rims to the bare spot should be identical. Through measuring the distance to the posterior rim and then to the defect edge anteriorly, one can accurately quantify the percent of glenoid bone loss.

Bone loss in shoulder instability is often not restricted to the glenoid. A potential finding at revision arthroscopy is the engaging Hill-Sachs lesion (see **Fig. 7**), which was defined by Burkhart and DeBeer[25] as a humeral head defect whose long axis is parallel to the anterior glenoid when the shoulder is in the functional position of abduction and external rotation. As this lesion engages the anterior cortex, it can cause the patient to experience symptoms similar to subluxation. This effective articular arc length mismatch has been reported to be a cause for failed instability repairs.[50]

Judicious attention to the soft tissues is as important as identification of bone defects. At revision arthroscopy, patients may be observed to have poor quality capsulolabral tissue or conversely capsular redundancy. Excessive capsular laxity was noted by Rowe and colleagues[41] in 83% of the patients undergoing revision shoulder stabilization. Other authors report the percentage as high as 86% to 91%.[39,51] Techniques should be used at primary surgery to optimize capsular tensioning and mobilization.

Unfortunately, asymmetric capsular repair and overtightening can also be a source of failure. This effect occurs by way of the *Erlenmeyer flask phenomena*, in which the patient tight anteriorly and superiorly but still has inferior instability from a neglected inferior glenohumeral ligament (IGHL) and inferior capsular pouch. In this situation, the patient will have restricted external rotation at the side clinically, but a positive sulcus sign. Levine and colleagues[39] noted these phenomena in 22% of their patients with recurrent instability at revision and suggested that an initial capsulorrhaphy should include an IGHL release to allow adequate reduction of the inferior capsular redundancy, thus potentially preventing failure of this mechanism.

Technical errors may also include failure of fixation from improper suture anchor insertion. Optimal position for suture anchors is at the margin of the articular surface along the anteroinferior glenoid rim to recreate the normal articular concavity.[43] Medialization of the repair through fixing the labral tissue proximal or medial to the glenoid margin results in the persistent loss of concavity and can lead to recurrent failure. This nonanatomic repair is found in 46% to 100% of failed instability procedures.[39,51–53]

SURGICAL TREATMENT

Open techniques have traditionally been the gold standard for treating recurrent traumatic anterior shoulder instability, with a postoperative recurrence rate of 2% to 17%.[5,54–58] Hobby and colleagues[59] recently published a meta-analysis on comparative studies of open versus arthroscopic repair for recurrent traumatic anterior instability and found the pooled failure rate of open repair to be 8.7%. They further analyzed arthroscopic studies using current arthroscopic techniques with suture anchor repair and capsular shift and noted a pooled recurrence rate of 8.9%, showing comparable results to open repair with modern arthroscopic techniques.

Although another meta-analysis by Lenters and colleagues[60] concluded that arthroscopic techniques were not as effective as open techniques in preventing recurrent instability (18% vs 8%), their analysis incorporated several outdated techniques and studies with lower levels of evidence. When they extrapolated just the data from level 1 studies using current arthroscopic techniques, they found no difference in recurrence between the techniques (5.7% open vs 7.9% arthroscopic).

Kim and colleagues[9] reported 95% good to excellent results in their case series of 167 patients with recurrent traumatic anterior instability of the shoulder treated with arthroscopic suture anchor repair and anteroinferior capsular shift, with 91% of patients returning to preinjury activity levels at a minimum 2-year follow-up. They noted a recurrence rate of 4%, which was related to an osseous defect of greater than 30% of the entire glenoid circumference. This study reiterates that identification and quantification of bone loss are essential to surgical planning of the optimal approach.

Outcome of revision surgery for instability is much less predictable. Levine and colleagues[39] reported a 17% failure rate after open revision stabilization in shoulders with one prior repair. This failure rate increased significantly to 44% in patients who had multiple prior surgeries, and the authors hypothesized that this was because of the presence of increased scar tissue, which was less effective at maintaining stability. Other investigators have found that the number of stabilizing attempts adversely affected outcome scores, motion, and patient satisfaction.[52]

ARTHROSCOPIC BANKART REVISION

In carefully selected patients, arthroscopic Bankart revision surgery can be a reliable procedure. Patients with good capsular tissues, minimal bone loss (<15%), and a deficiency of their primary repair from initial lack of recognition, nonanatomic repair, or recurrent trauma are good candidates for arthroscopic revision stabilization. Overhead, noncontact athletes are also good candidates, because open repair can lead to subscapularis muscle deficiency from the muscle needing to be detached during the procedure.[27]

Advantages of arthroscopic surgery include the ability to recognize and address the various soft-tissue pathologies encountered, minimization of iatrogenic damage to the tissues (especially the subscapularis tendon), decreased pain, and cosmesis.[61]

A limited body of quality evidence exists on the benefit of arthroscopic revision for failed shoulder instability. Most published studies are underpowered and represent heterogeneous patient populations. Kim and colleagues[53] reported on 23 patients with failed instability repairs (8 open with transosseous sutures or anchors, 15 arthroscopic with transglenoid or anchors) treated with arthroscopic Bankart repair with suture anchors, capsular placation, and capsular shift. They reported 83% good to excellent results, and 78% returned to greater than 90% of their preinjury activity level. Five patients (22%) experienced recurrent instability, and engagement in contact sports was found to be a significant risk factor. Published recurrence rates in other studies have ranged from 10% to 27%, with authors reporting greater than 73% good to excellent results after arthroscopic revision surgery.[61–66]

Patient selection and surgical technique are crucial in optimizing success of arthroscopic revision surgery for shoulder instability. Emphasis should be on not only anatomic suture anchor repair of the Bankart lesion but also adequate inferior and posterior–inferior capsular plication to eliminate the redundant inferior capsular pouch.[63]

Franceschi and colleagues[64] advised caution in patients with significant bone loss or shoulder hyperlaxity, and highlighted the importance of adequate mobilization of the often medialized labrum and proper decortication of the glenoid neck to encourage soft-tissue healing. In addition to suture anchor placement, the number of anchors seems to be important in revision surgery. Patel and colleagues[66] reported on 40 patients who underwent revision arthroscopic capsulolabral reconstruction and discovered that all their failures only had two anchors placed in the lower half of the glenoid. These findings are in concordance with the report by Boileau and colleagues[43] that the use of fewer than four suture anchors is a risk factor for anterior shoulder stabilization failure.

OPEN BANKART REVISION

Patient-specific factors and pathoanatomic factors should be taken into consideration when deciding on the surgical approach to revision anterior shoulder stabilization. Collision athletes and those with generalized hyperlaxity may be better candidates for open Bankart reconstruction.[45,46,64] Patients with bone loss greater than 15% should also be strongly considered for an open procedure. Another indication is poor capsulolabral tissue or capsular deficiency, such as may be seen in the setting of a prior thermal capsulorrhaphy. Patients with a HAGL are candidates for open surgery because access and repair of the lesion is often difficult arthroscopically. Patients who have exposed hardware or subscapularis deficiency should also undergo open stabilization procedures so that these associated issues can be adequately addressed.

As seen in arthroscopic revision surgery, the results of open revision shoulder stabilization are not as good as those for primary surgery. Levine and colleagues[39] found 78% good to excellent results in their group of 50 patients who underwent open revision surgery consisting of a Bankart repair and anteroinferior capsular shift. They discovered that although all of their traumatic revisions had excellent results, similar results were experienced by only 67% of the atraumatic instability patients. Risk factors for a poorer outcome included an atraumatic cause of failure, voluntary dislocations, and multiple prior stabilization attempts. These findings were further supported by Zabinski and colleagues[51] in their study of 43 patients who underwent revision shoulder stabilization for either traumatic or atraumatic causes. They noted good to excellent results in 78% of the patients with a traumatic cause, but in only 39% of those with an atraumatic cause. Sisto[67] reported 87% good to excellent results with no recurrences after revision open Bankart repair for failed arthroscopic stabilization after a traumatic event.

Recognition of bone defects and hyperlaxity is essential for a good outcome with open revision shoulder stabilization. A study by Cho and colleagues[68] of 26 shoulders that underwent open Bankart revision had 89% good to excellent results but an 11.5% recurrence of instability, which they associated with engaging Hill-Sachs lesions and shoulder hyperlaxity.

OSTEOARTICULAR PATHOLOGY

Surgeons should have a high index of suspicion for the presence of a glenoid bone defect in the recurrent dislocator. Although as many as 22% to 41% of acute dislocators have evidence of a glenoid defect, this value significantly rises to 73% to 86% in recurrent dislocators.[16,21,24,69] The amount of glenoid bone loss is important in determining the appropriate surgical approach in both initial and revision shoulder instability surgery. In the absence of bone loss, surgeons should account for other patient-specific factors when deciding on the most appropriate approach.

Relevant osteoarticular lesions can reduce stability and, according to the cadaveric study by Itoi and colleagues,[17] the limit on the glenoid is 21% of bony width. In the presence of less than 20% bone loss, good results can be obtained with soft-tissue arthroscopic capsulolabral stabilization.[33]

In the presence of osseous lesions 20% to 30% of glenoid width, Mologne and colleagues[70] published a 14% failure rate of arthroscopic Bankart repair, noting that all failures occurred in patients who had bony erosion where no bony fragment was identified. Improved results (92%–93% good to excellent) have been reported when a bony fragment was identified and could be incorporated into the repair, healing in a near-anatomic position.[71,72]

Bone replacement techniques should be considered when glenoid bone loss is greater than 25% to 30% of the width.[33,73] Various options and techniques have been described to treat glenoid deficiency.[24,33,73] The most popular and most often studied technique is the coracoid transfer, either a Bristow or a Latarjet, which involves the transfer of a portion of the coracoid to the anteroinferior glenoid defect.[74,75] Although the Bristow involves transferring just the coracoid tip, the Latarjet procedure transfers almost 3 cm of the coracoid to act as a substantial bone graft (**Fig. 8**).

In the Latarjet procedure, the coracoid is osteotomized with the conjoined tendon attached, leaving the coracoclavicular ligaments behind intact. The upper two thirds of the subscapularis are traditionally detached in an inverted L-shaped incision, allowing exposure of the anterior capsule. Because this approach has been reported to lead to subscapularis incompetence and a subsequent poor outcome in as many as 23% of patients, some surgeons now advocate a subscapularis split with two thirds superior and one third inferior.[27,76]

Maynou and colleagues[76] reported a significant decrease in muscle power of 42% for the L-shaped incision compared with only 8% for the subscapularis split. This finding correlated to a significant increase in fatty degeneration of the detached subscapularis muscle belly.

Accurate positioning of the coracoid on the glenoid rim is also essential to obtaining a good outcome. Lateralization can lead to early arthrosis of the joint and medialization can contribute to persistent instability. The coracoid graft is held with screw fixation and then the capsule is repaired. The capsular repair may either be directly to the glenoid, leaving the graft extra-articular, or it may be repaired to the coracoacromial ligament, making the graft intra-articular.

Burkhart and colleagues[77] published their results of Latarjet reconstruction for shoulder

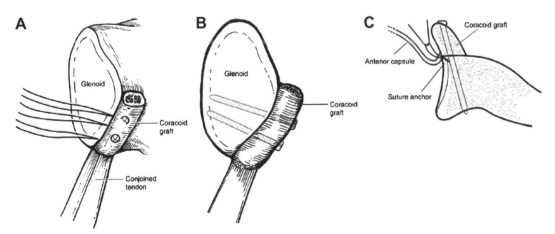

Fig. 8. (*A*) The coracoid graft is fixed to the glenoid with two bicortical screws. The raw bone surface where the pectoralis minor was removed will usually provide the best fit against the glenoid, and the graft can be further contoured with a power burr to fit the curve of the anteroinferior glenoid. (*B*) Note how the coracoid graft restores the pear shape of the glenoid by widening its inferior diameter. (*C*) The graft is placed so that it becomes an extra-articular platform that acts as an extension of the articular arc of the glenoid. (*Reproduced from* Burkhart SS, De Beer JF, Barth JR, et al. Results of modified Latarjet reconstruction in patients with anteroinferior instability and significant bone loss. Arthroscopy 2007;23(10):1033–41; with permission.)

instability in 102 patients with greater than a 25% loss of inferior glenoid bone width (inverted pear configuration) and reported a 4.9% recurrence rate. They concluded that Latarjet reconstruction can restore stability and function in more than 95% of patients with significant bone defects.

Glenoid reconstruction may also be accomplished with structural bone grafting. Warner and colleagues[78] reported excellent results on the use of intra-articular autogenous tricortical iliac crest bone graft in 11 patients with severe glenoid bone loss. No recurrences were seen at a mean follow-up of 33 months and all patients returned to preinjury activity levels. CT scans obtained 4 to 6 months postoperatively showed incorporation of the graft and maintenance of the joint space. Allogeneic bone grafting, using femoral head allograft, has also shown a high union rate and good stability in the management of large glenoid bone defects.[79]

Humeral head defects, or Hill-Sachs lesions, are identified in up to 100% of recurrent anterior dislocators.[21] They are often clinically asymptomatic if they are small (<20%) and treatment should be directed toward the restoration of soft-tissue integrity using Bankart repair.[24] Larger lesions, or those combined with anterior glenoid bone loss (engaging lesions), typically require treatment.[80]

Instability associated with engaging Hill-Sachs lesions can often be addressed with bony glenoid augmentation procedures by increasing the articular arc and thus preventing engagement of the humeral head defect.[77] In patients who have a Hill-Sachs defect that is greater than 30% of the articular surface and experience residual instability, bone grafting of the humeral defect with a structural allograft is an option. Miniaci and colleagues[81] reported good outcomes and no recurrences with this technique, using size-matched fresh-frozen humeral head or femoral head allografts in conjunction with anterior capsulolabral reconstruction. In older patients with posterolateral defects involving greater than 45% of the articular surface, arthroplasty should be considered, taking care to place the humeral component in 30° to 40° of retroversion to optimize stability.[24]

SUMMARY

The cause of failed treatment to correct anterior glenohumeral instability can usually be stratified as either a problem of patient selection, technical error, or recurrent trauma. A thorough clinical evaluation of the patient will help delineate the reason for failure and identify potential risk factors for recurrent instability after revision. Although arthroscopic stabilization procedures are often the preferred technique for addressing instability, surgeons should have a low threshold for considering an open approach in patients with significant bone defects or capsular insufficiency and those who participate in contact sports. Knowledge of the risk factors for failed instability surgery allows surgeons to appropriately counsel patients preoperatively and encourages more reasonable patient expectations.

REFERENCES

1. Romeo AA, Cohen BS, Carreira DS. Traumatic anterior shoulder instability. Orthop Clin North Am 2001; 32(3):399–409.
2. Arciero RA, Wheeler JH, Ryan JB, et al. Arthroscopic Bankart repair versus nonoperative treatment for acute, initial anterior shoulder dislocations. Am J Sports Med 1994;22(5):589–94.
3. Bottoni CR, Wilckens JH, DeBerardino TM, et al. A prospective, randomized evaluation of arthroscopic stabilization versus nonoperative treatment in patients with acute, traumatic, first-time shoulder dislocations. Am J Sports Med 2002;30(4):576–80.
4. Kirkley A, Werstine R, Ratjek A, et al. Prospective randomized clinical trial comparing the effectiveness of immediate arthroscopic stabilization versus immobilization and rehabilitation in first traumatic anterior dislocations of the shoulder: long-term evaluation. Arthroscopy 2005;21(1):55–63.
5. Tauber M, Resch H, Forstner R, et al. Reasons for failure after surgical repair of anterior shoulder instability. J Shoulder Elbow Surg 2004;13(3):279–85.
6. Law BK, Yung PS, Ho EP, et al. The surgical outcome of immediate arthroscopic Bankart repair for first time anterior shoulder dislocation in young active patients. Knee Surg Sports Traumatol Arthrosc 2008;16(2):188–93.
7. Valentin A, Winge S, Engstrom B. Early arthroscopic treatment of primary traumatic anterior shoulder dislocation. A follow-up study. Scand J Med Sci Sports 1998;8(6):405–10.
8. Carreira DS, Mazzocca AD, Oryhon J, et al. A prospective outcome evaluation of arthroscopic Bankart repairs: minimum 2-year follow-up. Am J Sports Med 2006;34(5):771–7.
9. Kim SH, Ha KI, Cho YB, et al. Arthroscopic anterior stabilization of the shoulder: two to six-year follow-up. J Bone Joint Surg Am 2003;85(8):1511–8.
10. Levine WN, Flatow EL. The pathophysiology of shoulder instability. Am J Sports Med 2000;28(6): 910–7.
11. Bigliani LU, Kelkar R, Flatow EL, et al. Glenohumeral stability. Biomechanical properties of passive and active stabilizers. Clin Orthop Relat Res 1996;330: 13–30.

12. Howell SM, Galinat BJ. The glenoid-labral socket. A constrained articular surface. Clin Orthop Relat Res 1989;243:122–5.

13. Bankart AS, Cantab MC. Recurrent or habitual dislocation of the shoulder-joint. 1923. Clin Orthop Relat Res 1993;291:3–6.

14. Urayama M, Itoi E, Sashi R, et al. Capsular elongation in shoulders with recurrent anterior dislocation. Quantitative assessment with magnetic resonance arthrography. Am J Sports Med 2003;31(1):64–7.

15. Sugaya H, Moriishi J, Dohi M, et al. Glenoid rim morphology in recurrent anterior glenohumeral instability. J Bone Joint Surg Am 2003;85(5):878–84.

16. Griffith JF, Antonio GE, Yung PS, et al. Prevalence, pattern, and spectrum of glenoid bone loss in anterior shoulder dislocation: CT analysis of 218 patients. AJR Am J Roentgenol 2008;190(5):1247–54.

17. Itoi E, Lee SB, Berglund LJ, et al. The effect of a glenoid defect on anteroinferior stability of the shoulder after Bankart repair: a cadaveric study. J Bone Joint Surg Am 2000;82(1):35–46.

18. Greis PE, Scuderi MG, Mohr A, et al. Glenohumeral articular contact areas and pressures following labral and osseous injury to the anteroinferior quadrant of the glenoid. J Shoulder Elbow Surg 2002;11(5): 442–51.

19. Buscayret F, Edwards TB, Szabo I, et al. Glenohumeral arthrosis in anterior instability before and after surgical treatment: incidence and contributing factors. Am J Sports Med 2004;32(5):1165–72.

20. Calandra JJ, Baker CL, Uribe J. The incidence of Hill-Sachs lesions in initial anterior shoulder dislocations. Arthroscopy 1989;5(4):254–7.

21. Taylor DC, Arciero RA. Pathologic changes associated with shoulder dislocations. Arthroscopic and physical examination findings in first-time, traumatic anterior dislocations. Am J Sports Med 1997;25(3): 306–11.

22. Rowe CR, Zarins B. Recurrent transient subluxation of the shoulder. J Bone Joint Surg Am 1981;63(6): 863–72.

23. Flatow EL, Warner JI. Instability of the shoulder: complex problems and failed repairs: Part I. Relevant biomechanics, multidirectional instability, and severe glenoid loss. Instr Course Lect 1998;47: 97–112.

24. Chen AL, Hunt SA, Hawkins RJ, et al. Management of bone loss associated with recurrent anterior glenohumeral instability. Am J Sports Med 2005;33(6): 912–25.

25. Burkhart SS, De Beer JF. Traumatic glenohumeral bone defects and their relationship to failure of arthroscopic Bankart repairs: significance of the inverted-pear glenoid and the humeral engaging Hill-Sachs lesion. Arthroscopy 2000;16(7):677–94.

26. Antonio GE, Griffith JF, Yu AB, et al. First-time shoulder dislocation: High prevalence of labral injury and age-related differences revealed by MR arthrography. J Magn Reson Imaging 2007;26(4): 983–91.

27. Sachs RA, Williams B, Stone ML, et al. Open Bankart repair: correlation of results with postoperative subscapularis function. Am J Sports Med 2005;33(10): 1458–62.

28. Beighton P, Horan F. Orthopaedic aspects of the Ehlers-Danlos syndrome. J Bone Joint Surg Br 1969;51(3):444–53.

29. Farber AJ, Castillo R, Clough M, et al. Clinical assessment of three common tests for traumatic anterior shoulder instability. J Bone Joint Surg Am 2006;88(7):1467–74.

30. Rokous JR, Feagin JA, Abbott HG. Modified axillary roentgenogram. A useful adjunct in the diagnosis of recurrent instability of the shoulder. Clin Orthop Relat Res 1972;82:84–6.

31. Itoi E, Lee SB, Amrami KK, et al. Quantitative assessment of classic anteroinferior bony Bankart lesions by radiography and computed tomography. Am J Sports Med 2003;31(1):112–8.

32. Pavlov H, Warren RF, Weiss CB Jr, et al. The roentgenographic evaluation of anterior shoulder instability. Clin Orthop Relat Res 1985;194:153–8.

33. Piasecki DP, Verma NN, Romeo AA, et al. Glenoid bone deficiency in recurrent anterior shoulder instability: diagnosis and management. J Am Acad Orthop Surg 2009;17(8):482–93.

34. Saito H, Itoi E, Sugaya H, et al. Location of the glenoid defect in shoulders with recurrent anterior dislocation. Am J Sports Med 2005;33(6):889–93.

35. Huysmans PE, Haen PS, Kidd M, et al. The shape of the inferior part of the glenoid: a cadaveric study. J Shoulder Elbow Surg 2006;15(6):759–63.

36. Gerber C, Nyffeler RW. Classification of glenohumeral joint instability. Clin Orthop Relat Res 2002; 400:65–76.

37. Probyn LJ, White LM, Salonen DC, et al. Recurrent symptoms after shoulder instability repair: direct MR arthrographic assessment–correlation with second-look surgical evaluation. Radiology 2007; 245(3):814–23.

38. Arciero RA, Spang JT. Complications in arthroscopic anterior shoulder stabilization: pearls and pitfalls. Instr Course Lect 2008;57:113–24.

39. Levine WN, Arroyo JS, Pollock RG, et al. Open revision stabilization surgery for recurrent anterior glenohumeral instability. Am J Sports Med 2000;28(2): 156–60.

40. Meehan RE, Petersen SA. Results and factors affecting outcome of revision surgery for shoulder instability. J Shoulder Elbow Surg 2005;14(1):31–7.

41. Rowe CR, Zarins B, Ciullo JV. Recurrent anterior dislocation of the shoulder after surgical repair. Apparent causes of failure and treatment. J Bone Joint Surg Am 1984;66(2):159–68.

42. Brophy RH, Marx RG. The treatment of traumatic anterior instability of the shoulder: nonoperative and surgical treatment. Arthroscopy 2009;25(3): 298–304.

43. Boileau P, Villalba M, Hery JY, et al. Risk factors for recurrence of shoulder instability after arthroscopic Bankart repair. J Bone Joint Surg Am 2006;88(8): 1755–63.

44. Balg F, Boileau P. The instability severity index score. A simple pre-operative score to select patients for arthroscopic or open shoulder stabilisation. J Bone Joint Surg Br 2007;89(11):1470–7.

45. Uhorchak JM, Arciero RA, Huggard D, et al. Recurrent shoulder instability after open reconstruction in athletes involved in collision and contact sports. Am J Sports Med 2000;28(6):794–9.

46. Pagnani MJ, Dome DC. Surgical treatment of traumatic anterior shoulder instability in American football players. J Bone Joint Surg Am 2002;84(5): 711–5.

47. Yiannakopoulos CK, Mataragas E, Antonogiannakis E. A comparison of the spectrum of intra-articular lesions in acute and chronic anterior shoulder instability. Arthroscopy 2007;23(9):985–90.

48. Lo IK, Parten PM, Burkhart SS. The inverted pear glenoid: an indicator of significant glenoid bone loss. Arthroscopy 2004;20(2):169–74.

49. Burkhart SS, Debeer JF, Tehrany AM, et al. Quantifying glenoid bone loss arthroscopically in shoulder instability. Arthroscopy 2002;18(5):488–91.

50. Burkhart SS, Danaceau SM. Articular arc length mismatch as a cause of failed Bankart repair. Arthroscopy 2000;16(7):740–4.

51. Zabinski SJ, Callaway GH, Cohen S, et al. Revision shoulder stabilization: 2- to 10-year results. J Shoulder Elbow Surg 1999;8(1):58–65.

52. Marquardt B, Garmann S, Schulte T, et al. Outcome after failed traumatic anterior shoulder instability repair with and without surgical revision. J Shoulder Elbow Surg 2007;16(6):742–7.

53. Kim SH, Ha KI, Kim YM. Arthroscopic revision Bankart repair: a prospective outcome study. Arthroscopy 2002;18(5):469–82.

54. Guanche CA, Quick DC, Sodergren KM, et al. Arthroscopic versus open reconstruction of the shoulder in patients with isolated Bankart lesions. Am J Sports Med 1996;24(2):144–8.

55. Karlsson J, Magnusson L, Ejerhed L, et al. Comparison of open and arthroscopic stabilization for recurrent shoulder dislocation in patients with a Bankart lesion. Am J Sports Med 2001;29(5):538–42.

56. Magnusson L, Kartus J, Ejerhed L, et al. Revisiting the open Bankart experience: a four- to nine-year follow-up. Am J Sports Med 2002;30(6):778–82.

57. Sperber A, Hamberg P, Karlsson J, et al. Comparison of an arthroscopic and an open procedure for post-traumatic instability of the shoulder: a prospective,

randomized multicenter study. J Shoulder Elbow Surg 2001;10(2):105–8.

58. Steinbeck J, Jerosch J. Arthroscopic transglenoid stabilization versus open anchor suturing in traumatic anterior instability of the shoulder. Am J Sports Med 1998;26(3):373–8.

59. Hobby J, Griffin D, Dunbar M, et al. Is arthroscopic surgery for stabilisation of chronic shoulder instability as effective as open surgery? A systematic review and meta-analysis of 62 studies including 3044 arthroscopic operations. J Bone Joint Surg Br 2007;89(9):1188–96.

60. Lenters TR, Franta AK, Wolf FM, et al. Arthroscopic compared with open repairs for recurrent anterior shoulder instability. A systematic review and meta-analysis of the literature. J Bone Joint Surg Am 2007;89(2):244–54.

61. Boileau P, Richou J, Lisai A, et al. The role of arthroscopy in revision of failed open anterior stabilization of the shoulder. Arthroscopy 2009;25(10):1075–84.

62. Barnes CJ, Getelman MH, Snyder SJ. Results of arthroscopic revision anterior shoulder reconstruction. Am J Sports Med 2009;37(4):715–9.

63. Creighton RA, Romeo AA, Brown FM Jr, et al. Revision arthroscopic shoulder instability repair. Arthroscopy 2007;23(7):703–9.

64. Franceschi F, Longo UG, Ruzzini L, et al. Arthroscopic salvage of failed arthroscopic Bankart repair: a prospective study with a minimum follow-up of 4 years. Am J Sports Med 2008;36(7):1330–6.

65. Neri BR, Tuckman DV, Bravman JT, et al. Arthroscopic revision of Bankart repair. J Shoulder Elbow Surg 2007;16(4):419–24.

66. Patel RV, Apostle K, Leith JM, et al. Revision arthroscopic capsulolabral reconstruction for recurrent instability of the shoulder. J Bone Joint Surg Br 2008;90(11):1462–7.

67. Sisto DJ. Revision of failed arthroscopic Bankart repairs. Am J Sports Med 2007;35(4):537–41.

68. Cho NS, Yi JW, Lee BG, et al. Revision open Bankart surgery after arthroscopic repair for traumatic anterior shoulder instability. Am J Sports Med 2009; 37(11):2158–64.

69. Rowe CR, Patel D, Southmayd WW. The Bankart procedure: a long-term end-result study. J Bone Joint Surg Am 1978;60(1):1–16.

70. Mologne TS, Provencher MT, Menzel KA, et al. Arthroscopic stabilization in patients with an inverted pear glenoid: results in patients with bone loss of the anterior glenoid. Am J Sports Med 2007;35(8):1276–83.

71. Sugaya H, Moriishi J, Kanisawa I, et al. Arthroscopic osseous Bankart repair for chronic recurrent traumatic anterior glenohumeral instability. J Bone Joint Surg Am 2005;87(8):1752–60.

72. Porcellini G, Campi F, Paladini P. Arthroscopic approach to acute bony Bankart lesion. Arthroscopy 2002;18(7):764–9.

73. Lynch JR, Clinton JM, Dewing CB, et al. Treatment of osseous defects associated with anterior shoulder instability. J Shoulder Elbow Surg 2009;18(2):317–28.

74. Allain J, Goutallier D, Glorion C. Long-term results of the Latarjet procedure for the treatment of anterior instability of the shoulder. J Bone Joint Surg Am 1998;80(6):841–52.

75. Helfet AJ. Coracoid transplantation for recurring dislocation of the shoulder. J Bone Joint Surg Br 1958;40(2):198–202.

76. Maynou C, Cassagnaud X, Mestdagh H. Function of subscapularis after surgical treatment for recurrent instability of the shoulder using a bone-block procedure. J Bone Joint Surg Br 2005;87(8):1096–101.

77. Burkhart SS, De Beer JF, Barth JR, et al. Results of modified Latarjet reconstruction in patients with anteroinferior instability and significant bone loss. Arthroscopy 2007;23(10):1033–41.

78. Warner JJ, Gill TJ, O'Hollerhan JD, et al. Anatomical glenoid reconstruction for recurrent anterior glenohumeral instability with glenoid deficiency using an autogenous tricortical iliac crest bone graft. Am J Sports Med 2006;34(2):205–12.

79. Weng PW, Shen HC, Lee HH, et al. Open reconstruction of large bony glenoid erosion with allogeneic bone graft for recurrent anterior shoulder dislocation. Am J Sports Med 2009;37(9):1792–7.

80. Millett PJ, Clavert P, Warner JJ. Open operative treatment for anterior shoulder instability: when and why? J Bone Joint Surg Am 2005;87(2):419–32.

81. Miniaci A, Hand C, Berlet G. Segmental humeral head allografts for recurrent anterior instability of the shoulder with large Hill-Sachs defects: a two to eight year follow-up. Presented at the 20th Annual Closed Meeting of the American Shoulder and Elbow Surgeons. Dana Point (CA), October 8–11, 2003.

Arthroscopic Bankart-Bristow-Latarjet (2B3) Procedure: How to Do It and Tricks To Make it Easier and Safe

Pascal Boileau, MD[a],*, Numa Mercier, MD[a],
Jason Old, MD, FRCSC[b,c]

KEYWORDS

- Shoulder • Instability • Arthroscopy • Stabilization
- Latarjet • Bristow

Technical advancements in arthroscopic shoulder surgery in the last 2 decades have dramatically altered the treatment of anterior shoulder instability. Arthroscopic labral repair, once considered an ineffective and impractical procedure is now considered routine and reliable, and in most situations is the treatment of choice for recurrent anterior shoulder instability.

Although the results of arthroscopic anterior labral repair using modern techniques have been shown to approach the success rates of open anterior stabilizations in most patients,[1–3] it has been recognized that it is much less effective in patients with risk factors for failure such as young age, hyperlaxity, competitive contact sport participation, and particularly severe glenoid or humeral bone loss.[4–7] In such patients coracoid transfer procedures have been shown to be more effective.[8]

This recognition combined with the trend toward minimally invasive shoulder surgery and incremental improvements in technology and technique have led some surgeons to push the boundaries of arthroscopic treatment even farther, developing techniques to treat severe instability with associated bone loss using arthroscopic coracoid transfer.[9–11] This approach may seem fanciful and impractical to many surgeons today, just as arthroscopic labral repair did 20 years ago. However, it is our belief that the rationale for the procedure is sound and that it provides certain advantages over the traditional open coracoid transfer procedures. Once certain technical challenges are overcome the authors believe that it will become a reliable and commonly performed procedure.

BACKGROUND

The open Bristow-Latarjet coracoid transfer, proposed as an alternative to capsulolabral repair in patients with significant glenoid bone loss, has been shown to be a reliable technique with a very low rate of recurrent instability, a high rate of return to sports at the preinjury level and a high rate of patient satisfaction.[8,12–18] However, placement of the transferred coracoid graft may be difficult because of the limited exposure, especially in young muscular athletes. Improper surgical placement of the coracoid bone block

Disclosure: Specific ancillary instruments have been developed in conjunction with Smith & Nephew, Andover, Massachusetts, USA.
[a] Department of Orthopaedic Surgery & Sports Traumatology, Hôpital de L'Archet 2, University of Nice-Sophia-Antipolis, 151 route de St Antoine de Ginestière, Nice, France 06202
[b] Section of Orthopaedic Surgery, University of Manitoba, Canada
[c] Pan Am Clinic, 75 Poseidon Bay, Winnipeg, Manitoba, Canada R3M 3E4
* Corresponding author.
E-mail address: boileau.p@chu-nice.fr

Orthop Clin N Am 41 (2010) 381–392
doi:10.1016/j.ocl.2010.03.005

and screw failures are common complications, which have been reported in up to 50% of patients, and may compromise the results of the procedure.[19,20] A coracoid bone block placed too medial or too high (over the glenoid equator) has been found to be associated with recurrent shoulder instability; late glenohumeral osteoarthritis may result from lateral placement of the bone block.[18,21,22]

In recent years the concept of performing the Bristow-Latarjet transfer procedure under arthroscopy has emerged. Our experience with an arthroscopic modified Bristow procedure started 10 years ago with the Bristow-Trillat procedure, which consists of an arthroscopic Bankart repair combined with a transfer of the tip of the coracoid process to a socket drilled in the glenoid neck over the subscapularis.[9] The authors have reported the results of this procedure, which supplements the Bankart repair with the sling effect of the conjoined tendon and allows stabilization of shoulders in hyperlax patients.[23–25] However, in patients with glenoid bone loss, the bone block effect is also needed, which means that the coracoid tip must be passed through the subscapularis muscle and fixed on the glenoid neck. Such a procedure is technically more difficult to perform arthroscopically.

Lafosse and colleagues[10] have recently proposed an arthroscopic technique similar to the original technique described by Latarjet in 1954. In this technique, the labrum and capsule are resected and the bone block is therefore positioned inside the glenohumeral joint. We have developed an all-arthroscopic approach that is different in at least 2 respects: (1) we do not resect the labrum and capsule but, instead repair them with suture and anchors; and (2) we place the bone block in the standing position outside the glenohumeral joint.[11]

The goal of our all-arthroscopic technique is to provide a nearly anatomic reconstruction of the glenohumeral joint by treating the soft tissue and the bony lesions, as well as to reinforce the weak anteroinferior capsule with the help of a musculotendinous sling. Our technique, which combines a Bristow-Latarjet coracoid transfer procedure with a Bankart repair, has been developed on cadaveric specimens by the senior author after 20 years of experience with the open technique. It provides a so-called triple-blocking effect (**Fig. 1**): (1) the labral repair recreates the anterior bumper and protects the humeral head from direct contact with the coracoid bone graft (bumper effect); (2) the transferred standing coracoid bone block compensates for anterior glenoid bone loss and conforms to the glenoid concavity (bony effect); and (3) the transferred

conjoined tendon creates a dynamic reinforcement of the inferior part of the capsule, by itself and by lowering the inferior part of the subscapularis, particularly when the arm is abducted and externally rotated (belt or sling effect). Our hope is that, by doing so, we can avoid some of the common complications reported with the standard Bristow-Latarjet procedure, such as residual instability (apprehension or subluxations), persistent shoulder pain, or glenohumeral osteoarthritis.[21,26–28]

SURGICAL TECHNIQUE

The patient is placed in the semi-beachchair position with the trunk elevated 30°. The arm is placed parallel to the floor in a support (Spider limb positioner, Tenet Medical, Canada) without traction.

In addition to the standard posterior portal, 5 anterior portals are used. Their locations are carefully marked on the skin (**Fig. 2**A). The central portal is located just lateral to the tip of the coracoid; the proximal portal (or north portal) is located above the coracoid process, just in front of the acromioclavicular joint; the distal portal (or south portal) is located in the axillary fold, 3 finger widths distal to the tip of the coracoid; the lateral portal (or west portal) is located 2 finger widths lateral to the tip of the coracoid; and the medial portal (or east portal) is located 3 to 4 finger widths medial to the tip of the coracoid, passing obliquely through the pectoralis major muscle (see **Fig. 2**B). Before starting, the soft tissues (skin, fat, and deltoid fascia) are elevated from the coracoid process and conjoined tendon by injecting 10 mL of xylocaine with adrenaline.

The surgical technique is comprised of 5 operative steps, all performed arthroscopically.

Step One: Glenoid Preparation and Drilling

With the arthroscope in the posterior portal, the rotator interval is opened using a radiofrequency device (VAPR, Depuy-Mitek, USA), and the coracoid process and conjoined tendon are identified. The anterior labrum is completely detached until the red fibers of the subscapularis muscle are clearly seen. A traction suture is passed through the labrum and used at the time of the Bankart repair to manipulate and shift it proximally. The anterior glenoid rim is debrided from 2 to 6 o'clock with a shaver and a burr. The scope is switched to the anterior central portal. A specific guide (glenoid guide, Smith & Nephew, USA), introduced through the posterior portal, is used to insert a guide pin through the glenoid neck from posterior to anterior. The glenoid guide is angled 15° from medial to lateral and has a stop at the distal end to prevent over-penetration of the guide pin (**Fig. 3**A). The guide pin is made of

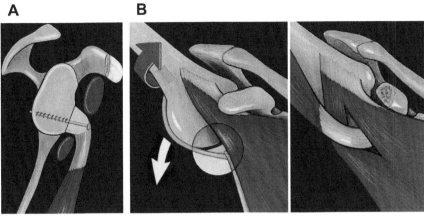

Fig. 1. (*A*) Principle of the Bristow-Latarjet procedure : the tip of the coracoid with the conjoint tendon is oste-tomized, passed through the subscapularis muscle, and fixed with a screw on the anterior neck of the scapula. (*B*) In the throwing (at risk) position, the conjoint tendon and the inferior part of the subscapularis, which is lowered, act as a dynamic sling, pushing the humeral head backward.

2 parts: a female part (2.8 mm in diameter) and a male part (1.5 mm in diameter). The guide pin should penetrate the glenoid neck anteriorly below the equator (at 5 o'clock) and 3 mm medial to the gle-noid surface (see **Fig. 3B**). The drilling depth is measured using the glenoid guide. Before leaving the glenohumeral joint a blunt switching stick is introduced through the posterior portal and pushed through the subscapularis muscle (under the labrum) to act as a landmark for the subscapularis split that will be performed later.

Step 2: Coracoid Harvesting

The scope is then placed in the anterior subdeltoid space through the lateral (west) portal and the coracoid process and subcapularis are identified, still using the VAPR. The distal (south) portal and medial (east) portal are created, using an outside-in technique with a blunt trochar directed to the tip of the coracoid process. When creating the east portal, care should be taken to keep the instruments superficial to the conjoined tendon to avoid injury to the brachial plexus and axillary vessels. The coracoacromial ligament is released from the lateral side of the coracoid and the pec-toralis minor insertion is released from its medial side. Because the brachial plexus lies just behind the pectoralis minor, the VAPR device is kept strictly in contact with the medial side of the cora-coid. The pectoralis minor and conjoined tendon are confluent at this level and should be separated with the VAPR, but only over a limited distance of 10 to 15 mm to prevent injury to the musculocuta-neous nerve and preserve the vascular pedicle of the coracoid graft.

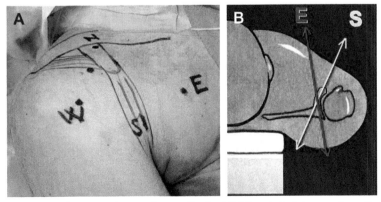

Fig. 2. (*A*) Five anterior portals are used to perform a Bankart-Bristow-Latarjet procedure; their locations were carefully marked on the skin: central, proximal (north), distal (south), lateral (west) and medial (east), the Cora-coid Compass. (*B*) The coracoid process, downward and laterally oriented, is accessible from the south portal (S), whereas screwing of the bone block parallel to the glenoid surface is only possible from the east (E) portal.

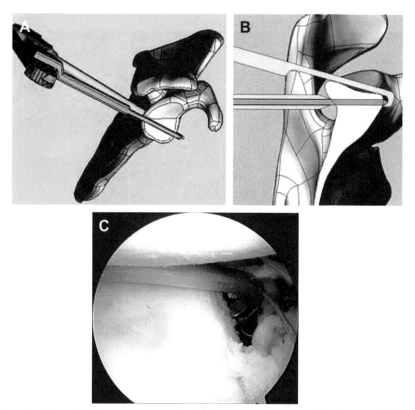

Fig. 3. (*A, B*) The glenoid guide allows accurate and safe placement of the cannulated screw. (*C*) With the scope in the anterior portal, the glenoid bone loss is evaluated and the glenoid guide is positioned below the equator.

Using a specific guide (coracoid guide, Smith & Nephew, USA), introduced through the distal (south) portal, a guide pin is inserted along the axis of the coracoid process (**Fig. 4**A). The coracoid is drilled along its axis using a cannulated drill. A 3.5-mm cannulated screw is then inserted centrally in the coracoid to a depth of 15 mm (see

Fig. 4B). The length of the screw that is selected is determined by adding the length of the coracoid graft to the glenoid drilling depth previously measured, and adding 2 mm to ensure that the posterior cortex is engaged.

The proximal (north) portal is then created just anterior to the acromioclavicular joint using a spinal

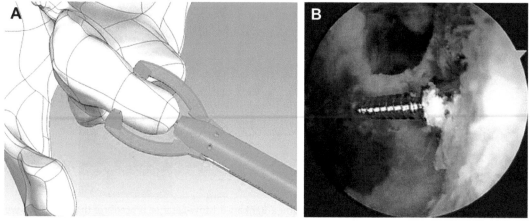

Fig. 4. (*A*) The coracoid guide allows accurate and safe placement of the guide wire and cannulated screw along the central axis of the coracoid. (*B*) After partial osteotomy of the coracoid process, the guide wire and cannulated screw are placed using the coracoid guide.

needle to ensure it is strictly perpendicular to the coracoid process. The coracoid is held using a grasper introduced through the central portal. Starting on its superior surface, the coracoid is osteotomized 15 mm from the tip using a zip burr or a saw via the proximal (north) portal. When half of the osteotomy is completed, the central location of the guide pin and screw is confirmed. The guide pin is then retrieved but the screwdriver is left in place. A metallic suture-passing wire is introduced through the screwdriver, screw, and bone block and retrieved through the medial (east) portal. The coracoid osteotomy is then completed in an oblique fashion, leaving more bone superiorly than inferiorly so that the cancellous surface of the bone block has an oblique shape matching the anterior glenoid neck.

Still holding the coracoid with the coracoid grasper, the screw is pushed further through the bone block. The screwdriver is disengaged from the screw and the other end of the suture-passing wire is retrieved with a grasper, also through the medial (East) portal. By pulling on both strands of the metallic wire from the medial (east) portal the bone block is flipped and medialized, thus giving free access to the subscapularis muscle belly.

Step 3: Axillary Nerve Identification and Subscapularis Splitting

At this stage of the procedure, the arm is placed in flexion and slight internal rotation to identify the axillary nerve. Using a blunt trocar, the nerve is located as it passes under the inferior rim of the subscapularis (**Fig. 5**A). The arm is then placed in neutral rotation to provide better access to the muscular part of the subscapularis. The bursa and fascia are removed from the anterior surface of the subscapularis muscle. Once the superior border of the subscapularis and its inferior border with the anterior axillary vessels (the 3 sisters) are identified, the switching stick is pushed fully through the subscapularis muscle. Using the VAPR via the medial (east) portal, the subscapularis muscle belly is then split in line with its fibers at the superior two-thirds and inferior one-third junction (at the level of the switching stick). The VAPR is moved from medial to lateral, away from the axillary nerve, which remains under constant visual control medially (see **Fig. 5**B). Hemostasis is carefully maintained as division of the muscle is slowly carried down to the glenoid neck.

A small U-shaped retractor is inserted in the subscapularis split via the proximal (north) portal and used to retract the upper part of the subscapularis superiorly. A second retractor is introduced through the distal (south) portal and placed under the neck of the scapula between the capsule and the subscapularis to retract the lower part of the muscle inferiorly (**Fig. 6**A). The lower part of the glenoid neck is exposed and the previously inserted glenoid guide wire is identified. To improve visualization of the anterior neck, the arthroscope can be then transferred to the distal (south) portal (together with the inferior retractor). Correct positioning of the pin is confirmed: below the equator and 3 mm medial to the glenoid surface. Decortication of the glenoid neck is completed using a burr, and a 2-mm deep socket created to receive and stabilize the bone block.

Step 4: Coracoid Transfer and Fixation

A swivel tip screwdriver is introduced via the medial (east) portal along 1 strand of the metallic wire (the one without the loop) and engaged in the previously

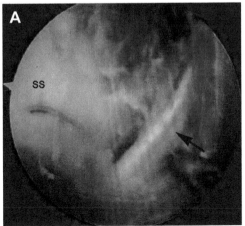
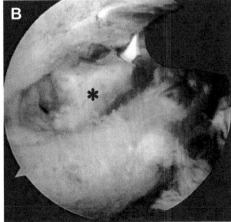

Fig. 5. (A) Identification of the axillary nerve as it passes beneath the inferior border of the subscapularis. (B) The subscapularis split is made, taking care to stay lateral to the axillary nerve.

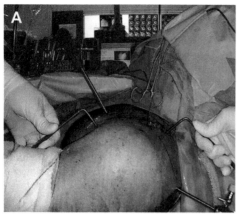
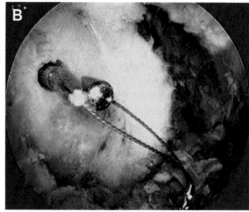

Fig. 6. (*A*) Retractors are placed via the north and south portals to keep the subscapularis split open and expose the anterior glenoid neck. The screwdriver is passed over the suture-passing wire via the medial (east) portal. (*B*) The suture retriever is introduced from posterior to anterior in the female guide wire to catch the loop of the suture-passing wire.

placed screw. A suture is placed trough the metallic loop and a knot pusher is introduced via the medial (east) portal over the suture to bring the wire's loop inside the shoulder. By pulling on the end of the metallic wire, the loop is brought to the tip of the screw. The screwdriver and the knot pusher are used to guide the bone block and wire's loop toward the glenoid neck. A hooked suture retriever (Captain Hook, Smith & Nephew, USA) is passed from posterior to anterior through the female guide pin and used to catch the loop and retrieve the metallic wire posteriorly (see **Fig. 6**B). Once the loop is caught by the hook, the knot pusher and suture are removed. By pulling on the Captain Hook, the nitinol wire is brought to the posterior aspect of the shoulder. Once the wire is retrieved posteriorly the female guide pin is removed using a pin puller. Two Kocher forceps are then clipped on each end of the nitinol wire (flush to the handle of the screwdriver anteriorly and flush to the skin posteriorly) to prevent disengagement of the screwdriver from the screw. With the subscapularis split maintained open with retractors and switching stick, the bone block and screw are guided into place on the glenoid neck by applying gentle traction on the suture-passing wire posteriorly and using the screwdriver as a joystick anteriorly. The switching stick can also be used as a lever to lift up the upper two-thirds of the subscapularis.

The screw is advanced through the bone block and into the hole in the glenoid neck guided by the metallic wire (**Fig. 7**A). After engaging the screw to a depth of approximately 10 mm, the scope is reintroduced into the glenohumeral joint through the posterior portal (using the switching stick) to obtain an intra-articular view. Pulling on the traction suture helps to lift up the labrum and

capsule to visualize the bone block from inside the joint. A grasper or spatula is introduced through the anterior central portal and used to rotate the coracoid graft 90° so that its concave surface conforms to the natural convexity of the glenoid. Compression of the bone block is controlled by direct visualization and any soft tissue interposed between the bone block and the glenoid neck is removed. Accurate initial positioning of the guide wire allows the bone block to be positioned flush to the glenoid surface and below the equator (see **Fig. 7**B).

Step 5: Capsulolabral (ie, Bankart) Repair

Still with the scope in the posterior portal, a classic arthroscopic Bankart repair is performed using 2 to 3 suture anchors (Lupine anchors or Knotless anchors, Depuy-Mitek, USA). The anchors are placed on the glenoid rim at 5, 4 and 3 (or 2) o'clock, which allows retensioning of the capsulo-ligamentous structures and recreation of the bumper effect of the labrum. The scope is reintroduced through the anterolateral (west) portal to observe the sling effect of the conjoined tendon passing through the subscapularis muscle. Range of motion is checked to ensure that complete mobility is maintained. The coracoid with the attached conjoined tendon maintains the subscapularis split open and no attempt is made to close the split because this would limit rotation. Postoperative radiographs are taken to confirm the correct positioning of the bone block (**Fig. 8**A–C).

POSTOPERATIVE CARE

The patient is discharged from the hospital on the second postoperative day. A sling is worn during

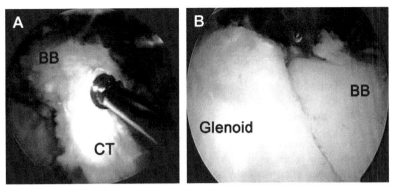

Fig. 7. (*A*) The coracoid bone block (BB) with attached conjoint tendon (CT) is transferred to the anterior glenoid neck and fixed with a 3.5-mm cannulated screw in the standing position. (*B*) Rotation and compression of the bone block are controlled with the scope introduced inside the glenohumeral joint through the posterior portal.

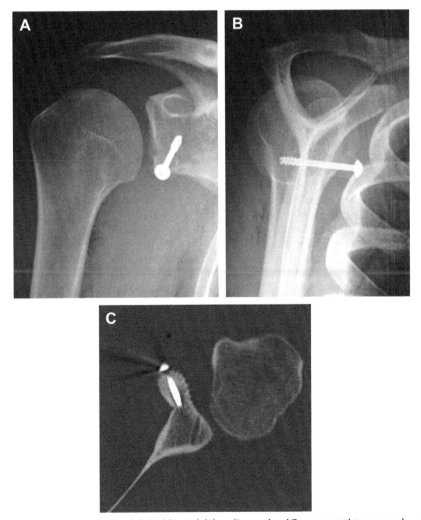

Fig. 8. Postoperative anterioposterior (*A*) and lateral (*B*) radiographs. (*C*) computed tomography scan confirms optimal positioning of the bone block below the equator and flush to the glenoid surface, restoring the concavity of the glenoid.

the first 3 to 4 weeks. Self-directed rehabilitation with pendulum exercises is started immediately (5 times a day, 5 minutes each session). The patient is encouraged to use their hand immediately for activities of daily living like eating, drinking, holding a newspaper or a book to read, typewriting, dressing, and so forth... After 4 weeks, formal rehabilitation with a physiotherapist is started and swimming pool therapy is recommended. No heavy lifting is allowed until 12 weeks to ensure that solid bony union is obtained. After 3 to 6 months, return to all types of sports activities is allowed, including collision and contact-overhead sports.

DISCUSSION

The authors propose a novel arthroscopic technique, combining a Bristow-Latarjet procedure with a Bankart repair, which can be an alternative in cases of recurrent anterior instability with glenohumeral bone deficiency and/or poor capsule. The combined arthroscopic procedure results in a "best of both worlds" stabilization, combining the Bankart repair's effect of retensioning the capsulolabral complex and recreating the labral bumper with the Bristow-Latarjet's effect of creating a dynamic musculotendinous sling and restoring the glenoid width and depth. In contrast to some other coracoid transfer procedures, the bone block remains extra-articular, mitigating the potential for poststabilization arthritis. The position of the bone block is also visualized intra-articularly, which helps to avoid the possibility of bone block malposition. But with these advantages come significant technical challenges and the potential for neurovascular injury, begging the question; can the theoretic advantages of the procedure be realized safely, reliably and efficiently?

To address these questions the authors undertook a prospective study using the described technique in 47 consecutive patients. The procedure was performed entirely arthroscopically in 41 of 47 patients (88%); conversion to open surgery was needed in 6 (12%). The conversions to open surgery occurred early in the series and were related to difficulties in passing the bone block through the subscapularis and/or fixing it to the glenoid neck. The axillary nerve and brachial plexus were identified in all cases and no nerve injuries were observed. The bone block was optimally positioned in at least 44 of 47 patients (94%). No dislocations have been observed in this series to date, however the average follow-up is only 14 months (6–28 months).[29] Although it is still too early to assess the clinical results of the procedure, these preliminary results

demonstrate that the procedure can be done safely and reliably with consistently accurate positioning of the bone block.

In developing this procedure, we have identified several key steps and concepts that the surgeon should keep foremost in mind to ensure the safety of the patient and to allow the procedure to be performed more easily:

Patient Positioning

Because much of the procedure is performed extra-articularly in the anterior subdeltoid space, we recommend performing the procedure in the beachchair position with the patient's trunk elevated 30° and the arm placed parallel with the floor on a support. This position opens the subdeltoid space by taking tension off the anterior deltoid and allowing the humeral head to sag posteriorly with the force of gravity.

Portal Placement

As with any arthroscopic procedure accurate portal placement is essential to the efficiency and safety of the procedure. Five separate anterior portals are used in this procedure and it is important to recognize that each has a specific role.

The central portal is a standard anterior portal located just lateral to the coracoid tip (see **Fig. 2**A). This portal is used to visualize the glenohumeral joint and ensure correct placement of the glenoid guide, and later to confirm correct bone block position and orientation. It is also used as a working portal for labral repair after the bone block has been fixed in place. The portal is created using a spinal needle to establish the correct orientation to allow anchor placement on the glenoid rim for labral repair.

The west portal is an anterolateral portal that is used as a viewing portal in the anterior subdeltoid space during coracoid harvest, transfer, and fixation. It is placed 2 finger widths lateral to the coracoid tip, and is established using the blunt trochar (see **Fig. 2**A). The working space in this part of the procedure is the anterior subdeltoid space, so care should be taken to keep the trochar in close contact with the humerus and to avoid violating the deep deltoid fascia, which may result in bleeding and excessive soft tissue swelling.

The north portal is an anterosuperior portal located just anterior to the clavicle (see **Fig. 2**A). The portal is used to osteotomize the coracoid process, and thus it is designed to be directly superior to it. The portal is established outside-in with a spinal needle used to ensure correct orientation for the osteotomy. The portal is subsequently used to place the superior retractor to open the subscapularis split.

The south portal is an anteroinferior portal placed in the axillary fold 3 finger widths inferior to the coracoid tip (see **Fig. 2**A). It is used as a working portal to expose the coracoid, and subsequently to drill and insert the screw in the coracoid. The trajectory of the portal must allow for insertion of the screw in the long axis of the coracoid, and a spinal needle is used to plan it.

The east portal is located 3 to 4 finger widths medial to the coracoid process and passes obliquely through the pectoralis major to arrive at the tip of the coracoid process (see **Fig. 2**A, B). The east portal is used initially as a working portal to expose the coracoid and later to retract the osteotomized coracoid bone block medially, however its principal function is to insert the screw that fixes the bone block to the glenoid, and it is this function that necessitates placing it medial to the coracoid process. If the portal is made more laterally its trajectory will not allow fixation of the bone block flush with the articular surface and will lead to an overhanging position (**Fig. 9**). To determine whether the east portal is safe, we measured the distance between nearby neurovascular structures and a 6-mm rod placed along the portal trajectory in 6 fresh frozen cadaveric shoulders. We found that as long as the trajectory was kept anterior to the conjoined tendon all neurovascular structures are at least 1 cm away.[30]

Bone Block Harvest

Great care must be taken to avoid damaging the brachial plexus when exposing the coracoid. It is essential to keep the dissection directly on the bone, particularly when elevating the pectoralis minor insertion from the medial side. Once the bone block is retracted medially using the wire, the brachial plexus is uncovered and no longer protected by the conjoined tendon.

The position of the screw in the bone block is critical to ensure adequate fixation while avoiding fracture. Early in our series we used a freehand technique to place the screw in the bone block and we experienced some early failures of fixation (5/47, 11%) including 1 case of bone block fracture (**Fig. 10**A, B).[29] We subsequently developed the coracoid guide, which has greatly improved the accuracy of screw placement (see **Fig. 3**A). Because it is difficult to control the bone block after it has been osteotomized, we recommend placing the screw before the osteotomy is completed (see **Fig. 3**B). We use a cannulated screw because it allows us to pass a wire through the screw, making manipulation and reduction of the bone block easier after the osteotomy is completed.

To ensure stable fixation, we believe that the bone block should be no longer than 12 to 15 mm. The attached conjoined tendon puts tension on the bone block, and it is our belief that the lever arm acting on the single cannulated screw used for fixation may be too great if the graft is any longer than this.

Another important surgical detail is shaping the base of the coracoid to conform to the slope of the worn anterior glenoid rim, because it increases the surface area and contributes to the stability of the construct. Because the coracoid is rotated 90° at the time of fixation, this means that the coracoid osteotomy must be done in an oblique fashion, resecting more bone superiorly than inferiorly.

Subscapularis Split

Splitting of the subscapularis must be performed at the correct level to adequately expose the glenoid neck and allow unhindered passage of the bone block. The switching stick is used from within the joint to establish the correct level for the split. The axillary nerve must be identified before commencing the split, and the instruments should always be working away from the nerve to prevent inadvertent injury (see **Fig. 5**A, B).

Bone Block Positioning and Fixation

Accurate bone block placement is the key to performing an effective Bristow-Latarjet procedure

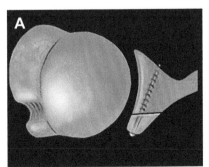
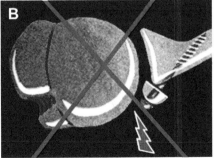

Fig. 9. (*A*) The correct screw trajectory leads to positioning of the bone block flush to the glenoid articular surface. (*B*) Screw trajectory directed too far medially results in an overhanging bone block.

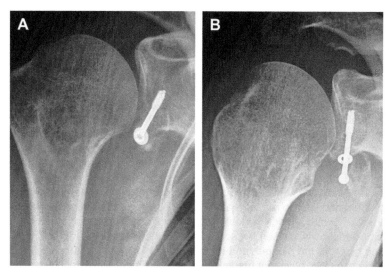

Fig. 10. (*A*) Early postoperative radiograph shows a bone block fixed with a screw placed eccentrically. (*B*) Radiograph at 3 months demonstrates failure of fixation as a result of bone block fracture.

that restores shoulder stability and avoids the complication of late arthrosis. For the bone block to positively influence glenohumeral joint stability it must reconstitute the size and shape of the glenoid articular surface. The bone block should be (1) below the equator, (2) as flush as possible to the articular surface, and (3) should conform to the natural convexity of the glenoid surface without overhanging excessively (see **Fig. 9**).

Positioning the block correctly depends on the distance from the screw's entry point to the articular surface and the axis of the screw's trajectory. The glenoid drill guide is designed to place the drill

hole 3 mm medial to the articular surface. The guide is angled 15° from medial to lateral to recreate the normal convexity of the glenoid surface without overhanging (see **Fig. 3**A–C). Blunt dissection is used to place the guide on the posterior glenoid neck to avoid injury to the suprascapular nerve. The guide should be positioned below the equator of the glenoid, reconstituting the deficient bone in the anteroinferior quadrant.

Drilling the screw hole is a potentially dangerous step, as the correct trajectory for the drill places the brachial plexus and associated vessels at risk anterior to the glenoid neck. A cadaveric study

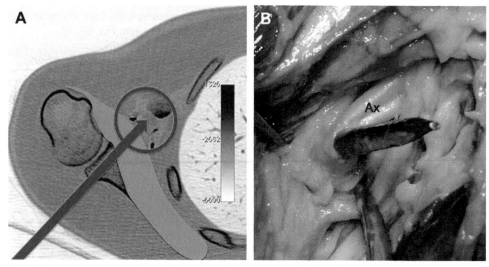

Fig. 11. (*A*) The correct screw trajectory intercepts the neurovascular bundle anterior to the glenoid. (*B*) Image from a cadaveric study shows the axillary artery (Ax) impaled by a 5-mm Steinmann pin that was advanced from posterior to anterior along this trajectory.

demonstrated that the correct trajectory for placing the glenoid screw passes directly through the brachial plexus (**Fig. 11**A, B).[30] For this reason drilling the glenoid arthroscopically from anterior to posterior is not advisable, because it is not possible to retract the neurovascular structures medially as is done in an open Bristow-Latarjet procedure. The surgeon is therefore forced to use a drill trajectory that diverges from the axis of the glenoid surface to avoid the medial neurovascular structures. The result is a bone block that exaggerates the convexity of the glenoid and may lead to later arthrosis, particularly if the bone block is placed intra-articularly (see **Fig. 8**B). For this reason the glenoid should be drilled from posterior to anterior, using a stop at the tip of the drill guide to prevent over-penetration of the drill, thus avoiding injury to the anterior neurovascular bundle (see **Fig. 3**A–C).

In coracoid transfer surgery the bone block may be placed either in the standing position, as in the classic Bristow procedure, or in the lying position, as in the Latarjet procedure. We believe that placing the bone block in the standing position is somewhat advantageous because (1) there is no need to abrade or burr it (and therefore to weaken it) as the bone cut is cancellous, (2) passing the bone block through the subscapularis muscle is easier to do, and (3) the inferior concave surface of the coracoid matches the natural concavity of the glenoid. We have found that the size of the standing coracoid is large enough to fill the glenoid bone defects encountered in all our cases. It has been our impression that the standing position of the bone block leaves more room for the inferior part of the subscapularis to slide during external rotation (ie, placing the bone block lying may squeeze the inferior part of the subscapularis muscle and could potentially limit external rotation).

Placement of the bone block is greatly aided by the suture-passing wire that is passed through the cannulated screw, as it guides the screw directly to the hole in the glenoid neck. Without the wire, the bone block and screw would have to be placed freehand, which would not only be technically difficult, but would place the brachial plexus and associated structures at risk. Once the screw is engaged in the glenoid, the intra-articular view is once again used to ensure correct rotation and adequate compression of the bone block (see **Fig. 7**B).

SUMMARY

The all-arthroscopic technique that we propose combines a Bristow-Latarjet procedure with a Bankart repair. This combined procedure provides a triple blocking of the shoulder (the so-called 2B[3] procedure): (1) the labral repair recreates the anterior bumper and protects the humeral head from direct contact with the coracoid bone graft (bumper effect); (2) the transferred coracoid bone block compensates for anterior glenoid bone loss (bony effect); and (3) the transferred conjoined tendon creates a dynamic sling that reinforces the weak anteroinferior capsule by lowering the inferior part of the subscapularis when the arm is abducted and externally rotated (belt or sling effect). This novel combined procedure allows the surgeon to extend the indications of arthroscopic shoulder reconstruction to another subset of patients with recurrent anteroinferior shoulder instability: those with glenoid bone loss and capsular deficiency. The procedure combines the theoretic advantages of the Bristow-Latarjet procedure and the arthroscopic Bankart repair, eliminating the potential disadvantages of each. The extra-articular positioning of the bone block together with the labral repair and capsule retensioning allow the surgeon to perform a nearly anatomic shoulder repair. It is an attractive surgical option to treat patients with a previous failed capsulolabral repair for which the surgical solutions are limited. Although the arthroscopic technique remains technically difficult, the magnification of the arthroscope and the use of specific instruments allow safe identification of the axillary nerve as well as safe harvesting and optimal positioning of the bone block, thus potentially reducing the risk of complications commonly associated with the open Bristow-Latarjet technique. Based on our experience, we advise surgeons to train first on cadaveric specimens and then to gradually transition from open, to mini-open, and then to all-arthroscopic, as is commonly done with rotator cuff repair. Our anatomic and preliminary clinical results are good and encourage us to continue using this arthroscopic technique in a selected patient population.

REFERENCES

1. Mohtadi NG, Bitar IJ, Sasyniuk TM, et al. Arthroscopic versus open repair for traumatic anterior shoulder instability: a meta-analysis. Arthroscopy 2005;21(6):652–8.
2. Hobby J, Griffin D, Dunbar M, et al. Is arthroscopic surgery for stabilisation of chronic shoulder instability as effective as open surgery? A systematic review and meta-analysis of 62 studies including 3044 arthroscopic operations. J Bone Joint Surg 2007;89(9):1188–96.

3. Lenters TR, Franta AK, Wolf FM, et al. Arthroscopic compared with open repairs for recurrent anterior shoulder instability. A systematic review and meta-analysis of the literature. J Bone Joint Surg 2007; 89(2):244–54.

4. Balg F, Boileau P. The Instability Severity Index Score. A simple pre-operative score to select patients for arthroscopic or open shoulder stabilisation. J Bone Joint Surg 2007;89:1470–7.

5. Boileau P, Villalba M, Hery JY, et al. Risk factors for recurrence of shoulder instability after arthroscopic Bankart repair. J Bone Joint Surg 2006; 88(8):1755–63.

6. Burkhart SS, De Beer JF. Traumatic glenohumeral bone defects and their relationship to failure of arthroscopic Bankart repairs: significance of the inverted-pear glenoid and the humeral engaging Hill-Sachs lesion. Arthroscopy 2000;16(7):677–94.

7. Millet PJ, Clavert P, Warner JJP. Current concepts review. Open operative treatment for anterior shoulder instability: when and why? J Bone Joint Surg 2005;87(2):419–31.

8. Burkhart SS, De Beer JF, Barth JR, et al. Results of modified Latarjet reconstruction in patients with anteroinferior instability and significant bone loss. Arthroscopy 2007;23(10):1033–41.

9. Boileau P, Bicknell RT, El Fegoun AB, et al. Arthroscopic Bristow procedure for anterior instability in shoulders with a stretched or deficient capsule: the "belt-and-suspenders" operative technique and preliminary results. Arthroscopy 2007;23(6):593–601.

10. Lafosse L, Lejeune E, Bouchard A, et al. The arthroscopic Latarjet procedure for the treatment of anterior shoulder instability. Arthroscopy 2007;23(11): 1242, e1241–e1245.

11. Boileau P, Roussanne Y, Bicknell R. Arthroscopic Bristow-Latarjet-Bankart procedure: the "triple locking" of the shoulder. In: Boileau P, editor. Shoulder concepts 2008. Arthroscopy & arthroplasty. Montpellier (France): Sauramps médical; 2008. p. 87–105.

12. Latarjet M. [Treatment of recurrent dislocations of the shoulder]. Lyon Chir 1954;49(8):994–7 [in French].

13. Helfet AJ. Coracoid transplantation for recurring dislocation of the shoulder. J Bone Joint Surg 1958;40:198–202.

14. May E, Ludde L, Holland C. [Treatment of habitual shoulder dislocations. (Late results following the Eden Hybinette surgical technic)]. Hefte Unfallheilkd 1975;126:118–20 [in German].

15. Patte D, Bancel P, Bernageau J. The vulnerable point of the glenoid rim. In: Bateman W, editor. Surgery of the shoulder. New York: Marcel Dekker; 1985.

16. Walch G, Boileau P. Latarjet-Bristow procedure for recurrent anterior instability of the shoulder. Tech Shoulder Elbow Surg 2000;1(4):256–61.

17. Lévigne C. [Long-term results of anterior coracoid abutments: a series of 52 cases with homogenous 12-year follow-up]. Rev Chir Orthop Reparatrice Appar Mot 2000;86(Suppl 1):114–21 [in French].

18. Hovelius L, Korner L, Lundberg B, et al. The coracoid transfer for recurrent dislocation of the shoulder. Technical aspects of the Bristow-Latarjet procedure. J Bone Joint Surg 1983;65(7):926–34.

19. Young DC, Rockwood CA Jr. Complications of a failed Bristow procedure and their management. J Bone Joint Surg 1991;73(7):969–81.

20. Zuckerman JD, Matsen FA 3rd. Complications about the glenohumeral joint related to the use of screws and staples. J Bone Joint Surg 1984;66(2):175–80.

21. Walch G. [Recurrent anterior shoulder instability.] La luxation récidivante antérieure de l'épaule. Rev Chir Orthop Reparatrice Appar Mot 1991;77(Suppl 1): 177–91 [in French].

22. Allain J, Goutallier D, Glorion C. Long-term results of the Latarjet procedure for the treatment of anterior instability of the shoulder. J Bone Joint Surg 1998; 80(6):841–52.

23. Trillat A, Dejour H, Roullet J. [Recurrent instability of the shoulder and glenoid labrum lesions]. Rev Chir Orthop Reparatrice Appar Mot 1965;51(6):525–44 [in French].

24. Walch G, Neyret P, Charret P, et al. [The Trillat procedure for anterior recurrent shoulder dislocations; Long term results of 250 cases with a mean follow-up of 11.3 years]. Lyon Chir 1989;85:25–31 [in French].

25. Torg JS, Balduini FC, Bonci C, et al. A modified Bristow-Helfet-May procedure for recurrent dislocation and subluxation of the shoulder. J Bone Joint Surg 1987;69(6):904–13.

26. Hovelius LK, Sandström BC, Rösmark DL, et al. Long term results with the Bankart and Bristow-Latarjet procedures: recurrent instability and arthropathy. J Shoulder Elbow Surg 2001;10(5):445–52.

27. Schroder DT, Provencher MT, Mologne TS, et al. The modified Bristow procedure for anterior shoulder instability. 26-year outcomes in Naval Academy midshipmen. Am J Sports Med 2006;5:778–86.

28. Collin P, Rochcongar P, Thomazeau H. Results of the Latarjet procedure for anterior chronic shoulder instability: a series of 74 cases. Rev Chir Orthop Reparatrice Appar Mot 2007;93:126–32 [in French].

29. Boileau P, Mercier N, Old J, et al. The arthroscopic Bristow-Latarjet-Bankart procedure for the treatment of recurrent anterior shoulder instability: is it reliable and safe? Arthroscopy 2010, in press.

30. Vargas P, Zumstein M, Rumian A, et al. The medial "East" portal for arthroscopic Bristow-Latarjet-Bankart procedure: an anatomical cadaveric study [abstract OP116]. In: Proceedings of the 22nd Congress of the European Society for Surgery of the Shoulder and the Elbow, Madrid: 2009. p. 119.

Arthroscopic Latarjet Procedure

Laurent Lafosse, MD[a], Simon Boyle, MSc, FRCS(Tr & Orth)[a,b,*],
Mikel Gutierrez-Aramberri, MD[a], Anup Shah, MD[a],
Rupert Meller, MD[a]

KEYWORDS

- Instability • Recurrence • Latarjet • Arthroscopy
- Stabilization • Bony defect

The increase in popularity of arthroscopic shoulder surgery in the past 20 years has led to an expansion in the operative treatment options available for shoulder instability. This in part can be explained by the arthroscopic exposure given to a new generation of shoulder surgeons throughout residency and fellowship training, and the enthusiasm with which many open surgeons have pioneered and embraced stabilizing techniques. In addition, the added scrutiny of the shoulder afforded by the use of the arthroscope has led to an improved understanding of previously unrecognized soft tissue lesions underlying many cases of instability. The role of glenoid and humeral head bone defects in recurrent instability has also been better appreciated arthroscopically, especially when these lesions are evaluated in combination with preoperative radiological studies.

Despite advances in techniques and instruments, and improvements in surgical training, there still remains a significant failure rate when stabilization procedures inadequately address the underlying pathology.[1] The open Latarjet procedure has shown excellent and reliable results in the recent literature.[2–6] The natural evolution of this procedure is an all-arthroscopic technique to confer all of the advantages of the open procedure while using a minimally invasive technique.

IS THERE A NEED FOR THE ARTHROSCOPIC LATARJET PROCEDURE?

Most shoulder surgeons are familiar with either an arthroscopic or open Bankart repair for recurrent shoulder instability largely because a capsulolabral avulsion from the glenoid rim is the most common lesion associated with shoulder dislocations.[7] This technique has demonstrated excellent results when used to treat isolated soft tissue Bankart lesions.[8,9] However, a problem emerges when this form of repair is used in patients who have more extensive soft tissue injuries such as complex labral disruptions, capsular attenuation, or humeral avulsion of glenohumeral ligament (HAGL) lesions. In these cases, reducing the labrum back on to the anterior glenoid is often not sufficient to restore shoulder stability,[1] particularly when the labral tissue is no longer functional or there is a capsular detachment on the humeral side.

Inferior results have also been associated with a capsulolabral repair when it is used in cases where bony deficiency is a major contributing factor to the recurrent instability.[10,11] This concern has been raised by many investigators after several years of follow-up, particularly with regard to young patients (<20 years) and those involved in overhead or contact sports.[12] In 2006, Boileau and colleagues[11] reviewed 91 consecutive patients

Financial disclosure: The authors, their immediate family, and any research foundation with which they are affiliated did not receive any financial payments or other benefits from any commercial entity related to the subject of this article. No outside funding or grants were received.
[a] Alps Surgery Institute, Clinique Generale, 4 Chemin Tour la Reine, Annecy 74000, France
[b] 4 De Ferrieres Avenue, Harrogate HG1 2AR, Yorkshire, UK
* Corresponding author. 4 De Ferrieres Avenue, Harrogate HG1 2AR, Yorkshire, UK.
E-mail address: siboyle@me.com

Orthop Clin N Am 41 (2010) 393–405
doi:10.1016/j.ocl.2010.02.004

who had undergone Bankart repairs for anterior shoulder instability, and found a 15.3% recurrence rate. The cause for recurrence was most commonly bone loss on the glenoid, bone loss on the humeral head, or inferior ligament hyperlaxity (as indicated by an asymmetric hyperabduction test). A combination of these abnormalities can result in up to 75% recurrence of instability after soft tissue repair, because the repair does not restore the glenoid articular arc that is reduced secondary to the glenoid bone loss or the engaging Hill-Sachs lesion.

There is an apparent need for an alternative surgical strategy to a standard Bankart repair to restore stability when the glenohumeral ligaments are torn or attenuated in combination with glenoid bone loss or an engaging Hill-Sachs lesion.

WHEN TO CONSIDER THE LATARJET PROCEDURE

All patients undergo a detailed history and clinical examination followed by radiography (including a Bernageau view) or computed tomography (CT)/magnetic resonance imaging (MRI) studies. This process usually identifies clinical situations in which a capsulolabral repair is thought to be insufficient and therefore a Latarjet procedure is believed to be superior. However, the situation can arise when the need for a Latarjet procedure becomes apparent only on initial arthroscopic inspection. For this reason it is necessary to consent patients accordingly.

The arthroscopic Latarjet procedure is considered in the following situations.

Complex Soft Tissue Injuries

Improvements in radiological investigations, especially when radiopaque dyes are used, has led to enhanced identification of HAGL lesions on preoperative CT or MRI scans. However, it is common to detect these lesions for the first time on arthroscopic inspection (**Fig. 1**). Multiple techniques are described for the arthroscopic repair of HAGL lesions, and most of these include only small case series with short follow-up periods.[13–15] The authors' experience using an all-arthroscopic soft tissue repair technique with anchors was disappointing because of postoperative stiffness experienced by some patients.

Where patients have had multiple dislocations, the intrinsic structure of the glenohumeral ligaments is usually found deranged, although this may not be evident macroscopically. Simply reopposing this damaged tissue back to the glenoid does not necessarily restore stability to the

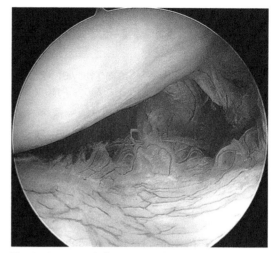

Fig. 1. An anteroinferior HAGL lesion.

shoulder. This practice has been likened to rehanging a baggy or incompetent hammock.

A further soft tissue injury is that of the irreparable labrum, especially in which there has been a complete radial tear thereby effectively breaking the ring. A repair of the labrum in this situation rarely provides sufficient strength of healing to restore stability.

In these situations, reattaching or repairing these structures leads to a suboptimal outcome either through stiffness or recurrence, and as such a Latarjet procedure would be performed.

Bony Defects

Glenoid bone loss

Glenoid bone loss as the cause for recurrent instability is frequently overlooked but is usually manifested by an avulsion type bony Bankart lesion, an impacted fracture, or erosion of the anteroinferior glenoid rim. Radiographs may show a fracture or a more subtle loss of contour of the anteroinferior glenoid rim.[16] A decrease in the apparent density of the inferior glenoid line often signifies an erosion of the glenoid rim between the 3- and 6-o'clock position. An axillary or Bernageau view may show flattening of this area of the glenoid when bone loss has occurred. CT provides a more detailed imaging modality, which is essential to quantify the bone loss preoperatively.[17] CT reconstructions also provide a more robust static measurement than those afforded by the arthroscopic view (**Fig. 2**).

The amount of glenoid bone loss can be assessed during preoperative evaluation or surgery. With adequate imaging, bone loss can be determined with the Bernageau view, sagittal and oblique CT scans, and 3-dimensional

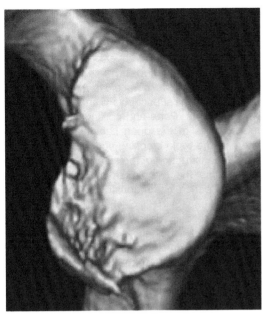

Fig. 2. Three-dimensional CT of significant anterior glenoid bone defect.

reconstructions. In addition, the amount of glenoid bone loss can be verified arthroscopically by measuring the distance from the glenoid rim to the bare spot,[18,19] thereby assisting the surgeon in identifying an inverted pear glenoid, and confirming substantial bone loss and the likely failure of an isolated soft tissue repair.[10] The threshold beyond which a soft tissue repair is likely to fail is difficult to define, and significantly increased glenohumeral instability has been suggested with defects anywhere between 21%[16] and 28.8%[18] of the glenoid (although caution should be exercised when comparing measurement methods).

Even when the bony fragment is present, replacing it is not always sufficient to restore the bony glenoid articular arc, especially when recurrent episodes of instability have further eroded the remaining glenoid edge.[17] There are also issues regarding healing in this potentially necrotic bone.[20] In these cases a bony reconstruction should be considered.

Humeral bone loss

The location and size of the Hill-Sachs lesion determines the degree to which the articular arc is reduced and when the lesion will engage on the glenoid. Dynamic arthroscopy with the shoulder in abduction and external rotation will demonstrate whether the lesion will engage during a functional or athletic overhead range of movement. To reduce the chances of recurrence, the

articular arc must be increased to prevent early engagement of the lesion on the glenoid rim when the arm is externally rotated; this can be achieved with the use of a bone block procedure. An alternative to this would be the "remplissage" procedure as described by Purchase and colleagues[21] (suturing of the infraspinatus and posterior capsule into the defect).

By enlarging the glenoid articular arc with a bone graft, the joint surface contact areas are increased and therefore the joint surface contact pressures are reduced during external rotation. The remplissage procedure does not alter the joint contact surface areas or increase the articular arc, and therefore has no effect on reducing the joint contact pressures, which may then have an effect on the development of future arthrosis. Advancing the infraspinatus and capsule into the humeral bony defect can also significantly decrease the amount of external rotation the patient may be able to achieve postoperatively.

Combinations of glenoid and humeral bone loss

These 2 lesions usually occur in tandem with varying degrees of severity. Preoperative radiographs (**Fig. 3**) and CT scans usually identify these lesions, but an arthroscopic dynamic evaluation of stability is necessary to determine the likely clinical effects of this combination (**Fig. 4**). The presence of an engaging Hill-Sachs lesion coexisting with a glenoid bone defect markedly reduces the defect size threshold at which recurrence will occur if the patient had only one soft tissue or bony defect in isolation. Latarjet procedure is found to be appropriate to address the abnormal anatomy.

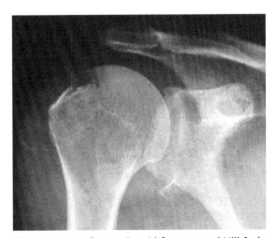

Fig. 3. Anteroinferior glenoid fracture and Hill-Sachs lesion.

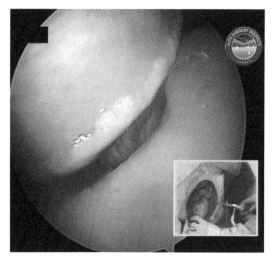

Fig. 4. Engaging Hill-Sachs lesion combined with a deficient anterior glenoid.

Revision Surgery for Instability

If the initial stabilizing procedure fails because of any of the reasons mentioned earlier, then a Latarjet procedure is ideally suited to restore stability. However, a second group of patients were observed who had seemingly successful Bankart repairs but went on to develop postoperative recurrent instability after 5 to 7 years. In this particular group, the soft tissue stabilization was adequate to return the patient to a sedentary lifestyle but it had not restored satisfactory stability for more active and sporting pastimes. This finding can in part explain the excellent results seen in series with a short follow-up. In these cases, although the initial operation was considered successful, the pathologic lesion was never truly corrected and the glenoid subsequently became increasingly eroded. These patients can be effectively managed with a Latarjet as well.

Patient Activity

Many patients now demand a quicker return to sports or their occupation, or they have a high risk of recurrence. This is particularly true for patients involved in collision sports (eg, rugby), overhead sports (eg, climbing), throwing sports, and high-demand physical overhead occupations (eg, carpentry). The ability to recreate a stable shoulder with a reduced rehabilitation time to return to full activity is another advantage of the arthroscopic Latarjet technique.

HOW DOES THE LATARJET PROCEDURE RESTORE STABILITY?

The procedure was first described by Latarjet in 1954[22] when he published his technique of transferring the horizontal part of the coracoid to the anteroinferior margin of the glenoid from the 2-o'clock to the 6-o'clock position. The original procedure required the upper part of the subscapularis to be detached, but this has since been modified to place the coracoid graft through a horizontal split in the subscapularis and fix it preferably with 2 screws. Patte and colleagues[23] explained the success of the open Latarjet procedure by virtue of the triple blocking effect. First, the triple bony reconstruction of the anterior glenoid serves to increase the glenoid articular arc (the bone block effect). This reconstruction prevents an otherwise engaging Hill-Sachs lesion from levering on the potentially deficient anteroinferior glenoid rim. Second, the split subscapularis tendon provides dynamic stability in abduction and external rotation due to the tension created by its intersection with the newly positioned conjoined tendon (the hammock effect). Finally, the capsule can be attached to the remnant of the coracoacromial ligament on the coracoid (the Bankart effect).

WHY NOT PERFORM A MODIFIED BRISTOW PROCEDURE?

The initial description of Bristow procedure by Helfet[24] entailed securing the detached tip of the coracoid to the repaired vertical split in muscle belly of subscapularis. This split was initially required to expose and decorticate the bone of the glenoid neck. Incorporating the coracoid in the suture closure of this defect was performed to appose the bony surfaces of the freshly osteotomized coracoid, and the glenoid neck and was later modified to employ a single screw fixation of the coracoid in a standing position. The Latarjet procedure instead applies the coracoid process in a lying position, which allows the natural shape of the inferior coracoid surface to follow the contour of the anterior glenoid. This position is then secured and compressed by 2 screws, giving the Latarjet procedure the advantage of providing an increased surface area of bone to bone contact to promote bony union. Furthermore, the use of 2 screws for fixation allows greater compression and gives excellent rotational stability, and minimizes graft micromotion with any conjoined tendon contraction. These differences in technique allow a significantly accelerated postoperative rehabilitation, and favor graft union and stability for the Latarjet procedure.

WHY PERFORM A LATARJET PROCEDURE INSTEAD OF A FREE BONE GRAFT?

It has been previously demonstrated that the sling effect of the conjoined tendon crossing the subscapularis has a significant effect on shoulder stability.[25] This effect is best understood by considering that the further the shoulder goes into external rotation, the more the newly placed conjoined tendon will stabilize the shoulder through its increased tension and sling effect over the inferior subscapularis muscle. The added important soft tissue stabilizing effect does not occur when free bone block transfers are performed.

A free bone graft does have a role in restoring the glenoid articular arc in cases of large anterior glenoid bony deficiencies,[26] and for posterior instability when there has been posterior glenoid bone loss or a reverse Hill-Sachs lesion; this is because there is no local osseo-tendinous structure that can be transferred posteriorly. A free bone graft is also a useful tool in the management of the failed or revision Latarjet procedure.

SHOULD I CHANGE FROM AN OPEN TO AN ARTHROSCOPIC PROCEDURE?

Although the open Latarjet procedure has proven to be successful in restoring shoulder stability, performing the procedure arthroscopically offers many advantages. These include the following.

Graft Placement

Placement of the bone graft is more accurate under arthroscopic control. Several different views can be afforded by the arthroscopic technique that not only improve graft placement but also reduce the chances of overhang and impingement. Lateral graft placement has been associated with the subsequent development of glenohumeral arthritis.[27]

Management of Associated Shoulder Pathologies

Open surgery does not easily allow the treatment of concomitant pathologies, particularly of the superior and posterior shoulder, such as superior labrum anterior posterior (SLAP) tears and posterior labral lesions. These lesions can be missed or prove challenging to treat. and can be addressed much more readily with an arthroscopic approach.

Bidirectional Instability

Concurrent anterior and posterior instability is uncommon and difficult to diagnose. However, when this does occur it can be treated during the same surgical procedure by using anterior and posterior bone blocks using arthroscopic methods. This treatment is not possible through a single open approach.

Shoulder Stiffness

Even though the strength of the bone block fixation allows early mobilization, the risk of adhesions and shoulder stiffness is higher with an open technique than with arthroscopy.

Ease of Conversion

If during an intended Bankart repair the tissue is determined to be nonreconstructable, the surgeon can perform an arthroscopic bone block stabilization without potentially having to reposition the patient or convert to open surgery. This technique is especially useful to arthroscopists who use the beach chair position for stabilization surgery.

Faster Rehabilitation

As in other joints, arthroscopy offers the advantages of less postoperative pain, earlier mobility, and quicker rehabilitation, and return to sports.

Cosmesis

The arthroscopic Latarjet procedure uses small skin incisions that are esthetically superior to a single larger open incision.

HOW DO I INTRODUCE THE ARTHROSCOPIC LATARJET INTO MY SURGICAL PRACTICE?

Initially, the operating surgeon should be familiar and experienced with performing the procedure using an open technique because it permits a more global understanding of the anatomy involved and the potential difficulties of the procedure. It also serves as a safety net when performing the arthroscopic procedure to allow the surgeon to convert to the open technique if necessary. Before embarking on the arthroscopic procedure, the first step in this transition requires the surgeon to be acquainted with the arthroscopic instruments. The familiarity can be achieved by performing the open Latarjet using the arthroscopic instruments.

Once the surgeon is proficient in using the instruments for the open procedure, he or she can then make the transition to perform the arthroscopic Latarjet procedure. The transition should proceed in a stepwise fashion, and the surgeon is encouraged to convert to the open procedure at any stage if necessary to ensure the optimal result. With training and experience it is possible to perform the entire procedure arthroscopically. Of paramount importance is an optimally placed graft to provide bony union and shoulder stability without complications. The surgeon should not hesitate to open the shoulder at any stage if this is the best way of achieving the optimal placement of graft.

The technique is conveniently broken down into 5 stages.

Joint Evaluation/Achieving Exposure

The consented and prepared patient is positioned in the beach chair position with the arm in gentle traction. Preoperatively an interscalene block is performed before the induction of general anesthesia.

The intra-articular evaluation is started through the standard "soft spot" and posterior A portal is made and a probe is introduced through the rotator interval (RI). This probe uses the anterior E portal, which is established using an outside-in technique (the anterior portals can be seen in **Fig. 5**). A dynamic stability assessment is made and the internal structures are further assessed with the probe (glenoid defects, humeral defects, HAGL and so forth).

Open the rotator interval and subscapularis exposure

The glenohumeral joint is opened at the upper border of subscapularis (**Fig. 6**), and the anteroinferior labrum and middle glenohumeral ligament are resected between the 2- and 5-o'clock position to expose the glenoid neck using electrocautery. The intended graft site is marked, and the capsule between the glenoid neck and subscapularis is split. To provide a healthy base for graft

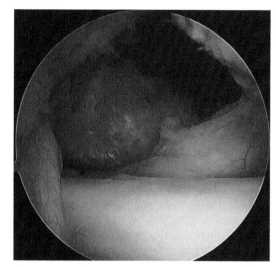

Fig. 6. Rotator interval opened, revealing the coracoid.

healing, the glenoid neck is abraded with the burr. Both sides of the subscapularis tendon are then exposed, with particular attention to the articular side of subscapularis. These releases are necessary to facilitate the transfer of the coracoid graft.

If there is any other intra-articular pathology, it can be dealt with at this stage (eg, a SLAP repair). If the inferior glenohumeral ligament or posterior labrum is damaged but reparable, this can be achieved with suture anchors.

Once this intra-articular preparation is completed, extra-articular preparation is done.

Coracoid soft tissue preparation

The coracoacromial ligament (CAL) is located and is followed down to the coracoid, where it is detached. The anterior aspect of the conjoined tendon is liberated from the fascia on the deep aspect of the deltoid, and the lateral side of the conjoined tendon is released, the inferior limit of which is the pectoralis major tendon.

There is a tissue barrier medial to the conjoined tendon that separates the plexus from the subcoracoid bursa (**Fig. 7**). This barrier is opened to reveal the nerves to the subscapularis, and further gentle inferior dissection exposes the axillary nerve. It is important to identify these nerves and appreciate their location when it comes to placing future portals. Any further soft tissue attachments to the coracoid in the bursa are released to free the coracoid for its later transfer.

The scope is moved from the posterior A portal to the anterolateral D portal to give a better viewing perspective of the anterior structures. This portal lies 1 cm inferior and lateral to the anterolateral

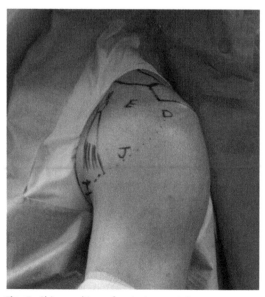

Fig. 5. Skin marking of anterior portals.

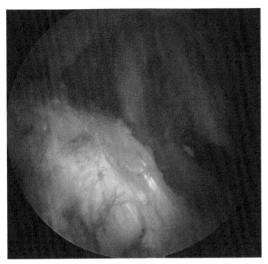

Fig. 7. Plexus seen from the D portal with the coracoid in the foreground.

corner of the acromion, and is also created using an outside-in technique.

Subscapularis Split

Establish the I portal in apex of axillary fold
This portal gives excellent access to the anterior glenoid neck in the correct direction to place the screws for the graft. First, a spinal needle is placed in the apex of the anterior axillary fold and is guided under direct vision to pass lateral to the conjoined tendon and above the subscapularis. The needle is advanced to the glenoid neck at the intended graft site and a 2-cm incision is made in the skin for the I portal.

Determine the level of the subscapularis split
The switching stick is inserted through the A portal and passed across the glenohumeral joint at the level of the glenoid defect. It is then advanced through the subscapularis to establish the level of the split. The conjoined tendon and plexus are retracted medially to prevent neurologic injury on further advancement of the switching stick. The switching stick now holds the plexus and conjoined tendon medially while penetrating the subscapularis at the level of the split.

Establish the J portal
This portal is placed midway on an arc between the I and the D portals using an outside-in technique. It gives a more heads-on view of the coracoid whereas the D portal gives a better lateral view. Two perpendicular views are necessary to ensure optimum coracoid preparation.

Subscapularis split
The subscapularis is elevated with the switching stick, introducing the electrocautery through the J portal, and the split is commenced (**Fig. 8**). The scope is moved to the J portal and the electrocautery to the I portal to complete the split. The split is completed down to the glenoid neck in the line of the subscapularis fibers, extending from the lateral insertion of the subscapularis on the lesser tuberosity, passing medially close to the axillary nerve.

At this point, if this is revision surgery, alternatively an iliac crest graft can be placed as the subscapularis split is done and the glenoid neck exposed.

Harvesting the Coracoid Graft

At this point the scope is in the J portal and the electrocautery is in the I portal. A trocar is placed in the D portal and the space is elevated above the coracoid (like using a retractor in open surgery).

Define the H Portal

The H portal is necessary to allow instrument access to the superior coracoid. Two needles are placed to locate the tip and the midpoint of the coracoid. Next, the arthroscope (J portal) is rotated to give a perpendicular view of the coracoid to ensure correct needle alignment. This step serves to guide the position of the coracoid drill guide. Once satisfactory, a superior incision is made for the H portal.

The pectoralis minor tendon on the medial border of the coracoid is now released, taking care to remain on bone at the coracoid level (**Fig. 9**). Below this, the conjoined tendon can be

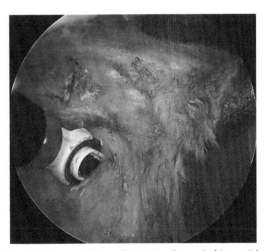

Fig. 8. Subscapularis split. Note the switching stick elevating the muscle.

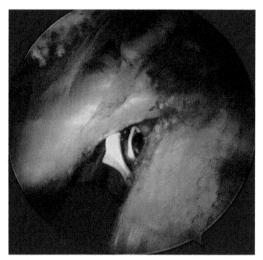

Fig. 9. Pectoralis minor tendon being released from the coracoid.

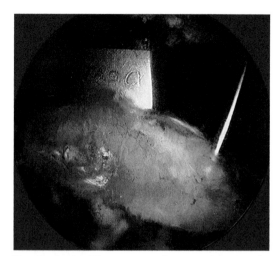

Fig. 10. K-wire alignment on the coracoid using the coracoid drill guide.

released medially using blunt dissection, taking special care to prevent damage to the musculocutaneous nerve and plexus.

With this dissection completed and having an awareness of the position of the nerves, the surgeon can proceed with the knowledge that everything lateral to the conjoined tendon is safe.

Drilling the coracoid
It is important to regularly change the viewing angle of the arthroscope by rotation to ensure mediolateral alignment of the coracoid drill guide. The guide is placed over the junction of lateral two-thirds and medial one-third of the coracoid, and α hole (inferior and distal) is drilled with a k wire. It is important while doing this to visualize under the coracoid to verify that the direction of the k wires is perpendicular to the superior surface of the coracoid, and to prevent subscapularis penetration. The coracoid drill guide is rotationally aligned around the α wire and then the second k wire is inserted into the β (proximal) hole (**Fig. 10**).

The drill guide is removed and the wire positions are checked with the scope in the D and J portals. A coracoid step drill is used to overdrill both holes, and the drills and k wires are removed.

Inserting the top hats
The drill holes are now tapped to prepare for the top hat and glenoid screws (5.0/3.5 mm). The taps are cannulated and allow placement of the coracoid-securing flexible Chia wire. This wire is passed through the tapped drill holes in the coracoid and out through the H portal. It serves to allow the cannulated introduction of the top hat washers and also later transfer control of the

coracoid between portals. The top hats are then inserted over the Chia wire and (see **Fig. 10**) a portal plug placed in the H portal to prevent water escaping.

The Subscap Channeler is a large trocar placed through the subscapularis split via the I portal onto the glenoid neck in the intended graft location. This step serves to judge whether the earlier soft tissue split is adequate to allow transfer of the coracoid to the glenoid neck.

Retrieving the Chia wires through the I portal
The coracoid will ultimately be controlled and directed from the I portal and as such the Chia wires must be transferred there. To do this the crochet hooks are passed through the coracoid positioning cannula in the axillary I portal to retrieve these (**Fig. 11**). Once retrieved, slotted pegs with specific narrow channels are placed over both Chia wires to prevent water being lost through the cannula (**Fig. 12**).

Coracoid osteotomy
Once the coracoid is prepared, osteotomy is performed. The burr is used on the superior, inferior, and lateral aspects of the coracoid, proximal to the β hole, to create a stress riser. The medial aspect of the osteotomy site can be burred through the H portal. The osteotome is now placed in the H portal and a controlled osteotomy is carried out (**Fig. 13**).

Coracoid Transfer

To gain rigid control of the graft, it must be reduced onto the coracoid positioning cannula. This step is achieved by placing gentle traction on both limbs of the Chia wire (**Fig. 14**), then

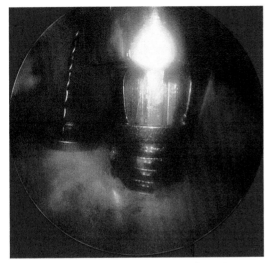

Fig. 11. Top hats being inserted over Chia wire.

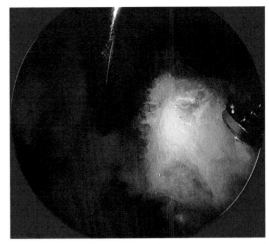

Fig. 13. Coracoid osteotomy with osteotome proximal to the β hole.

passing the coracoid 3.5 screw over the Chia wires. The screw advances through the top hat and into the coracoid, where it engages the bone. The coracoid should now be secure on the coracoid positioning cannula.

Graft trimming

The freshly harvested graft is mobilized, and all remaining adhesions of the pectoralis minor and the medial fascia are removed. Particular attention must be paid to prevent injury to the musculocutaneous nerve while this is done. The mobilized coracoid usually has a medial spike arising from its base that must be trimmed to permit good bony contact with the glenoid. To do this the scope is held by the assistant, and with the

surgeon using a 2-handed technique, the graft is controlled on the cannula with one hand and trimmed with the burr with the other. Ideally, the burr is held stationary while the coracoid is manipulated around the burr to allow the accurate debridement of the graft and to minimize any risk to the plexus.

The graft is now ready for transfer and fixation to the glenoid. The coracoid on the coracoid positioning cannula (I portal) is manipulated to the glenoid neck. This action is made easier by elevating the subscapularis split with the switching stick.

Coracoid Fixation

Once the graft is sited on the glenoid neck in the desired position, fixation is undertaken. Two long

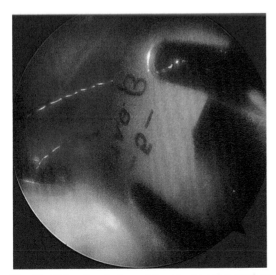

Fig. 12. Chia wires being retrieved using the crochet hooks.

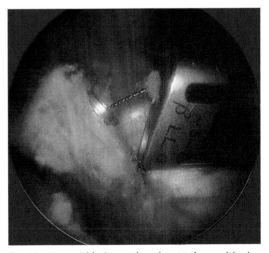

Fig. 14. Coracoid being reduced onto the positioning cannula.

k wires are inserted through the coracoid positioning cannula, passing through the graft and then the glenoid to gain temporary fixation. The scapula must be pulled posteriorly by the assistant using a posterior drawer on the upper arm to decrease the relative glenoid anteversion. The handle of the cannula must be pushed medially to ensure there is minimum angulation between the k wires and the glenoid surface. These wires will emerge through the skin of the posterior shoulder, at which stage a clip is placed on them.

The position of the graft is then checked from different portals to ensure the best vertical and horizontal position. It is preferred to place the graft from the 3- to 5-o'clock position and flush with the glenoid.

Drill and screw the graft

The α coracoid 3.5 screw (inferior) is removed and the 3.2 glenoid drill passed over the k wire. The length of the definitive screw can be read from the depth gauge on the drill. The drill is removed (k wire remains) and the screw is placed in the α hole. The same action is repeated for the β hole after which the inserted screws are alternately tightened to reduce the graft in compression onto the glenoid neck (**Fig. 15**). The k wires can then be removed posteriorly.

Final check

The graft and screw position are checked through the D (**Fig. 16**), J, and A portals, and any final trimming can be done at this stage with the burr.

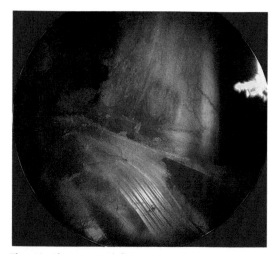

Fig. 16. The coracoid fixation can be seen with the conjoined tendon passing over the subscapularis. Note the close proximity of the plexus medially.

POSTOPERATIVE MANAGEMENT

Postoperatively the patients require no immobilization and may begin full active range of movements immediately. Patients can return to work as soon as pain allows and play low-risk sports at 3 weeks. For high-risk (throwing) and collision sports, the authors recommend that patients do not resume these activities before 6 weeks (**Figs. 17** and **18**).

CLINICAL RESULTS

The all-arthroscopic Latarjet procedure has been performed on more than 180 shoulders since its inception in December 2003. Preoperative, perioperative, and postoperative data on all these patients have been prospectively collected.

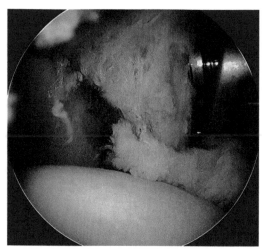

Fig. 15. Coracoid transfer and fixation onto the glenoid neck.

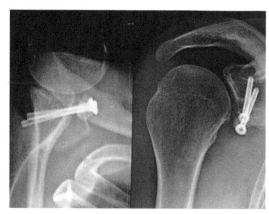

Fig. 17. Six weeks post operation.

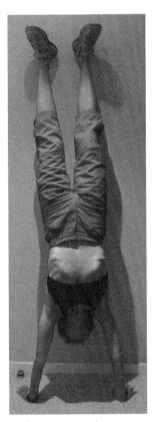

Fig. 18. Six weeks post operation.

The demographics of the first 100 shoulders comprised 98 patients, with 46 right shoulders and 54 left shoulders. The male to female patient ratio was 4:3 and the average age of the patients was 27.5 (range, 17–54) years. Of these patients, 88% were involved actively in sports, 38% of these at a competitive level.

All patients had sustained dislocations (1–3, 40%; 4–10, 50%; >10, 10%) with 97% of these being traumatic in nature. Of the patients, 15% had undergone previous surgery for instability, all of whom had undergone Bankart repairs. The average delay from the initial dislocation to the Latarjet procedure was 54 months (range, 1 month to 20 years).

Radiographic evaluation revealed Hill-Sachs lesions in 89% of shoulders, and 25% had evidence of a glenoid fracture.

All procedures were performed by one surgeon (L.L.), with operative time reduced from 4 hours at the inception of the procedure to an average of 45 to 50 minutes. Concomitant lesions were found in 7% of patients (6 SLAP tears, 1 posterior Bankart lesion) that were treated during the same procedure.

Eighteen-Month Follow-Up

Of the 98 patients, 62 were available for direct clinical review, 27 were reviewed by telephone conversation and structured questionnaire, and 11 patients were lost to follow-up.

Eighty percent of patients described their result as excellent and 18% as good, with 2% disappointed with their outcome. All patients had returned to work at a mean of 2 months (range, 7 days to 4 months) and returned to sport at 10 weeks (range, 21 days to 6 months).

Radiographic Results

Radiographic evidence of arthrosis was assessed and compared with preoperative films according to the criteria of Samilson and Prieto.[28] 11% had progressed 1 stage only (stage 0: 24 patients [69%], stage 1: 9 [26%], stage 2: 2 [6%]).

Coracoid graft position was reviewed using CT scanning. The graft was flush with the glenoid in 80%, medially placed in 8%, and there was lateral overhang in 12%. Vertically positioning was 78% perfect (3 to 5 o'clock), too high in 7%, and too low in 5%. Screw angle in relation to the glenoid face was on average 29° (range, 2°–50°).

Complications

Perioperative complications included 2 hematomas, 1 intraoperative fracture of the graft, and 1 transient musculocutaneous nerve palsy that fully recovered. Late complications included 4 cases of coracoid nonunion, and of these 4 cases, 2 had originally undergone coracoid fixation using just 1 screw. A further 3 shoulders were found to have lysis around the screws leading to prominence. In total, 4 patients required late arthroscopic screw removal.

At 26 months, 35 patients were available for review and on average, patients had lost 18° external rotation as compared with the opposite shoulder. There were no cases of recurrent dislocation.

These results represent all the available patients from the first 100 procedures performed, and therefore those procedures performed at the start of the learning curve.

SUMMARY

Soft tissue Bankart repairs yield good results when used for capsulolabral avulsions and tears. However, patients with more complex pathologic instability require a surgical option that addresses the underlying abnormalities to ensure a low rate of recurrence postoperatively. The use of arthroscopy and radiological investigations has identified more complex soft tissue and bony lesions that can be more successfully treated using a Latarjet procedure. The authors have advanced this technique to make it possible arthroscopically, and therefore confer the benefits that this type of surgery offers.

Before embarking on surgery of this complexity, it is important that the surgeon becomes familiar with the open technique and the arthroscopic instruments it uses. To introduce this into practice, a stepwise progression of the technique is recommended in the stages as described, whereby the surgeon converts to the open procedure at any point to ensure an optimal result. With training and experience, this procedure can then be performed entirely arthroscopically.

The arthroscopic Latarjet technique has shown excellent results at short- to mid-term follow-up, with minimal complications and good graft positioning. As such, this procedure is recommended to surgeons with good anatomic knowledge, advanced arthroscopic skills, and familiarity with the instrumentation.

REFERENCES

1. Tauber M, Resch H, Forstner R, et al. Reasons for failure after surgical repair of anterior shoulder instability. J Shoulder Elbow Surg 2004;13(3):279.
2. Hovelius LK, Sandstrom BC, Rosmark DL, et al. Long-term results with the Bankart and Bristow-Latarjet procedures: recurrent shoulder instability and arthropathy. J Shoulder Elbow Surg 2001;10(5):445.
3. Allain J, Goutallier D, Glorion C. Long-term results of the Latarjet procedure for the treatment of anterior instability of the shoulder. J Bone Joint Surg Am 1998;80(6):841.
4. Collin P, Rochcongar P, Thomazeau H. [Treatment of chronic anterior shoulder instability using a coracoid bone block (Latarjet procedure): 74 cases]. Rev Chir Orthop Reparatrice Appar Mot 2007;93(2):126 [in French].
5. Hovelius L, Sandstrom B, Sundgren K, et al. One hundred eighteen Bristow-Latarjet repairs for recurrent anterior dislocation of the shoulder prospectively followed for fifteen years: study I—clinical results. J Shoulder Elbow Surg 2004;13(5):509.
6. Spoor AB, de Waal Malefijt J. Long-term results and arthropathy following the modified Bristow-Latarjet procedure. Int Orthop 2005;29(5):265.
7. Hintermann B, Gachter A. Arthroscopic findings after shoulder dislocation. Am J Sports Med 1995;23(5):545.
8. Gartsman GM, Roddey TS, Hammerman SM. Arthroscopic treatment of anterior-inferior glenohumeral instability. Two to five-year follow-up. J Bone Joint Surg Am 2000;82(7):991.
9. Kim SH, Ha KI, Cho YB, et al. Arthroscopic anterior stabilization of the shoulder: two to six-year follow-up. J Bone Joint Surg Am 2003;85(8):1511.
10. Burkhart SS, De Beer JF. Traumatic glenohumeral bone defects and their relationship to failure of arthroscopic Bankart repairs: significance of the inverted-pear glenoid and the humeral engaging Hill-Sachs lesion. Arthroscopy 2000;16(7):677.
11. Boileau P, Villalba M, Hery JY, et al. Risk factors for recurrence of shoulder instability after arthroscopic Bankart repair. J Bone Joint Surg Am 2006;88(8):1755.
12. Balg F, Boileau P. The instability severity index score. A simple pre-operative score to select patients for arthroscopic or open shoulder stabilisation. J Bone Joint Surg Br 2007;89(11):1470.
13. Page RS, Bhatia DN. Arthroscopic repair of humeral avulsion of glenohumeral ligament lesion: anterior and posterior techniques. Tech Hand Up Extrem Surg 2009;13(2):98.
14. Parameswaran AD, Provencher MT, Bach BR Jr, et al. Humeral avulsion of the glenohumeral ligament: injury pattern and arthroscopic repair techniques. Orthopedics 2008;31(8):773.
15. Wolf EM, Cheng JC, Dickson K. Humeral avulsion of glenohumeral ligaments as a cause of anterior shoulder instability. Arthroscopy 1995;11(5):600.
16. Itoi E, Lee SB, Amrami KK, et al. Quantitative assessment of classic anteroinferior bony Bankart lesions by radiography and computed tomography. Am J Sports Med 2003;31(1):112.
17. Sugaya H, Moriishi J, Dohi M, et al. Glenoid rim morphology in recurrent anterior glenohumeral instability. J Bone Joint Surg Am 2003;85(5):878.
18. Lo IK, Parten PM, Burkhart SS. The inverted pear glenoid: an indicator of significant glenoid bone loss. Arthroscopy 2004;20(2):169.
19. Burkhart SS, Debeer JF, Tehrany AM, et al. Quantifying glenoid bone loss arthroscopically in shoulder instability. Arthroscopy 2002;18(5):488.
20. Roberts CP, Huysmans P, Cresswell T, et al. The histopathology of glenoid bone lesions and its relevance to surgery for glenohumeral instability. J Bone Joint Surg Br 2005;90(Suppl II):213.
21. Purchase RJ, Wolf EM, Hobgood ER, et al. Hill-Sachs "remplissage": an arthroscopic solution for the engaging hill-sachs lesion. Arthroscopy 2008;24(6):723.

22. Latarjet M. [Treatment of recurrent dislocation of the shoulder]. Lyon Chir 1954;49(8):994 [in French].

23. Patte D, Bernageau J, Bancel P. The anteroinferior vulnerable point of the glenoid rim. New York (NY): Marcel Dekker; 1985.

24. Helfet AJ. Coracoid transplantation for recurring dislocation of the shoulder. J Bone Joint Surg Br 1958;40(2):198.

25. Wellmann M, Petersen W, Zantop T, et al. Open shoulder repair of osseous glenoid defects: biomechanical effectiveness of the Latarjet procedure versus a contoured structural bone graft. Am J Sports Med 2009;37(1):87.

26. Warner JJ, Gill TJ, O'Hollerhan JD, et al. Anatomical glenoid reconstruction for recurrent anterior glenohumeral instability with glenoid deficiency using an autogenous tricortical iliac crest bone graft. Am J Sports Med 2006;34(2):205.

27. Hovelius L, Sandstrom B, Saebo M. One hundred eighteen Bristow-Latarjet repairs for recurrent anterior dislocation of the shoulder prospectively followed for fifteen years: study II—the evolution of dislocation arthropathy. J Shoulder Elbow Surg 2006;15(3):279.

28. Samilson RL, Prieto V. Dislocation arthropathy of the shoulder. J Bone Joint Surg Am 1983;65(4):456.

Glenoid Bone Defects—Open Latarjet with Congruent Arc Modification

Joe F. de Beer, MBChB, MMed(Orth)[a],*,
Christopher Roberts, FRCS(Tr & Orth)[b]

KEYWORDS

• Shoulder • Instability • Latarjet • Bone defects

Recurrent anterior shoulder instability is commonly associated with glenoid bone defects. Significant untreated glenoid bone defects are one cause of failed instability repairs. It is, therefore, important to recognize and treat glenoid bone defects appropriately. The size of the defect together with concomitant pathologies and patient demands determine the significance of the bone loss. When the glenoid bone defect is deemed significant, the authors recommend treating it with the congruent arc modification of the Latarjet procedure.

BONY RECONSTRUCTION OF THE GLENOID

Bony reconstruction of the glenoid was popularized in English-speaking countries after the publication of the Bristow procedure by Helfet[1] in 1958. He described a technique that was taught to him by Rowley Bristow approximately 19 years previously. The technique involved "transplanting the terminal half-inch of the coracoid." This was affixed adjacent to an area of roughened glenoid neck with sutures through a split in the subscapularis. This technique was modified to fixation of the coracoid with a screw. This modification was first described by McMurray[2] in 1961. The technique and results were then published by May in 1970.[3] Only the terminal portion of the coracoid

was used, however. May also described that the stabilizing mechanism of this procedure was attributable to the bracing role played by the conjoined tendon and the subscapularis tendon in abduction and external rotation rather than by the bone block itself.

Michel Latarjet,[4] however, first described his procedure in 1954. Latarjet described affixing the horizontal limb of the coracoid process with a screw flush to the anteroinferior margin of the glenoid, making a horizontal incision through the fibers of the subscapularis.

The Latarjet procedure has undergone some modifications over the years. Patte and Debeyre[5] suggested modifying the procedure by suturing the anterior joint capsule to the stump of the coracoacromial ligament. They termed this the "triple-blocking procedure." The term, *blocking*, is misleading, however, because articular incongruity with this procedure should be avoided to prevent rapid-onset arthropathy.

The triple effect described was as follows. The first effect was the glenoidplasty effect with restoration or lengthening of the glenoid arc. The second effect was the hammock effect of the sling created by the intact lower third of the subscapularis, which is inferiorized by the positioning of the block with its intact conjoint tendon. This is especially evident as the arm is brought into abduction

a Cape Shoulder Institute, 43 Bloulelie Crescent, Cape Town 7505, South Africa
b Ipswich Hospital NHS Trust, Heath Road, Ipswich, Suffolk IP4 5PD, UK
* Corresponding author.
E-mail address: joe@shoulderinstitiute.co.za

Orthop Clin N Am 41 (2010) 407–415
doi:10.1016/j.ocl.2010.02.008
0030-5898/10/$ – see front matter © 2010 Published by Elsevier Inc.

and external rotation. The third effect was the Bankart effect, from resuturing the capsule to the coracoacromial ligament. In addition, the conjoint tendon has a tensioning effect on the inferior part of the subscapularis, adding to the stabilization effect and virtually counteracting the ligamentous laxity, which is often part of the instability.

In order for the coracoid to be used in the manner described by Latarjet, the inferior surface of the coracoid must be decorticated to encourage bony union. Once placed, a graft may need to be contoured with a burr to ensure articular congruity and to prevent articular overhang. It has been shown, although not published, that the radius of curvature of the inferior surface of the coracoid is an excellent match for the radius of curvature of the glenoid. It is, therefore, possible by rotating the coracoid through 90° about the axis to match the 2 surfaces. By removing the pectoralis tendon with a sliver of bone, a ready decorticated surface is obtained for optimum integration of the bone block. These modifications have created the congruent arc Latarjet.

Critical to long-term success of bony reconstruction of the glenoid is optimization of glenohumeral contact forces. Rotation of the coracoid in this modification of the traditional technique has been shown to optimize these contact forces.[6] The optimal position for the graft is flush with the glenoid surface. Grafts placed medially result in increased pressures with high edge loading. Bone grafts placed in a proud position not only increase the peak contact forces anteroinferiorly but also increase the posterosuperior glenoid pressure, indicating a shift posteriorly. An accurately placed graft using this technique should, therefore, minimize the rate of late-onset arthropathy.

PATIENT SELECTION

The Latarjet procedure is generally reserved for patients with significant bone loss. The significance of any glenoid bone loss is dependant, to some degree, on patient demand. There is an inverse relationship between the amount of bone loss tolerated and the demands placed on the shoulder (ie, the higher the demand, the less bone loss that is tolerated). The authors, therefore, feel that even small bony deficiencies in contact athletes are often significant.

Previous work has identified a high failure rate associated with bone loss in contact athletes,[7] leading to the inverted pear glenoid concept. This represents a 25% bone loss of the inferior pole of the glenoid.[8] The effect of sizeable glenoid defects on shoulder instability has been confirmed in cadaveric studies. Itoi and colleagues[9] performed sequential glenoid osteotomies to determine their effect on humeral head translation. They determined that glenoid deficiencies of a width greater 21% of the glenoid length may be best served by restoration of the glenoid arc for reasons of stability and range of movement. The same was found by Yamamoto and colleagues,[10] who performed a biomechanical cadaver study on anterior glenoid defects.

The size of the defect can be determined by CT, MRI, or arthroscopy. Preoperative CT scanning also helps with the operative planning. Although it is most common for the cleavage plane of the bone loss to be perpendicular to the plane of the glenoid, this is not always the case. If the cleavage plane is shallower, then it may be necessary to burr this flat or modify the pectoralis minor osteotomy to compensate.

Balg and Boileau[11] have provided a useful index to further clarify the decision-making process as to who would most likely benefit from a Latarjet procedure. The instability severity index score takes into account 6 significant preoperative factors: age under 20 (2 points), competitive sports (2 points), contact or forced overhead activity (1 point), anterior or inferior hyperlaxity (1 point), and on the anteroposterior radiograph a visible Hill-Sachs lesion in external rotation (2 points) and loss of normal inferior glenoid contour (2 points). A score of 3 or less is associated with a recurrence rate of 5% with arthroscopic stabilization and 6 or less with a 10% recurrence rate; with a score greater than 6, the recurrence rate escalates to 70%. The investigators suggested that a patient with a score of more than 6 is better served by open surgery (ie, a Latarjet procedure).

An arthroscopic evaluation provides invaluable information that may prove crucial to the final decision as to which procedure to perform if the other evaluations, especially the static imaging results, are inconclusive. If a patient has a moderate Hill-Sachs with small glenoid bone loss but the Hill-Sachs engages (**Fig. 1**) on air arthroscopy, then a Latarjet is more appropriate than a soft tissue arthroscopic reconstruction.

The Latarjet procedure, however, is not a panacea. It is not a substitute for sound clinical judgment. Patients with multidirectional instability, muscle patterning, and voluntary dislocators are not suitable for this procedure.

TECHNIQUE

The patient is placed in a beach chair position and brought to the edge of the table, or a table with a shoulder cutout is used. The scapula must be

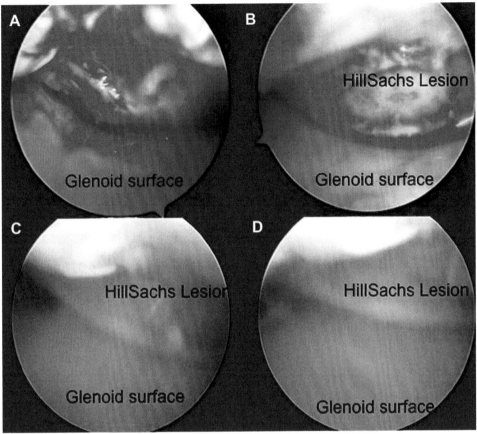

Fig. 1. Intraoperative view of a right shoulder. (*A* and *B*) Air arthroscopy. (*A*) In engaged position. (*C* and *D*) After infusion of saline solution, due to the distension of the capsule, the engaging position cannot be reached anymore. (*From* de Beer JF, Roberts CP, Huijsmans P. Anterior shoulder instability in the elite athlete. Shoulder & Elbow 2010;2:63–70; with permission.)

well supported but overprotracting the scapula avoided because this makes exposure and graft positioning and fixation more difficult. The head is supported and the arm is draped free.

An examination of the shoulder is performed to confirm the degree of anterior laxity. Any posterior laxity and laxity of the other shoulder are also noted.

An initial arthroscopic evaluation of the shoulder is performed. The arthroscope is introduced through a standard posterior portal and a 20-mL syringe is connected to the inflow tap on the scope and 20 to 40 mL of air is introduced into the joint. The joint is examined arthroscopically and special attention is paid to the glenoid, anterior labrum (Bankart lesion), and degree of bone loss. The humeral head is examined for the Hill-Sachs lesion, and if the latter is difficult to view, the arm is externally rotated. Most importantly, the absence or presence of a humeral avulsion of the glenohumeral ligaments (HAGL) lesion is noted. The arm is then moved into abduction and external rotation and the Hill-Sachs lesion is followed to

note if engagement of the defect takes place over the edge of the glenoid (see **Fig. 1**). This dynamic view is one of the most decisive factors to confirm that a deficient articular arc is present and that bone augmentation is indicated.

The scope is then moved to the anterosuperior portal and air is again introduced into the joint because the air pressure may have been lost with the changeover of the scope to the anterior portal. Through this portal the anterior edge of the glenoid can be viewed better than through the posterior portal (**Fig. 2**). Bone loss from the glenoid can be evaluated most accurately from this portal, and it is this view that led the authors to first describe the inverted pear appearance of the glenoid.[7] The glenoid is measured as described by Lo and colleagues.[8] The presence of an HAGL lesion is also best appreciated through the anterior portal.

There are advantages to using air arthroscopy as opposed to viewing with water inflow. The dynamic view of an engaging Hill-Sachs lesion is

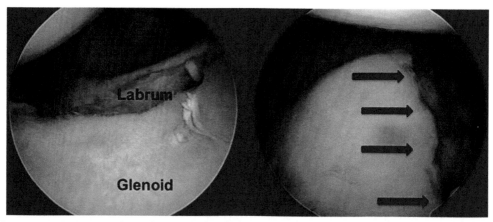

Fig. 2. Intraoperative view of a Left shoulder. (*Left*) Through posterior portal (glenoid seems intact). (*Right*) Through anterosuperior portal; large bony defect (same patient). (*From* de Beer JF, Roberts CP, Huijsmans P. Anterior shoulder instability in the elite athlete. Shoulder & Elbow 2010;2:63–70; with permission.)

best with air; after water is instilled into the joint under pressure, this phenomenon disappears due to the tightening of the capsule from the pressure. Also, if a Latarjet procedure is performed after the scope, tissue swelling from water inflow is avoided.

When a decision is made to proceed with a Latarjet procedure, the patient is reclined to 30° to 40°. With the arm slightly abducted, a low bra-strap incision is made with a wide subcutaneous dissection to the top of the clavicle. This is facilitated by flexing the arm. The conjoint tendon is exposed through the deltopectoral interval and a self-retainer inserted. A lever retractor, such as a glenoid lever, is placed above the coracoid.

The fascial interval between the pectoralis minor and coracobrachialis is opened. In the underlying fatty layer, the musculocutaneous nerve is identified. It is typically found entering the coracobrachialis muscle approximately 4 cm below the tip of the coracoid. The nerve is marked. The identity of the nerve can be checked using a nerve stimulator. It is useful to mark the nerve at this stage because once the coracoid is osteotomized and the surrounding structures detensioned, the nerve is more difficult to identify. The nerve marks the inferior extent of the soft tissue release and mobilization of the coracoid.

The coracoacromial ligament is removed from the lateral side of the coracoid. It is useful to use cutting diathermy for this because the acromial branch of the thoracoacromial trunk is often encountered here.

The pectoralis minor is then removed from the medial side of the coracoid using a sharp chisel (**Fig. 3**). The plane and thickness of this osteotomy are critical to the later glenoid reconstruction. Adequate exposure and premarking of the line of

the osteotomy are critical. The goal is to remove the pectoralis minor tendon with a thin sliver of bone. The bone sliver should be slightly thicker inferiorly than superiorly because this increases the contact surface area, inclines the graft correctly, and facilitates screw insertion (**Fig. 4**).

The entire horizontal limb of the coracoid back to the attachment of the coracoclavicular ligaments is available to be osteotomized. The aim is to perform an osteotomy from this point into the elbow of the coracoid (**Fig. 5**). Flexion of the arm again facilitates best coracoid exposure for the osteotomy. Through a low bra-strap incision it is not possible to use a saw for the osteotomy. A sharp curved osteotome is used for this purpose.

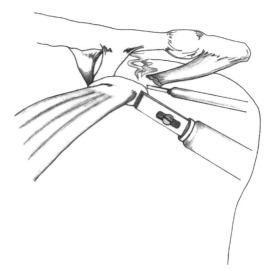

Fig. 3. On the medial side of the coracoid, the pectoralis minor is detached with a silver of bone and laterally the coracoacromial ligament is detached with eletrocautery.

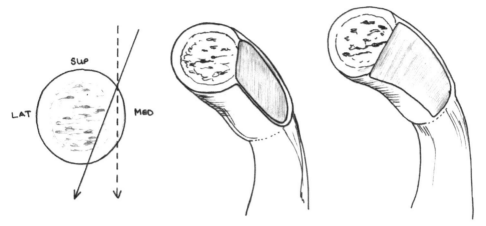

Fig. 4. The surface of the area on the coracoid to be applied to the glenoid neck can be enlarged by cutting it obliquely (based on the concavity of the coracoid).

The coracoid is then released from the remaining soft tissue attachments and mobilized. If the osteotomy is not perfect and a spike from the inferior surface is attached, it is removed at this stage. The coracoid is then predrilled with 2 parallel 2.5-mm holes. The drill holes should be made from closer to the convex side laterally into the center of the contact area. This keeps the screw heads further from the articular surface and keeps the exit drill holes and tips of the screws further from the suprascapular nerve (**Fig. 6**). To make the holes easily visible for later use, they are marked and cleared of soft tissue with cutting diathermy. A stay suture is passed through one of the drill holes and the coracoid is then stored in the wound.

The arm is then brought out from the side and rested on a Mayo table in abduction. A split is then made through the subscapularis at the junction of its superior and middle thirds. Anterior subluxation of the humeral head often makes this exposure difficult. It is, therefore, advantageous to have an assistant hold the head reduced while

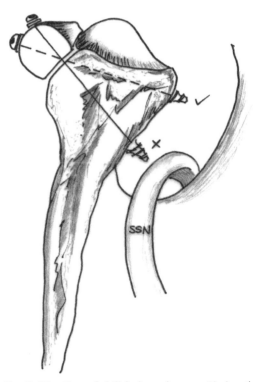

Fig. 6. Direction of drill hole and screw. Aiming the screw too medially endangers the suprascapular nerve in the spinoglenoid notch. It also causes the head of the screw to sit proud of the articular surface. SSN, supra-scapular nerve.

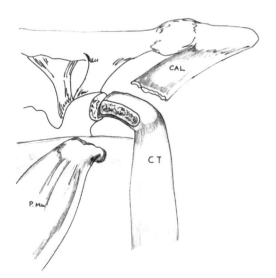

Fig. 5. After detaching the coracoacromial ligament and pectoralis minor, the coracoid is detached just distal to its vertical part. CAL, coraco-acromial ligament; CT, conjoint tendon.

the split and capsular dissection take place. The split is started through the muscular fibers because the plane between the muscle and the capsule is most easily identified medially. The split is then extended laterally. A common mistake is to split the subscapularis too high or too low, making coracoid positioning difficult (**Fig. 7**). The plane is further developed by pushing a swab under the muscle fibers until it lies medial to the glenoid rim. The capsule must be separated from the subscapularis to the 6-o'clock position inferiorly. The subscapularis split can be held apart using a deep Gelpi retractor, and a Hohmann retractor is placed inferiorly to protect the axillary nerve. A lever retractor is placed medial to the glenoid rim. An alternative approach is to release the upper one-third of the subscapularis from its origin.

The capsule is then released medially. To lengthen the capsule as much as possible, the capsule is elevated subperiosteally from the glenoid neck, elevating with it the labrum. The capsular release must be as far as the 6-o'clock position. The capsulotomy may be extended superiorly to make an L shape (**Fig. 8**). The exposure is completed by inserting a humeral head retractor into the joint.

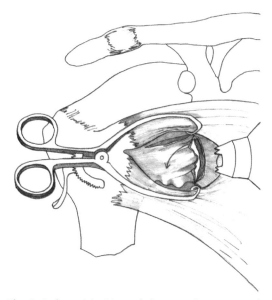

Fig. 8. L-shaped incision of the capsule. Arrow indicates the direction the capsular flap is retracted to reveal the gleno-humeral joint.

To facilitate anatomic reconstruction of the glenoid and optimize union rates, the bed of the bone loss must be made flat and decorticated. This may be accomplished with a rasp or high-speed burr (**Fig. 9**). The next stage is the most critical step. Optimum exposure is critical to allow for accurate placement of the coracoid. The coracoid is then retrieved and rotated about its long axis. The concavity of the coracoid is lined up with the joint surface. It must be placed flush with or slightly medial to the glenoid rim using a bone holder (**Fig. 10**), ensuring that the inferior part of the graft also overlies bone and is not placed too inferior. A standard 2.5-mm drill is inserted through the inferior drill hole and left in situ to stabilize the graft

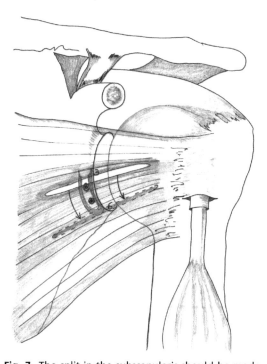

Fig. 7. The split in the subscapularis should be made at the level of the junction of the superior third and middle third—this leads the horizontal split to the 3-o'clock position on the neck of the glenoid. If the split is made too inferiorly, it leads to below the inferior pole of the glenoid. Arrows indicate direction of displacement of inferior 2/3rds of subscapularis.

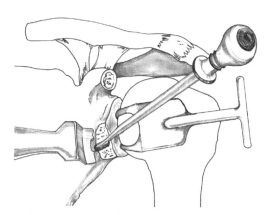

Fig. 9. The rasp is used to prepare the glenoid neck for attachment of the coracoid graft.

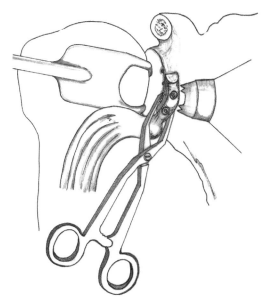

Fig. 10. Coracoid: the coracoid bone clamp holding the coracoid in place for drilling and inserting the screws.

while the next hole is drilled. A long 2.5-mm drill is then placed through the superior hole, removed, and the drill hole measured. A partially threaded 4-mm small fragment screw is then inserted finger tight. The inferior drill then is removed and exchanged for a similar screw. The screws can then be alternately tightened. During screw insertion, ensure that the screw is engaging the glenoid because if it does not it may elevate the graft causing it to crack. If it is difficult to engage the glenoid, cannulated screws may be used. Washers may be used but not if they protrude above the joint surface.

Two or 3 suture anchors are placed on the edge of the original glenoid around the screws and used to repair the capsule, thus placing the graft in an extra-articular position (**Figs. 11** and **12**).

The subscapularis split is not closed. The pectoralis minor can be reattached to the coracoid stump using a screw-in anchor into the osteotomy site with the aim of maximizing functional recovery (**Fig. 13**). Although this restores the anatomy, in those cases in which this is not performed, no functional deficit has been discernible.

POSTOPERATIVE REHABILITATION

Patients tend to have little pain after the procedure and the authors perform it as an outpatient procedure. Owing to lack of damage to the subscapularis and lengthening of the capsule, there is no soft tissue repair to protect postoperatively and the rehabilitation can be accelerated. Return to activity and ultimately sport is only limited by the rate of bony union of the coracoid block. Contact athletes are usually advised to return to full activity at 3 months. At present, research is being undertaken into CT techniques to determine the exact time of bony union of the coracoid graft to the edge of the glenoid—once that is demonstrated, it is safe to allow players back to their full activities.

Range of motion with the hand in vision, thus avoiding abduction and external rotation, is encouraged from day 1. The sling is used only for comfort and usually discarded in the first couple of weeks. Early rehabilitation and gym work, not placing undue strain on the bone graft, is started when discomfort allows. Noncontact ball work is allowed from 8 weeks with return to full contact after 3 months.

RESULTS

The results of this modification of the Latarjet procedure for shoulder instability associated with an inverted pear glenoid (bone loss of at least 25% of the width of the inferior glenoid) or an engaging Hill-Sachs lesion have been previously reported.[12] From March 1996 to December 2002,

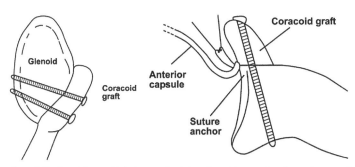

Fig. 11. Coracoid is placed flush with or slightly medical to glenoid margin. Capsular repair results in the graft being extra-articular.

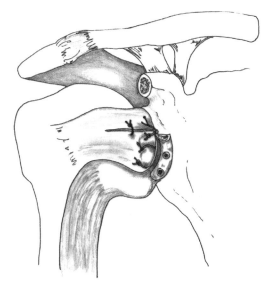

Fig. 12. The capsule is reattached to the edge of the glenoid with bone anchors and the horizontal split repaired, thus placing the coracoid in an extra-articular position.

102 patients underwent an open Latarjet procedure for shoulder instability with significant bone loss, 47 of whom were available for follow-up physical examination. The remaining 55 patients were contacted by telephone or letter to see if they had had recurrent dislocation or subluxation. The mean age of the patients was 26.5. Of the patients available for physical examination, there

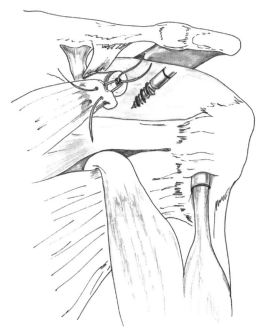

Fig. 13. An anchor into the stump of the coracoid is used to reattach the *pectoralis* minor.

were 46 male patients and 1 female patient. The mean follow-up time was 59 months. The postoperative functional scores were a mean Constant score of 94.4 and a mean Walch-Duplay score of 91.7. Five of the 102 who underwent this modification of the Latarjet procedure had a recurrence (4 dislocations and 1 subluxation), representing a 4.9% recurrence rate. There were no cases of infection or neurologic injury in this series.

COMPLICATIONS

Although this is a technically demanding procedure, complications are rare. The key to avoiding complications is meticulous attention to detail.

Nerve injuries are rare—specifically, musculocutaneous nerve injury is preventable by early nerve identification, allowing for safe coracoid mobilization and preventing undue tension on the nerve after coracoid transplantation. Rare cases of neurapraxia usually resolve over time without specific intervention.

Soft tissue complications similarly can be avoided. Subscapularis rupture is unlikely with this technique because the tendon (and muscle) are split rather than tenotomized.

Failure of the coracoid to unite is relatively uncommon. In the series of 160 Latarjet-Bristow procedures reported by Walch and Boileau,[13] pseudarthrosis of the coracoid process occurred in 2.4% of cases. Banas and colleagues[14] reported an 82% union rate with 14% fibrous unions.

Screw breakage or coracoid displacement occurs rarely and usually relates to overaggressive rehabilitation, especially early return to contact sports. Walch and Boileau[13] reported fracture of the coracoid process in 2.4% of cases, always occurring within 3 months of surgery as a result of intraoperative overtightening of the screws. In their series, neither pseudarthrosis nor coracoid fracture had a statistical influence on the clinical result. Union of the coracoid using this modified technique is maximized by ensuring maximum surface area, decortication of the bony surfaces, and compression by using partially threaded screws.

Partial resorption of the coracoid occurs in 9% of patients. If bony resorption involves greater than two-thirds of the coracoid, persistent apprehension and decreased athletic participation have been reported.[13]

Recurrent instability, which in this demanding category of patients has previously been reported as high with arthroscopic soft tissue repair, is between 1% and 5%.[12,13]

Range of motion is well preserved after this procedure and in particular external rotation is not as limited as it is after other open procedures. The loss of external rotation in the series previously reported[12] was only 5°. Others have reported greater loss of range of motion.[14] Maximizing capsular length with this technique is probably responsible for the preservation of external rotation.

Arthrosis is a concern after this procedure but there are currently no long-term follow-up data for this modification of the Latarjet procedure. Published data are largely for the modified Bristow procedure; arthrosis rates in some series are high and usually relate to malpositioning of the graft. Allain and colleagues[15] reported malpositioning in 35 of 58 (58%) coracoid transfers in their series. Hovelius and colleagues[16] reported on a series of 118 patients at 15 years' follow-up. When all radiographic views were included, moderate or severe dislocation arthropathy was found in 14% of the shoulders and a further 35% had mild arthropathy. The authors believe that because this procedure results in optimized glenohumeral contact forces, the arthropathy rates for this procedure may be lower.

Infection is rare but should be considered in cases of ongoing and otherwise unexplainable pain in the perioperative period.

Occasionally there is need to remove the screws in cases of persistent pain and symptoms. If the screws are too long, they can be associated with posterior shoulder pain. More rarely, prominent screw heads or washers anteriorly necessitate removal.

SALVAGE SURGERY

If the Latarjet procedure fails, then the available options depend on the integrity of the coracoid block. In acute failures where the coracoid block is intact, reattachment of the bone is possible in some cases. When failures occur later, however, particularly when they are caused by coracoid resorption, then another source of bone graft is required. The most common procedure used in this circumstance is the Eden-Hybinette procedure, where a piece of iliac crest is used in place of the coracoid.

REFERENCES

1. Helfet AJ. Coracoid transplantation for recurring dislocation of the shoulder. J Bone Joint Surg Br 1958;40:198–202.

2. McMurray TB. Recurrent dislocation of the shoulder (proceedings). J Bone Joint Surg Br 1961;43:402–5.

3. May VR. A modified Bristow operation for anterior recurrent dislocation of the shoulder. J Bone Joint Surg Am 1970;52:1010–6.

4. Latarjet M. A propos du traitement des luxations récidivantes de l'épaule. Lyon Chir 1954;49:994–1003.

5. Patte D, Debeyre J. Luxations recidivantes de l'epaule. Paris-Technique chirurgicale. Orthopedie. Encycl Med Chir 1980;44265:44–52.

6. Ghodadra N, Shewman E, Goldstein J, et al. Normalization of glenohumeral articular contact pressures after either Latarjet or iliac crest bone grafting procedure: impact of graft type, position, and coracoid orientation. J Bone Joint Surg Am, in press.

7. Burkhart SS, De Beer JF. Traumatic glenohumeral bone defects and their relationship to failure of arthroscopic Bankart repairs: significance of the inverted-pear glenoid and the humeral engaging Hill-Sachs lesion. Arthroscopy 2000; 16(7):677–94.

8. Lo IK, Parten PM, Burkhart SS. The inverted pear glenoid: an indicator of significant glenoid bone loss. Arthroscopy 2004;20(2):169–74.

9. Itoi E, Lee SB, Berglund LJ, et al. The effect of a glenoid defect on anteroinferior stability of the shoulder after Bankart repair: a cadaveric study. J Bone Joint Surg Am 2000;82(1):35–46.

10. Yamamoto N, Itoi E, Abe H, et al. Effect of an anterior glenoid defect on anterior shoulder stability: a cadaveric study. Am J Sports Med 2009;37(5): 949–54.

11. Balg F, Boileau P. The instability severity index score. A simple pre-operative score to select patients for arthroscopic or open shoulder stabilisation. J Bone Joint Surg Br 2007;89(11):1470–7.

12. Burkhart SS, De Beer JF, Barth JR, et al. Results of modified Latarjet reconstruction in patients with anteroinferior instability and significant bone loss. Arthroscopy 2007;23(10):1033–41.

13. Walch G, Boileau P. Latarjet-Bristow procedure for recurrent anterior instability. Tech Shoulder Elbow Surg 2000;1:256–61.

14. Banas MP, Dalldorf PG, Sebastianelli WJ, et al. Long-term followup of the modified Bristow procedure. Am J Sports Med 1993;21(5):666–71.

15. Allain J, Goutallier D, Glorion C. Long-term results of the Latarjet procedure for the treatment of anterior instability of the shoulder. J Bone Joint Surg Am 1998;80(6):841–52.

16. Hovelius L, Sandström B, Saebö M. One hundred eighteen Bristow-Latarjet repairs for recurrent anterior dislocation of the shoulder prospectively followed for fifteen years: study II-the evolution of dislocation arthropathy. J Shoulder Elbow Surg 2006;15(3):279–89.

Humeral Head Bone Defects: Remplissage, Allograft, and Arthroplasty

Marshal S. Armitage, MD, FRCSC[a],
Kenneth J. Faber, MD, MHPE, FRCSC[a],
Darren S. Drosdowech, MD, FRCSC[a],
Robert B. Litchfield, MD, FRCSC[b],
George S. Athwal, MD, FRCSC[a],*

KEYWORDS

- Hill-Sachs • Remplissage • Instability
- Bone defect • Shoulder

Traumatic unidirectional glenohumeral joint instability is common and typically occurs in conjunction with labral or capsular injury; however, it can also be associated with bony lesions. Successful treatment requires recognition of all aspects of simple and complex instability to determine the most appropriate treatment algorithm. Management of glenohumeral instability includes nonoperative rehabilitation, soft-tissue repair or reconstruction, osseous reconstruction, or prosthetic replacement. This review outlines treatment options to restore or reconstruct osseous anatomy and shoulder stability in patients with humeral head bone defects.

In the nineteenth century, Flower[1] and Broca and Hartmann[2] described a posterior superior humeral head defect sustained after glenohumeral joint dislocation. In 1941, Hill and Sachs[3] further described the eponymous lesion of humeral articular impaction that resulted from contact with the dense cortical bone of the anterior inferior glenoid rim during anterior subcoracoid dislocation. Palmer and Widén[4] and Burkhart and DeBeer[5] described an engaging Hill-Sachs lesion that occurs when the glenoid falls into the humeral head defect. To truly engage, the long axis of the humeral head defect must be parallel to the anterior glenoid rim with the arm in a position of abduction and external rotation. Engagement outside of this functional arc, with the arm at the side for example, is termed nonfunctional engagement or functionally nonengaging. If the humeral defect is not parallel to the glenoid rim, it may provide a sensation of subluxation when the lesion rolls over the anterior glenoid, but the rim will not fall into the defect and lever the humeral head from the glenoid socket.

Anterior inferior glenoid bone loss and engaging Hill-Sachs lesions have been implicated as factors leading to higher failure rates following soft-tissue stabilization procedures.[5–8] Although osseous lesions are recognized factors associated with shoulder instability, there is little information describing surgical indications and optimal techniques to restore osseous anatomy and joint stability.

EPIDEMIOLOGY

Humeral head impression fractures are found in 65% to 71% of initial glenohumeral dislocations,[9,10]

a Department of Orthopedic Surgery, St Joseph's Health Care, HULC, University of Western Ontario, 268 Grosvenor Street, London, Ontario, N6A 4L6, Canada
b Department of Orthopedic Surgery, Fowler-Kennedy Sports Medicine Clinic, 3M Centre, University of Western Ontario, London, Ontario, N6A 3K7, Canada
* Corresponding author.
E-mail address: gathwal@uwo.ca

Orthop Clin N Am 41 (2010) 417–425
doi:10.1016/j.ocl.2010.03.004
0030-5898/10/$ – see front matter © 2010 Elsevier Inc. All rights reserved.

orthopedic.theclinics.com

and in up to 100% of patients with recurrent instability.[7] A correlation between the presence of humeral head lesions and bony Bankart lesions exists and increases with recurrent instability. In a study of 61 patients, Widjaja and colleagues[11] found that after a first dislocation, 64% of patients with a bony Bankart lesion also had a Hill-Sachs, and 70% of those with a Hill-Sachs lesion also had a Bankart lesion. Seventy-nine percent of patients with recurrent instability and a bony Bankart lesion also had a Hill-Sachs, and 81% of those with a Hill-Sachs had a bony Bankart lesion.

IMAGING AND ANATOMY

Hill and Sachs[3] attributed the humeral impression fracture to the impact of the posterior humeral head onto the dense cortical bone of the anterior glenoid rim. They described the compression of softer cancellous bone of the humeral head as a radiographically discernable line of increased radiodensity along the medial wall of the lesion. The best technique for visualizing the defect has been debated. Reports have evaluated the integrity of the posterolateral humeral head with an internally rotated anteroposterior radiograph of the shoulder, an apical oblique view of Garth and colleagues,[12] a Stryker notch view, a modified Didiee view,[13] and through use of orthographic projection as described by Ito and colleagues.[14] The Ito technique produces an undistorted image of the posterolateral notch by positioning the patient supine with the arm in 135° of flexion and 15° of internal rotation with the cassette directly under the shoulder joint and the central x-ray beam angled vertically through the humeral head.

The size and location of the lesion are important factors to consider when assessing the degree of instability and the risk of engagement of the defect on the glenoid rim during humeral abduction and external rotation. It is theorized that the size of a lesion is related to the force of the injury and the extent of joint laxity of the shoulder. A deep defect is more common following 2 or more dislocations, whereas patients with recurrent subluxations and apprehension following a dislocation are more likely to have a shallow lesion.[14] A possible explanation for this observation is that greater force is required to dislocate a stable shoulder and a larger defect in the humerus results. However, less force is required to precipitate instability in individuals with ligament laxity and less impaction of the humeral head occurs.

Cross-sectional imaging is routinely used to evaluate humeral bone loss. Two-dimensional axial, sagittal, and coronal oblique reconstructions help to quantify the size and location of a defect, especially if it seems to involve greater than 20% of the humeral head. In a computerized tomography (CT) study, Saito and colleagues[15] reported that Hill-Sachs lesions exist from 0 to 24 mm from the top of the humeral head, oriented from 6:46 cephalad to 8:56 caudal on a clock face with 12:00 defined as the intertubercular sulcus. The caudal extent is not to be mistaken for the bare spot or natural humeral groove that is regularly found between 19 and 21 mm from the top of the humeral head in the same location.[16] Yamamoto and colleagues[17] proposed the glenoid track as the zone of glenoid contact on the posterior humeral head from inferiormedial to superiorlateral, and postulated that a Hill-Sachs lesion extending medial to this area would likely engage the glenoid rim and risk recurrent dislocation. They defined the glenoid track as the region on the humeral head that begins at the rotator cuff insertion site on the greater tuberosity and extends medially on the humeral head for a distance equal to 84% of the glenoid width. Any anterior glenoid bone loss will reduce the glenoid width, increase the likelihood that the humeral defect is located medial to the glenoid track, and increase the risk of engagement and redislocation. When the humeral lesion is located medial to the glenoid track, Bankart repair alone may be insufficient to prevent lesion re-engagement. Thus, factors affecting the influence of a Hill-Sachs lesion on glenohumeral stability include the size, location, and orientation of the humeral defect but also the amount of anterior glenoid bone loss.

Miniaci and Gish[18] recommend three-dimensional reconstructions of the bony anatomy to better map the size, location, and especially the orientation of humeral bone loss. He notes that the humeral defects are often oblique to the axial plane and thus not well represented and often underappreciated with two-dimensional imaging.

Ultrasound has also been successfully used to image Hill-Sachs lesion. Cicak and colleagues[19] prospectively showed sonography to be 96% sensitive, 100% specific, and 97% accurate in diagnosing Hill-Sachs lesions compared with surgical findings in 61 patients with average lesions 19.2 mm long, 16.0 mm wide, and 4.1 mm deep. However, the diagnostic value of ultrasound may be lessened by the challenges associated with accurately identifying the lesion location and orientation.

Magnetic resonance imaging (MRI) is often used as an alternative to CT to assess osseous deformity when additional soft-tissue pathologies such as rotator cuff injuries, chondral defects, labral tears, and capsular laxity are suspected.

CLASSIFICATION

Rowe and colleagues[8] categorized humeral lesions according to size, as follows: mild, 2×0.3 cm; moderate, 4×0.5 cm; severe, 4×1 cm or larger. In their series of solely Bankart repairs, recurrence rates were 0/30 (0%) for mild lesions, 3/64 (4.7%) for moderate, and 1/16 (6%) for severe. From these data, Rowe and colleagues[8] recommended that severe lesions be addressed surgically because those shoulders were at risk for recurrent dislocation.

The size of the defect can also be calculated as a percentage loss of articular length relative to the entire humeral articular surface. General guidelines for surgical treatment based on percentage of articular involvement have been developed based on these criteria.[20]

INDICATIONS

The indications for humeral head reconstruction are controversial. Kropf and Sekiya[21] proposed that recreating normal humeral articular length would reduce tension on anterior capsulolabral structures and protect a Bankart repair. However, many[20,22] consider humeral reconstruction secondary or even superfluous to anterior inferior glenoid bone grafting for recurrent instability. Traditionally, Hill-Sachs lesions have been corrected only after failure of a primary soft-tissue stabilizing procedure. More recently, surgical reconstruction of a humeral defect is advocated as a primary procedure when patients experience ongoing symptomatic shoulder instability including painful apprehension, popping, or catching accompanied by a significant (>25% of the humeral head) engaging bone defect or a defect medial to the glenoid track.[18] Patients at high risk for surgical failure, such as contact athletes or those with seizure disorders, may benefit from early primary humeral head reconstruction. More importantly, Grondin and Leith[23] stress that the surgeon should be prepared to address glenoid and humeral bone loss when preoperative CT examination reveals more than 30% surface loss of each. Despite these recommendations, there have been no definitive studies defining the specific size, location, or orientation of a lesion that must be addressed surgically. Whether patients require surgical treatment of the humeral head alone, in conjunction with anterior reconstruction, or not at all for unidirectional anterior shoulder instability with associated humeral bone loss has yet to be clearly defined.

SURGICAL TREATMENT OPTIONS

Treatment options to reconstruct symptomatic Hill-Sachs lesions can be broadly categorized into 4 groups. The defect may be disimpacted, filled with soft tissue or allograft bone, rotated away, or partially or completely replaced.

Humeralplasty/Disimpaction

The technique for acutely elevating an impaction fracture without significantly altering normal anatomic structures has been termed humeralplasty.[24] In a cadaveric study, Kazel and colleagues[24] described a technique to reduce the volume of freshly created humeral defects using curved bone tamps inserted retrograde through a distal cortical window. One year later, Re and colleagues[25] reported a humeralplasty technique performed on 4 patients in whom the lesion was localized using an anterior cruciate ligament (ACL) drill guide, elevated with retrograde tamping and filled with cancellous bone graft. Three patients were also treated with anterior capsulolabral reconstruction, and the fourth patient underwent a concomitant Latarjet procedure. There were no recurrences or other complications at 1 year follow-up. Although Re and colleagues[25] did not specifically comment on the acuity of their cohort, humeralplasty is likely most reproducible and beneficial following an acute injury. An advantage of this technique is the ability to restore the normal proximal humeral geometry without internal fixation or extensive surgical alteration of normal anatomy (**Fig. 1**). There is scant information on the indications and outcomes of this technique,

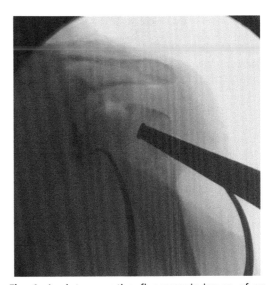

Fig. 1. An intraoperative fluoroscopic image of an acute disimpaction of a moderate-sized Hill-Sachs lesion after open reduction and internal fixation of an associated anterior glenoid rim fracture.

but general guidelines for humeralplasty include defects that are less than 3 weeks old and involve less than 45% of the humeral articular surface.[26]

Remplissage

Remplissage, which means filling in French, refers to the insetting of the infraspinatus tendon and posterior capsule into the Hill-Sachs lesion.[27] The lesion is filled with soft tissue and converted to an extra-articular lesion incapable of engaging with the glenoid. The procedure initially involves preparation and repair of the associated anterior labral lesion. To conduct the remplissage procedure, the Hill-Sachs lesion is viewed with the camera placed through an anterior portal. Superior and inferior suture anchors, inserted percutaneously or through a posterior cannula, are placed into the bony defect. A sharp penetrating device is used to create horizontal mattress sutures through the infraspinatus and joint capsule. These sutures are then tied in the subdeltoid space, which secures the infraspinatus and posterior capsule to the Hill-Sachs lesion, thereby filling the bony defect. To facilitate suture tying, the subdeltoid space may be cleared before suture passage (**Fig. 2**).

Purchase and colleagues[28] reported a recurrence rate of 7% (2 of 24), no complications, and no loss of shoulder motion in any plane following remplissage. Both recurrences occurred following traumatic incidents. As Connolley[29] noted in a review of 15 patients treated with open infraspinatus and posterior capsule filling of large Hill-Sachs lesions, maximum stabilization occurs as a result of forced restriction of humeral gliding on the glenoid but not humeral rotation. However, Deutsch and Kroll[27] reported 1 case of significant external rotation restriction following remplissage that was alleviated after takedown of the fixating sutures. In this case, the preoperative external rotation of 70° was reduced to 45° postoperatively despite a 2-year course of physical therapy. In 90° abduction, there was 90° external rotation that sustained obligate internal rotation with the impact of the tenodesed infraspinatus on the posterior glenoid during adduction, again causing a firm limit of 45° external rotation with the arm at the side. The remplissage procedure has several advantages. The procedure can be performed in acute and chronic scenarios, and it can be preformed arthroscopically and without interruption of

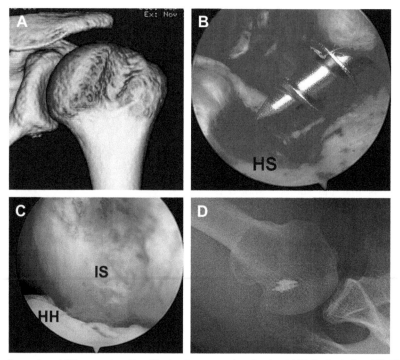

Fig. 2. A three-dimensional CT reconstruction illustrating a moderate-sized Hill-Sachs lesion (*A*). The patient was managed with arthroscopic Bankart repair and remplissage. An arthroscopic image (*B*) with the camera placed through the anterior portal visualizing the Hill-Sachs defect and a suture anchor being inserted percutaneously through the infraspinatus tendon. The sutures, once tied in the subdeltoid space, inset the infraspinatus tendon and posterior joint capsule into the Hill-Sachs defect (*C, D*). HH, humeral head; HS, Hill-Sachs; IS, infraspinatus.

a previous anterior repair or reconstruction. In contrast, remplissage is a nonanatomic technique that can lead to restrictions in motion and provocation of instability in other directions. Further studies on indications, outcomes, and the biomechanical effects of this technique are needed.

Allograft Reconstruction

Osteoarticular allograft reconstruction of the humeral head can also be performed to prevent symptomatic engagement of a Hill-Sachs lesion. Structural allograft replacement has been described for posterior locked dislocations with associated bone loss[30,31] and recurrent anterior instability.[32] Yagishita and Thomas,[32] Kropf and Sekiya,[21] and Chapovsky and Kelly[33] each reported a single case of allograft reconstruction of humeral head defects. Yagishita and Thomas used structural femoral allograft for a large, deep lesion (4 × 2 × 2.5 cm), whereas Kropf and Sekiya and Chapovsky and Kelly used a mosaicplasty technique with humeral head allograft to restore humeral head anatomy. In each case, internal fixation was not used and all patients maintained joint stability and had no evidence of graft resorption at 1 to 2 years follow-up.

Miniaci and colleagues[18] produced the most comprehensive report on the use of allograft for reconstruction of humeral head defects. They reported on 18 cases treated with fresh frozen or irradiated humeral head structural osteoarticular allografts. All patients had failed previous instability repairs and had defects involving greater than 25% of the humeral head. Partial graft collapse occurred in 2 of 18, early evidence of osteoarthritis in 3, and mild posterior subluxation in 1 patient. Two patients complained of pain in external rotation that resolved after hardware removal. At an average of 50 months follow-up, the Western Ontario Shoulder Instability (WOSI) index,[34] a validated, disease-specific quality-of-life measurement tool for those with shoulder instability, had improved. The average constant score was 78.5, 89% had returned to work, and there were no reported incidents of recurrent instability.

Specific indications for allograft reconstruction that have been outlined for posterior dislocations[33] may also apply to anterior instability with Hill-Sachs lesions. These include young patients with large defects in their humeral heads without osteoporosis or degenerative joint disease. Osteoporotic bone may not reliably support allograft, leading to collapse and redislocation, and the presence of arthritis is more appropriately treated with an arthroplasty.[30] Further advantages of allograft reconstruction of Hill-Sachs lesions include anatomic repair that theoretically allows for improved motion and stability.

Tjoumakaris and colleagues[35] described a case of primary combined anterior glenoid and humeral head allograft reconstruction in a 19-year-old male marine 3-time dislocator with 30% humeral bone loss and painful apprehension at 60° of external rotation. By addressing the humeral head defect and the anterior inferior glenoid bone deficiency, a near anatomic glenohumeral arc of motion was retained, allowing this high-demand patient to regain motion and return to a high level of activity without recurrent instability at short-term follow-up. This procedure is in contrast to that of Kropf and Sekiya[21] who advocated a staged approach to humerus and glenoid surgery. They argued that addressing the humeral lesion from a limited posterior approach prevents compromise of the anterior reconstruction, avoids excessive humeral head rotation and retraction, and minimizes vascular insult. Another advantage of a staged procedure is the ability to determine graft size based on an arthroscopic evaluation of defect engagement, size, and shape.

The authors typically conduct humeral head allograft reconstruction through an anterior approach (**Fig. 3**). A side-matched and size-matched allograft humeral head is used because it is usually a better fit than a femoral head or a contralateral humeral head graft. Fixation of the structural graft may be conducted antegrade or retrograde. The advantage of retrograde compression screw fixation from the intact metaphyseal segment into the graft allows easier removal of hardware if the graft resorbs and the hardware becomes prominent. Hardware removal can be conducted through a limited approach rather than re-entering the shoulder joint, potentially compromising a successful stabilization surgery.

Rotational Osteotomy

Although numerous studies have been published on proximal humeral rotational osteotomy for the treatment of Hill-Sachs–associated shoulder instability in the German literature,[36–39] there are few reports in English language journals.[38,39] According to Weber and colleagues,[40] the primary indication for a rotational osteotomy was an active young patient with recurrent instability and a moderate to severe Hill-Sachs lesion on the Rowe scale (>4.0 cm long and 0.5 cm deep). The technique, initially described for the late treatment of perinatal brachial plexus palsy, involves a subcapital humeral osteotomy with 25° medial rotation of the humeral head and imbrication of the subscabularis and anterior capsule. The technique

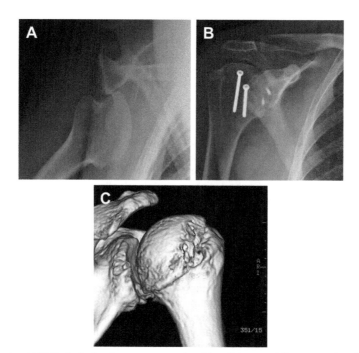

Fig. 3. A moderate-sized Hill-Sachs lesion in a recurrent shoulder dislocator (*A*) managed with side-matched and size-matched humeral head osteochondral allograft (*B*) via an anterior deltopectoral approach. (*C*) Follow-up three-dimensional CT shows articular reconstruction with graft healing.

prevents engagement by limiting external rotation of the joint while preserving external rotation of the arm through the osteotomy.

Weber and colleagues[40] reviewed the results of 180 rotational osteotomies performed at a mean age of 29.5 years during a 14-year period from 1967 to 1981 and found a 5.7% redislocation rate. However, of 207 patients, a combined rotational osteotomy and Bankart repair was performed only 3 times. They reported 162 patients (90%) with good to excellent results on the Rowe scale. Complications requiring reoperation included 2 patients (1%) with recurrent instability, 6 patients (3%) with delayed or nonunion, 2 patients (1%) needing early manipulation under anesthesia to regain motion, and 1 patient (0.5%) with over-rotation

of the osteotomy. In 7 (3.9%) patients, a loss of more than 10° of external rotation or abduction was documented. All athletes in the series returned to previous levels of function, including 14 professionals.

Partial Resurfacing

Partial resurfacing has not been widely reported as a solution for humeral head defects in shoulder instability. This technique uses a round caplike cobalt-chrome articular component to fill the Hill-Sachs lesion and reestablish joint congruity, thus preventing defect engagement. There are multiple sizes and offsets to reproduce the widely varying geometry of the humeral head and the defect (**Fig. 4**).

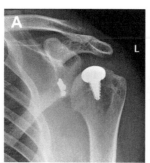
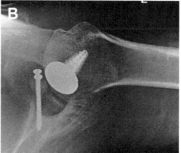

Fig. 4. Partial humeral head resurfacing used to manage a moderate-sized engaging Hill-Sachs lesion (*A, B*).

In 2009, Grondin and Leith[23] and Moros and Ahmad[41] detailed their techniques of focal humeral arthroplasty to regain stability of the shoulder. Grondin and Leith[23] reported on 2 patients with estimated humeral defects of 40% and inverted pear glenoids with 33% bone loss. In each case the HemiCAP (Arthrosurface, Franklin, MA) implant alone did not provide sufficient stability and a Latarjet-style coracoid transfer to reconstruct the glenoid defect was also performed. Each patient had an improved WOSI index and neither had recurrence or motion loss at 1-year follow-up. Moros and Ahmad[41] used a similar technique to restore stability in a patient with multiple dislocations following an open stabilization procedure. At 2-year follow-up, the patient had a stable pain-free shoulder and had returned to work.

The advantages of a partial resurfacing, as listed by Grondin and Leith,[23] include absence of donor site morbidity compared with autograft; more accurate contouring, shorter operative time, no associated graft resorption and subsequent hardware removal, and lack of disease transmission. Disadvantages of partial resurfacing for instability as described by Moros and Ahmad[41] include inadequate fixation of the implant, a mismatch between the implant and defect geometry that requires reaming and resurfacing of unaffected humeral cartilage, and an inability to accurately align the surface of the prosthesis with the adjacent articular surface.

Complete Resurfacing/Hemiarthroplasty

Although classic teaching and management algorithms designate humeral hemiarthroplasty or total shoulder arthroplasty for humeral articular lesions greater than 40% to 45%,[21] there are few data for this specific population. In an older patient group, osteopenic bone often leads to large defects after dislocation and makes the previously discussed solutions significantly more difficult to conduct successfully. This patient group is also more likely to have preexisting degenerative arthritis and place lesser demands on their shoulders. Therefore, elderly patients with large defects and osteoporotic bone or arthritic shoulders are ideal candidates for hemi- or total arthroplasty (**Fig. 5**). Flatow and colleagues[42] reported on 9 patients (mean age 65 years) treated with arthroplasty (8 total, 1 humeral hemiarthroplasty) for locked chronic anterior dislocations with an average duration of 3 years. Four had humeral lesions greater than 40%, but all had destroyed humeral articular cartilage and 4 required structural glenoid bone grafting. Humeral component retroversion was increased as needed for stability and at 3.9 years follow-up there were 4 excellent and 4 satisfactory results with no patient reporting functional limitation. They reported that the operative group was clearly superior to the 7 nonoperatively managed patients. Pritchett and Clark[43] reported on a similar group. They also reported that increased humeral retroversion, of up to 50°, was needed to achieve a satisfactory, stable, total shoulder arthroplasty.

In younger, active patients there are obvious drawbacks to complete resurfacing that should have the surgeon considering humeralplasty, remplissage, allograft, or focal prosthetic reconstruction. For those young patients with greater than 45% humeral articular defects and disuse osteopenia or early degenerative joint disease, no optimal solution exists. In this instance, the decision between surgical tactics is difficult and there is no good-quality literature to support 1 specific approach.

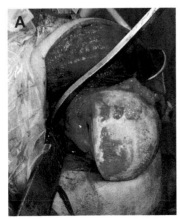
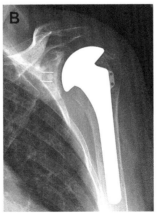

Fig. 5. Cartilage damage and a 40% Hill-Sachs lesion viewed through a deltopectoral approach in a 62-year-old woman (A) managed with a total shoulder arthroplasty (B).

SUMMARY

The Hill-Sachs lesion is a well-known entity that threatens recurrent instability, but the treatment options are multiple and the surgical indications remain undefined. The evidence for each operative technique is limited to retrospective reviews and small case series without controls. Therefore, the decision of which technique to use resides with the comfort level and expertise of the surgeon. However, there are some useful guidelines. Older, osteopenic patients, especially those with underlying arthritis and large defects, should be managed with complete humeral resurfacing. Humeralplasty is best used in younger patients with good-quality bone in an acute setting with small-to moderate-sized bone defects. Partial resurfacing and remplissage are best used with small to moderate lesions, and both require further study. Allograft humeral reconstruction is the workhorse technique for patients with moderate to large defects, and is best applied to nonosteopenic bone. Surgeons must be able to recognize the presence of humeral bone loss via specialized radiographs or cross-sectional imaging and understand its implications as it relates to increased failure of soft-tissue-only stabilization procedures. The techniques to manage humeral bone loss are evolving and further biomechanical and clinical studies are required to define the indications and treatment algorithms.

REFERENCES

1. Flower WH. On the pathological changes produced in the shoulder joint by traumatic dislocation, as derived from an examination of all specimens illustrating this injury in the museums of London. Trans Pathol Soc London 1861;12:179.

2. Broca A, Hartmann H. Contribution à l'étude des luxations de l'épaule. Bull Soc Anat Paris 1890;4: 416–23 [in French].

3. Hill HA, Sachs MD. The groove defect of the humeral head. A frequency unrecognized complication of dislocations of the shoulder joint. Radiology 1940;35:690.

4. Palmer I, Widén A. The bone block method for recurrent dislocation of the shoulder joint. J Bone Joint Surg Br 1948;30:53–8.

5. Burkhart SS, DeBeer JF. Traumatic glenohumeral bone defects and their relationship to failure of arthroscopic Bankart repairs: significance of the inverted-pear glenoid and the humeral engaging Hill-Sachs lesion. Arthroscopy 2000;16:677–94.

6. Flatow EL, Warner JJP. Instability of the shoulder: complex problems and failed repairs. J Bone Joint Surg Am 1998;80:122–40.

7. Taylor D, Arciero R. Pathologic changes associated with shoulder dislocations. Am J Sports Med 1997; 25:306–11.

8. Rowe CR, Zarins B, Ciullo JV. Recurrent anterior dislocation of the shoulder after surgical repair. Apparent causes of failure and treatment. J Bone Joint Surg Am 1984;66:159–68.

9. Calandra J, Baker C, Uribe J. The incidence of Hill-Sachs lesions in initial anterior shoulder dislocations. Arthroscopy 1989;5:254–7.

10. Antonio GE, Griffith JF, Yu AB, et al. First-time shoulder dislocation: high prevalence of labral injury and age-related differences revealed by MR arthrography. J Magn Reson Imaging 2007;26:983–91.

11. Widjaja AB, Tran H, Bailey M, et al. Correlation between Bankart and Hill-Sachs lesions in anterior shoulder dislocation. ANZ J Surg 2006;76:436–8.

12. Garth WP Jr, Slappey CE, Ochs CW. Roentgenographic demonstration of instability of the shoulder: the apical oblique projection. J Bone Joint Surg Am 1984;66:1450–3.

13. Danzig LA, Greenway G, Resnick D. The Hill-Sachs lesion: an experimental study. Am J Sports Med 1980;8:328–32.

14. Ito H, Takayama A, Shirai Y. Radiographic evaluation of the Hill-Sachs lesion in patients with recurrent anterior shoulder instability. J Shoulder Elbow Surg 2000;9:495–7.

15. Saito H, Itio E, Minagawa H, et al. Location of the Hill-Sachs lesion in shoulders with recurrent anterior dislocation. Arch Orthop Trauma Surg 2009 [Epub ahead of print].

16. Richards RD, Sartoris DJ, Pathria MN, et al. Hills Sachs lesion and normal humeral groove: MR imaging features allowing their differentiation. Radiology 1994;190:665–8.

17. Yamamoto N, Itoi E, Abe H, et al. Contact between the glenoid and the humeral head in abduction, external rotation, and horizontal extension: a new concept of glenoid track. J Shoulder Elbow Surg 2007;16:649–56.

18. Miniaci A, Gish M. Management of anterior glenohumeral instability associated with large Hill-Sachs defects. Tech Shoulder Elbow Surg 2004;5:170–5.

19. Cicak N, Bilic R, Delimar D. Hill-Sachs lesion in recurrent shoulder dislocation: sonographic detection. J Ultrasound Med 1998;17(9):557–60.

20. Chen AL, Hunt SA, Hawkins RJ, et al. Management of bone loss associated with recurrent anterior glenohumeral instability. Am J Sports Med 2005;33:912.

21. Kropf EJ, Sekiya JK. Osteoarticular allograft transplantation for large humeral head defects in glenohumeral instability. Arthroscopy 2007;23(3):322.e1–5.

22. Lynch JR, Clinton JM, Dewing CB, et al. Treatment of osseous defects associated with anterior shoulder instability. J Shoulder Elbow Surg 2009;18:317–28.

23. Grondin P, Leith J. Combined large Hill-Sachs and bony Bankart lesions treated by Latarjet and partial

humeral head resurfacing: a report of 2 cases. Can J Surg 2009;52:249–54.

24. Kazel MD, Sekiya IK, Greene JA, et al. Percutaneous correction (humeroplasty) of posterolateral humeral head defects (Hill-Sachs) associated with anterior shoulder instability: a cadaveric study. Arthroscopy 2005;21:1473–8.

25. Re P, Gallo RA, Richmond JC. Transhumeral head plasty for large Hill-Sachs lesions. Arthroscopy 2006;22:798e1–4.

26. Gerber C. Chronic locked anterior and posterior dislocations. In: Warner JJP, editor. Complex revision problems in shoulder surgery. Philadelphia: Lippincott Williams & Wilkins; 1997. p. 99–116.

27. Deutsh AA, Kroll DG. Decreased range of motion following arthroscopic remplissage. Orthopedics 2008;31:492.

28. Purchase RJ, Wolf EM, Hobgood ER, et al. Hill-Sachs "remplissage": an arthroscopic solution for the engaging Hill-Sachs lesion. Arthroscopy 2008;24:723.

29. Connolly JF. Humeral head defects associated with shoulder dislocation—their diagnostic and surgical significance. Instr Course Lect 1972;21:42–54.

30. Martinez AA, Calvo A, Domingo J, et al. Allograft reconstruction of segmental defects of the humeral head associated with posterior dislocation of the shoulder. Injury 2008;39:319–22.

31. Gerber G, Lambert SM. Allograft reconstruction of segmental defects of the humeral head for the treatment of chronic locked posterior dislocation of the shoulder. J Bone Joint Surg Am 1996;78:376–82.

32. Yagishita K, Thomas BJ. Use of allograft for large Hill Sachs lesion associated with anterior glenohumeral dislocation. A case report. Injury 2002;33(9):791–4.

33. Chapovsky BS, Kelly JD. Osteochondral allograft transplantation for treatment of glenohumeral instability. Arthroscopy 2005;21:1007.

34. Kirkley A, Griffin S, McLintock H, et al. The development and evaluation of a disease-specific quality of life measurement tool for shoulder instability. The Western Ontario Shoulder Instability Index (WOSI). Am J Sports Med 1998;26(6):764–72.

35. Tjoumakaris FP, Humble B, Sekiya JK. Combined glenoid and humeral head allograft reconstruction for recurrent anterior glenohumeral instability. Orthopedics 2008;31:497.

36. Hardegger F. Technik und Ergebnisse der subcapitalen Humerusdrehosteotomie bei vorderer habitueller Schulterluxation. Orthopade 1978;77:147–53 [in German].

37. Hardegger F, Kappeler U. Die Teillsäionen bei der traumatischen Erstluxation des Schultergelenkes. Zeitschr Orthop 1980;118:553–4 [in German].

38. Marti R, Weber BG, Afchampour P. Technik und Ergebnisse der Humerusosteotomie bei habitueller Schultergelenksluxation. Z Unfallmed Berufskr 1973; 66:130–6 [in German].

39. Müller-Färber J, Müller KH, Scheuer I. Die differenzierte Therapie der rezidivierenden Schulterluxation. Unfallheilkunde 1983;86:87–95 [in German].

40. Weber BG, Simpson LA, Hardegger F. Rotational humeral osteotomy for recurrent anterior dislocation of the shoulder associated with a large Hill-Sachs lesion. J Bone Joint Surg Am 1984;66:1443–50.

41. Moros C, Ahmad CS. Partial humeral head resurfacing and Latarjet coracoid transfer for treatment of recurrent anterior glenohumeral instability. Orthopedics 2009;32:602.

42. Flatow EL, Miller SR, Neer CS. Chronic anterior dislocation of the shoulder. J Shoulder Elbow Surg 1993; 2:2–10.

43. Pritchett JW, Clark JM. Prosthetic replacement for chronic unreduced dislocations of the shoulder. Clin Orthop Relat Res 1987;216:89–93.

Open Capsular Shift: There Still Is A Role!

Karen J. Boselli, MD[a], Elizabeth A. Cody, BA[b],
Louis U. Bigliani, MD[a],*

KEYWORDS

- Open • Instability • Revision • Multidirectional
- Recurrence • Plication

Open shoulder stabilization is a proven means of preventing recurrent instability, reliably restoring function and quality of life to near preinjury levels.[1–8] Although open repair has produced consistently favorable results, arthroscopic management has recently gained popularity as techniques have evolved and surgeons have acquired increased experience. Most instability surgery can now be successfully performed with an arthroscopic approach, and recent results have been comparable to historic treatment with open capsulolabral repair.[9–12] In spite of these advances in arthroscopic technique, there is still an essential role for open capsular shift in the management of anterior instability; the choice of surgical treatment should therefore be based on surgeon experience and individual patient pathology.[13] The goal of this article is to review the indications, technique, and clinical results of open capsular shift, specifically addressing the cases in which open stabilization shift remains the treatment of choice.

RATIONALE FOR REPAIR

The rationale for open shoulder stabilization is based on knowledge of the pathoanatomy associated with anterior instability. Advances in our understanding of shoulder anatomy and biomechanics have led to improvements in procedure selection, as well as an evolution in the techniques used for stabilization.[14]

Historically, the essential lesion of shoulder instability was described as an avulsion of the anterior-inferior glenoid labrum.[15] Recurrent instability has since been attributed to concomitant capsular deformation at the time of dislocation.[15,16] In fact, biomechanical studies have demonstrated that complete dislocation cannot occur after the creation of a Bankart lesion unless capsular disruption is also present.[17] It is now recognized that the primary pathology of instability encompasses labral detachment, along with a capsular abnormality, which may include macroscopic capsular rupture, capsular deformation or stretch,[18–20] capsular redundancy or laxity,[20] periosteal capsular stripping, or any combination of these.[20,21] Subsequent to the primary capsulolabral disruption, there is loss of tension on the glenohumeral ligaments with resultant instability.[22]

The goal of any surgical stabilization procedure is to address the specific pathology of a patient with recurrent subluxation or dislocation. Surgical intervention is therefore aimed at addressing the labral avulsion, as well as the exact type of capsular abnormality present. When these two primary pathologic features of instability are not addressed, higher rates of failure have been reported.[22–26] Failure to address capsular laxity has also been suggested as a potential explanation for the higher reported recurrence rates after arthroscopic stabilization.[21,22] Open capsular shift effectively addresses both labral disruption and capsular abnormalities, restoring the native static stabilizers of the shoulder joint.

a Center for Shoulder, Elbow and Sports Medicine, Department of Orthopaedic Surgery, Columbia University Medical Center, 622 West 168th Street, PH 11, New York, NY 10032, USA
b Columbia University College of Physicians and Surgeons, 630 West 168th Street, New York, NY 10032, USA
* Corresponding author.
E-mail address: lub1@columbia.edu

Orthop Clin N Am 41 (2010) 427–436
doi:10.1016/j.ocl.2010.03.002

INDICATIONS

Surgical intervention is generally recommended for those patients who continue to experience pain or instability in spite of adequate nonoperative treatment.[27] More specifically, the choice of stabilization procedure should be based on the pathology of the patient, the preferences of the patient, and the experience of the surgeon.[21] Patient history and activity or sport requirements are also important considerations in the selection of surgical approach. There is significant overlap between the relative indications for open and arthroscopic stabilization and, therefore, the choice of approach must be individualized. In many cases, both arthroscopic and open repair can be successful, as long as (1) both labral injury and capsular disruption are addressed, and (2) surgeon technical expertise allows for either.

Arthroscopic instability treatment has recently gained popularity, as it is minimally invasive, avoids release of the subscapularis, poses limited morbidity to the patient,[28] and provides an improved ability to identify and treat associated pathologic conditions.[13,29] Most indications for arthroscopic stabilization, however, are relative and not absolute. Ideal candidates have a history of traumatic instability with a documented labral or capsular detachment, without significant capsular laxity or deficiency.[21] Arthroscopic management is also indicated in patients who wish to avoid the increased morbidity of open stabilization,[28] and is relatively indicated in patients with concomitant intra-articular abnormalities.[21] In high-performance overhead athletes, arthroscopic management may offer a faster return to activity and decreased loss of external rotation.[30,31] Recent literature has presented conflicting evidence on postoperative range of motion following instability repair; some reports have demonstrated equivalent external rotation after open and arthroscopic treatment, making this indication somewhat controversial.[9]

In spite of advances in the arthroscopic management of instability, numerous relative contraindications exist. Among these are humeral avulsions of the glenohumeral ligaments (HAGL), capsular ruptures, revision stabilization procedures in which capsular deficiency is a concern, and prior failed thermal capsulorrhaphy procedures. Generally speaking, arthroscopic treatment is relatively contraindicated in all cases in which there is concern for severely compromised tissue quality. More importantly, it is absolutely contraindicated if the surgeon does not have the expertise or advanced equipment necessary for this technically demanding procedure. The surgeon should always be prepared to convert an arthroscopic procedure to a traditional open capsular shift if deemed necessary to treat the specific pathology, and reduce the risk for postoperative recurrence of instability.[13]

Although arthroscopic repair may enable faster recovery and avoid the morbidity of open surgery,[31] open capsular shift remains effective in treating a wide spectrum of symptomatic instability patients. Furthermore, it may be specifically indicated over arthroscopic treatment in certain patient populations. Open treatment is generally indicated for revision of failed prior open or arthroscopic stabilization procedures, cases of significant glenoid or humeral bone loss,[14] capsular deficiency or midsubstance rupture, and chronic irreparable deficiency of the rotator cuff, specifically the subscapularis.[13] It is absolutely indicated in irreducible or open dislocations, and in cases when arthroscopic techniques cannot appropriately address the pathology present. Atraumatic and multidirectional instability present another compelling indication for open capsular shift, with favorable subjective and objective results demonstrated at mid- and long-term follow-up.[3,6,32,33] With few exceptions, open surgery is also relatively indicated for humeral avulsions of the glenohumeral ligaments.

Recently, Balg and Boileau[34] investigated the risk factors for redislocation after arthroscopic repair, in an attempt to develop a simple method for identifying patients who would be better served by open stabilization. The investigators identified 131 consecutive patients who underwent arthroscopic treatment for recurrent anterior instability with suture anchors. Risk factors for postoperative instability included: age less than 20 at the time of surgery, involvement in competitive or contact sport, shoulder hyperlaxity, and bony defects of the humerus or glenoid. Each of these factors should be carefully considered during preoperative evaluation and procedure selection.

Some advocate the selection of open repair based on specific findings at the time of surgery, after examination under anesthesia and assessment of the pathology present during diagnostic arthroscopy.[9] The presence of marked anterior or multidirectional laxity on physical examination, or the absence of a discrete Bankart lesion and well-defined inferior glenohumeral ligament (IGHL), are thought to make arthroscopic management less advisable. Cole and colleagues[9] reported the results of 63 surgical patients with traumatic anterior instability, in whom the decision on arthroscopic Bankart repair versus open capsular shift made after examination under anesthesia and diagnostic arthroscopy. Thirty-nine patients had pure anterior translation with a discrete Bankart lesion; 24 had anterior and inferior translation, along with capsular laxity seen at the time of arthroscopy. The former group was managed with arthroscopic Bankart repair, while the latter was managed with open anterior-inferior capsular shift. At a mean of 54 months postoperatively, there were no significant differences between the groups in Rowe, American Shoulder and Elbow Surgeons (ASES), or SF-36 scores. With the exception of a slight loss of forward elevation in the capsular shift group, measured losses in range of motion between the groups were minimal. Overall, 75% of the patients in each group returned to their preinjury activity levels with minimal or no limitations. The investigators concluded that favorable results can be achieved if the choice of surgical management is made based on the pathologic findings present at the time of surgery.

Patients with attenuated anterior ligamentous structures are ideal candidates for open stabilization; this severe capsular deficiency is often seen in a revision setting following previous failed open or arthroscopic repair. Tauber and colleagues[25] performed a retrospective review of 41 patients with recurrent instability, highlighting the indication for open treatment in revision instability repair. At the time of revision surgery, a bony defect was present in 56% of patients, an enlarged or overstretched capsule in 22%, and a laterally torn capsule in 5%. Each of these pathologic findings has not traditionally been considered as amenable to arthroscopic management. Furthermore, only 17% of patients had typical Bankart lesions with good capsular tissue quality that might otherwise be considered for arthroscopic repair. In the revision setting, open treatment may better address the capsular insufficiency, or multiple causes of instability in these complex individuals.[13,23,25,35]

It has been suggested that all patients who require absolute stability, or those who present an excessively high risk for postoperative dislocation, are indicated for open stabilization. Recently, this indication has become more controversial. Some argue that collision athletes present a clear indication for open surgery, given the favorable results and minimal recurrence rates shown in the literature.[36,37] Others contend that with good patient selection and modern surgical techniques, arthroscopic treatment can offer similar results.[38–40]

Cho and colleagues[36] compared the results of arthroscopic stabilization in 29 collision and noncollision athletes, finding that arthroscopic treatment reliably restored shoulder function and range of motion, with consistent return to sports activity. An overall 17.2% rate of recurrent instability was reported, however, with five patients (28.6%) in the collision group versus one patient (6.7%) in the noncollision group. More recently, Rhee and colleagues[41] compared open and arthroscopic stabilization in 48 shoulders of 46 collision athletes, 16 who underwent arthroscopic stabilization and 32 with open repairs. At a mean follow-up of 72 months, visual analog scale (VAS), Rowe, and Constant scores improved in all patients, with no significant difference in scores between the two repair groups. There was, however, a 25% rate of recurrent instability in the arthroscopic group, compared with a 12.5% rate in the open group. Given the higher failure rate after arthroscopic repair, the investigators concluded that open stabilization was a more reliable method for the management of anterior shoulder instability in collision athletes.

OPEN CAPSULAR SHIFT

Historically, Rowe and colleagues[8] popularized the classic Bankart repair as an anatomic technique of restoring shoulder stability. Results were excellent, with only a 3.5% recurrence rate over 30 years. Later, the open capsular shift was proposed by Neer and Foster[6] as a treatment for multidirectional instability. The procedure was designed to reduce capsular volume and subsequently restore tension in the glenohumeral ligaments, through a superior shift of the inferior capsule. The procedure allows the surgeon to adjust the degree of shift depending on the direction and extent of capsular laxity. Most modern techniques for the management of instability are modifications of previously described procedures, involving a combination of Bankart repair and capsular shift, with a selective determination of ligamentous tension.[27] The concept of a selective shift is based on an understanding that the capsuloligamentous structures of the shoulder act predictably as checkreins to translation based on arm position.[42] Selective restoration of ligamentous tension is, therefore, able to restrict anterior and inferior translation in a position of apprehension.

The anterior-inferior capsular shift uses a T-capsulorrhaphy to decrease the volume of the joint capsule, thereby restoring tension on the glenohumeral ligaments. The decreased capsular volume increases responsiveness of the intra-articular pressure to downward loading, decreasing the amount of inferior displacement expected with any given load.[43] The shift allows tightening of the capsule in two directions, both superior-inferior and medial-lateral. To preserve external rotation, however, over-tightening in the medial-lateral direction must be avoided.[42] A careful titration of the shift will stabilize the joint without compromising external rotation and maximum forward elevation, thus avoiding overconstraint.[44,45]

The technique for capsular shift presented in this article is favored by the senior author because of its anatomic reattachment of the displaced labrum, in addition to a capsular plication. The key pathologic elements of instability are addressed with this procedure, enabling an effective correction of most forms of anterior and multidirectional instability.

Surgical Technique

The procedure is performed with the patient in a modified beach chair position, with the head of the bed elevated to 30°. Through an axillary incision, the deltopectoral interval is identified. The cephalic vein is preserved and retracted laterally with the deltoid. If needed to obtain additional inferior exposure, the upper 0.5 to 1 cm of the pectoralis major insertion can be released and tagged for later repair. Superiorly the coracoid is identified, and the clavipectoral fascia is incised just lateral to the strap muscles. Deep retractors are placed, taking care to avoid injury to the musculocutaneous nerve. For improved superior exposure, a small crescent of the coracoacromial ligament can be excised at its anterolateral edge.

A complete anterior bursectomy is performed to expose the subscapularis muscle and its borders. The tendon is then incised 1 cm medial to its insertion onto the lesser tuberosity. The subscapularis is detached from the underlying joint capsule, which can be technically difficult owing to attachments between the capsule and tendon at its superior border.[46] The plane between muscle and capsule should therefore be identified inferiorly by blunt dissection (**Fig. 1**). Working from inferior to superior, an elevator and Mayo scissors can be used to tease the muscle from the capsule. During this dissection, the axillary nerve should be identified and protected; adduction and external rotation of the arm will move the nerve farther from the site of dissection. The subscapularis is tagged for later repair.

Following release of the subscapularis, the capsule is incised. The preferred approach for the capsular shift is humeral-based, as a glenoid-based shift is more likely to endanger the axillary nerve and may result in a greater loss of external rotation.[47] This approach is also better suited to identify and repair humeral avulsion of the capsule. Specific instability patterns, however, may require variation in the exact site of capsular incision.[47] The incision is generally planned at a site 5 mm medial to the subscapularis stump, beginning

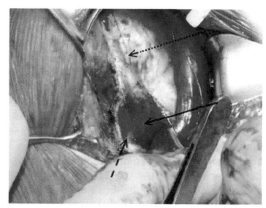

Fig. 1. Separating subscapularis from the underlying capsule may be difficult at the superior margin, where the two structures are confluent (*dotted arrow*). Inferiorly, a plane is more easily developed (*dashed arrow*) and the undersurface of the subscapularis (*solid arrow*) can be visualized. (*From* Bahu MJ, Covey AS, Bigliani LU, et al. Open instability repair: the anterior-inferior capsular shift. Operat Tech Orthop 2008;18:62; with permission.)

superiorly at the rotator interval and moving inferiorly to the neck of the humerus. A cuff of capsular tissue is left attached to the humeral neck for later repair. Traction sutures are placed at the free medial edge of the capsule.

Once the neck of the humerus is reached, the arm is externally rotated to increase exposure of the inferior capsule. The capsular release is continued inferiorly to a level appropriate to the degree of capsular redundancy; the release is considered adequate if superolateral tension on the capsular traction stitches obliterates the inferior capsular pouch (**Fig. 2**). It is important to note that the inferior capsule has two layers that attach separately to the humeral neck, both of which must be released (**Fig. 3**).[46] After completion of the release, the external surface of the capsule should be closely examined. Any residual attachments to the subscapularis should be incised, as they can hinder mobility of the capsule during the shift.

The humerus is next retracted posteriorly to expose the glenoid. If detachment of the anterior-inferior labrum or inferior glenohumeral ligament is identified, it is repaired. The glenoid rim is prepared with a curette until bleeding bone is encountered, and the labrum is repaired at the junction of the articular cartilage and scapular neck using suture anchors.

Attention is then turned to the capsular shift and reattachment. The arm should be placed in 20° to 30° of abduction and 20° to 30° of external rotation to avoid overconstraint after the shift is completed.

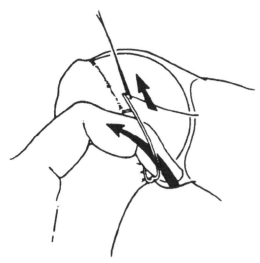

Fig. 2. Superolateral tension on the capsular traction stitch should obliterate the inferior capsular redundancy. To assess the degree of inferior capsular release, if a surgeon's finger is pushed out of the pouch when traction is applied, the release is considered sufficient. (*From* Pollock RG, Owens JM, Flatow EL, et al. Operative results of the inferior capsular shift procedure for multidirectional instability of the shoulder. J Bone Joint Surg Am 2000;82-A(7):920; with permission.)

In overhead athletes, more abduction and external rotation can be used to prevent overtightening of the capsule. In contrast, less abduction and external rotation should be used in patients with large deficiencies of the humeral head or glenoid. By placing traction on the tag sutures, the inferior portion of the capsule is drawn up and reattached

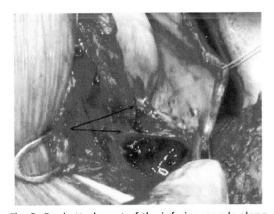

Fig. 3. Dual attachment of the inferior capsule along the surgical neck of the humerus. Both layers must be released to allow for a complete shift of the capsule. (*From* Bahu MJ, Covey AS, Bigliani LU, et al. Open instability repair: the anterior-inferior capsular shift. Operat Tech Orthop 2008;18:62; with permission.)

superiorly. If any residual capsular redundancy exists, a horizontal incision is made in the capsule between the inferior and middle glenohumeral ligaments, producing a T-shaped capsulotomy. The superior capsular segment can then be overlapped across the inferior segment in a pants-over-vest fashion, further reducing capsular volume (**Fig. 4**). For patients with an extremely large inferior pouch, a T-shaped capsulotomy is more likely necessary; in these individuals, the horizontal incision can be performed initially, before attempting the capsular shift.

A significant percentage of patients may present with anteromedial capsular redundancy or anterior glenoid labral deficiency. This pathology is more commonly seen in those with a longer duration of preoperative symptoms and recurrent dislocations.[48] Often, this pathology cannot be fully addressed with an isolated laterally-based capsulorrhaphy. In these individuals, a crimping barrel stitch technique can be used. A suture is passed into the capsule at the superior margin of the redundancy near the capsulolabral junction. It exits at the inferior margin of the redundancy, and is then tied outside of the capsule. Tightening the stitch obliterates the localized medial redundancy and bolsters the anterior glenoid labrum (**Fig. 5**).[48] Once the barrel stitch has been tied, the capsular shift (as previously described) is performed, with a T-shaped capsulorrhaphy if necessary.

The rotator interval is repaired if the preoperative sulcus sign was positive in external rotation. The subscapularis and pectoralis major are then repaired, and the wound is closed in layers. Drains are not routinely required. An intraoperative assessment of motion is performed to determine the safe range for postoperative rehabilitation. After conclusion of the procedure, a sling and swathe are applied.

Rehabilitation

Sling use is continued for the first 6 weeks postoperatively. Passive pendulum exercises are initiated at 10 days. Although the limits for range of motion are dependent on the intraoperative assessment, forward elevation to 100° and external rotation to 15° are generally allowed at 10 to 14 days. By 2 to 4 weeks, forward elevation is increased to 140°, with external rotation to 30°. Active and gentle resistive exercises are also permitted. At 4 to 6 weeks, range of motion is again increased to 165° of forward elevation and 40° of external rotation, along with a slight increase in resistive exercises. Six weeks postoperatively, the arm may be positioned in maximum forward elevation. The

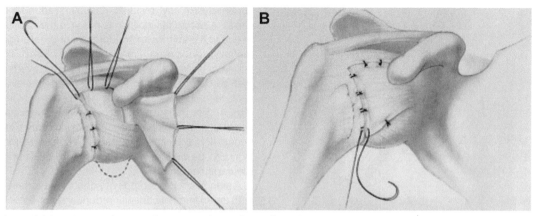

Fig. 4. (*A*) Traction on the capsular tag stitches reduces the inferior redundancy; the inferior capsule is reduced and reattached in a more superior and lateral position. (*B*) If a horizontal split was made in the capsule, the inferior segment is first reduced as shown in **Fig. 4**A. The superior segment is then overlapped in a pants-over-vest fashion, further reducing capsular volume. (*From* Pollock RG, Owens JM, Flatow EL, et al. Operative results of the inferior capsular shift procedure for multidirectional instability of the shoulder. J Bone Joint Surg Am 2000;82-A(7):921; with permission.)

goal of early range of motion must be balanced against the risk of compromising the repair by hasty advances in rehabilitation. Return to contact sports is not recommended before 6 months.

RESULTS

Open stabilization procedures have been used for many years with various modifications; most have excellent results when performed in properly selected patients with good surgical technique. In the classic article by Rowe and colleagues,[8] open Bankart repair was performed on 145 shoulders, with a 3.5% recurrence rate from 1 to 30 years (mean 6 years). More recently, Gill and colleagues[4] have reported long-term results after Bankart repair in 56 patients. After a mean of

11.9 years postoperatively, good or excellent results were obtained in 93% of patients.

The open anterior-inferior capsular shift was initially described as a treatment for multidirectional instability, with failure rates of less than 10%.[1,3,6,7,32] Neer and Foster[6] reported the preliminary results of 40 shoulders with involuntary multidirectional instability treated with an inferior capsular shift. Of the 14 patients with an anterior approach, 10 had more than 1 year of follow-up with no unsatisfactory results. Pollock and colleagues[7] reported the results of 52 shoulders treated with a laterally based capsular shift, with good or excellent results obtained in 94% of patients at a mean of 61 months postoperatively.

Cooper and Brems[3] reported similar favorable results in 43 shoulders with multidirectional instability, treated with inferior capsular shift through

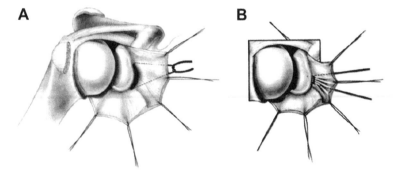

Fig. 5. In patients with anteromedial capsular redundancy, a barrel stitch can be employed. A suture is passed through the capsule at the superior and inferior margins of the redundancy (*A*), which crimps the capsule when tightened (*B*). The stitch obliterates the localized redundancy and bolsters the anterior glenoid labrum. (*From* Ahmad CS, Freehill MQ, Blaine TA, et al. Anteromedial capsular redundancy and labral deficiency in shoulder instability. Am J Sports Med 2003;31(2):249; with permission.)

an anterior approach. At a minimum of 2 years postoperatively, range of motion was well maintained and 91% of patients reported a subjective satisfactory outcome, with no recurrent episodes of instability.

For those patients with anteromedial capsular redundancy, an isolated anterior-inferior capsular shift may be inadequate to restore glenohumeral stability. The barrel stitch technique, as previously described, is an effective means of imbrication to achieve stability when incorporated into a capsular shift procedure.[48] In a retrospective review of 78 patients undergoing open anterior-inferior capsular shift for recurrent instability, Ahmad and colleagues[48] reported a 49% incidence of anteromedial capsular redundancy. Patients with redundancy were found to have a significantly greater number of dislocations and a longer duration of symptoms before surgery. At a mean follow-up of 6.1 years, good or excellent postoperative results were obtained in 92% of the patients requiring a barrel stitch, with 97% of patients reporting no episodes of recurrent instability.

In athletes, recurrence rates after capsular shift have been similarly favorable. The ability to return to competitive throwing, however, has been less consistent. Bigliani and colleagues[1] evaluated 68 shoulders in 63 athletes treated with an anterior-inferior capsular shift. A concomitant repair of a Bankart lesion was performed in 21 individuals. Overall, 94% experienced good or excellent results, with only two (2.9%) redislocations. Ninety-two percent of patients were able to return to sport, but only 50% of elite throwing athletes returned at the same competitive level. Altchek and colleagues[32] treated 42 shoulders with a modified Bankart procedure using a glenoid-based T-shaped capsulotomy. Postoperative subjective satisfaction rate was 95%, with an average loss of external rotation of only 5°. However, in spite of an overall 83% rate of return to full sports participation, the three throwing athletes in the series reported only "moderate participation" secondary to a decrease in throwing velocity.

In a revision setting, reasonable results have been reported with the use of capsular shift following failed previous instability surgery.[23,35] Levine and colleagues[35] retrospectively evaluated 50 patients who underwent open revision stabilization surgery with anterior-inferior capsular shift for a failed anterior instability procedure. The most common reason identified for recurrent instability was a failure to address the pathology present at the time of initial surgery: a redundant anteroinferior capsular pouch, an avulsed labrum, or both. At a mean of 4.7 years postoperatively, good or

excellent results were reported in 78% of patients. Poor results were seen in atraumatic recurrent or voluntary dislocators, and in those patients with multiple prior stabilization attempts.

Recent studies also support the long-term reliability of the open capsular shift.[2,49] Cheung and colleagues[2] reported results after 22 years of follow-up in 34 patients undergoing laterally-based T-shaped capsular shift. Although 4 patients experienced recurrent subluxation and 11 had positive apprehension, no dislocations occurred, and no further additional instability surgeries were required. Clinically significant arthritis developed in only 2 patients, ultimately requiring total shoulder arthroplasty.

Early arthroscopic techniques were consistently associated with high recurrence rates.[30,50–53] Freedman and colleagues[50] performed a meta-analysis of all studies comparing open to arthroscopic Bankart repair with bioabsorbable tacks or transglenoid sutures. The rate of recurrent dislocation was significantly higher in the arthroscopic group (12.6%) than in the open (3.4%). The total rate of recurrence (including subluxation or dislocation) was also significantly higher in the arthroscopic group (20.3%) than in the open (10.3%). The proportion of good or excellent postoperative Rowe scores was significantly higher in the open repair group.

With the use of modern arthroscopic techniques, postoperative recurrence rates have significantly decreased.[11,12,54,55] In fact, some investigators have demonstrated equivalent or better results using arthroscopic suture anchor techniques compared with open repair.[10] Unfortunately, many of the studies that directly compare open and arthroscopic approaches are difficult to interpret owing to the use of varied techniques in patients with mixed pathologies.[9,10,28,50,51,53,54,56]

Mohtadi and colleagues[57] performed a meta-analysis of all clinical studies directly comparing arthroscopic and open repair for traumatic recurrent anterior shoulder instability. Eleven studies were included in the analysis, only one of which was a randomized trial. The odds ratio for recurrent instability was 2.04 in favor of the open repair. For return to activity, odds ratio was 2.85 again in favor of open repair. More recently, Lenters and colleagues[52] conducted a review of 18 published or presented studies comparing the relative effectiveness of the two surgical approaches. Meta-analysis demonstrated that arthroscopic repairs had a significantly higher risk of recurrent instability, recurrent dislocation, and reoperation. Even with modern arthroscopic suture anchor techniques, there was a higher risk of recurrent instability than with traditional open methods. In spite of these results, arthroscopic repair was associated with higher Rowe scores than open stabilization. These results suggest that, although arthroscopic techniques may result in improved function, they are less effective in the prevention of recurrent instability.

A recent Cochrane review has been published comparing effectiveness of arthroscopic versus open instability repair in adults.[58] Three randomized controlled trials involving 184 patients were included in this systematic review. The pooled results showed no statistically significant difference between the two groups in regards to recurrent instability or subsequent instability-related surgery. Furthermore, there were no clinically significant differences between the groups for all other outcomes including shoulder function. The review highlights a lack of sufficient evidence from randomized controlled trials to conclude that either arthroscopic or open instability repair is superior; future high-quality studies will be needed to further define the appropriate indications for each procedure.

SUMMARY

The treatment of anterior shoulder instability continues to evolve. As our understanding of the pathoanatomy of glenohumeral instability has improved, surgical techniques have progressed. Current surgical treatments effectively address the two key contributors to shoulder instability: labral disruption and capsular abnormality. Although many instability repairs are now successfully performed arthroscopically, open repair continues to play an important role in the management of instability in certain patients with specific pathology. Complex instability patterns, revision of previous stabilization attempts, and collision athletes should all be considered for open instability repair. The open capsular shift provides an accurate and selective capsular plication tailored to the degree of laxity found at surgery. When performed with proper surgical technique, shoulder range of motion can be preserved. Reported recurrence rates are extremely low and subjective satisfaction with the procedure is high, making it a durable and effective option in the modern management of shoulder instability.

REFERENCES

1. Bigliani LU, Kurzweil PR, Schwartzbach CC, et al. Inferior capsular shift procedure for anterior-inferior shoulder instability in athletes. Am J Sports Med 1994;22:578.
2. Cheung EV, Sperling JW, Hattrup SJ, et al. Long-term outcome of anterior stabilization of the shoulder. J Shoulder Elbow Surg 2008;17:265.
3. Cooper RA, Brems JJ. The inferior capsular-shift procedure for multidirectional instability of the shoulder. J Bone Joint Surg Am 1992;74:1516.
4. Gill TJ, Micheli LJ, Gebhard F, et al. Bankart repair for anterior instability of the shoulder. Long-term outcome. J Bone Joint Surg Am 1997;79:850.
5. Meller R, Krettek C, Gosling T, et al. Recurrent shoulder instability among athletes: changes in quality of life, sports activity, and muscle function following open repair. Knee Surg Sports Traumatol Arthrosc 2007;15:295.
6. Neer CS 2nd, Foster CR. Inferior capsular shift for involuntary inferior and multidirectional instability of the shoulder. A preliminary report. J Bone Joint Surg Am 1980;62:897.
7. Pollock RG, Owens JM, Flatow EL, et al. Operative results of the inferior capsular shift procedure for multidirectional instability of the shoulder. J Bone Joint Surg Am 2000;82:919.
8. Rowe CR, Patel D, Southmayd WW. The Bankart procedure: a long-term end-result study. J Bone Joint Surg Am 1978;60:1.
9. Cole BJ, L'Insalata J, Irrgang J, et al. Comparison of arthroscopic and open anterior shoulder stabilization. A two to six-year follow-up study. J Bone Joint Surg Am 2000;82:1108.
10. Fabbriciani C, Milano G, Demontis A, et al. Arthroscopic versus open treatment of Bankart lesion of the shoulder: a prospective randomized study. Arthroscopy 2004;20:456.
11. Kim SH, Ha KI. Bankart repair in traumatic anterior shoulder instability: open versus arthroscopic technique. Arthroscopy 2002;18:755.
12. Kim SH, Ha KI, Cho YB, et al. Arthroscopic anterior stabilization of the shoulder: two to six-year follow-up. J Bone Joint Surg Am 2003;85:1511.
13. Millett PJ, Clavert P, Warner JJ. Open operative treatment for anterior shoulder instability: when and why? J Bone Joint Surg Am 2005;87:419.
14. Miniaci A, Hayes DE, Williams GR, et al. Anterior and anteroinferior instability: open and arthroscopic management, vol. 1. Philadelphia: Lippincott Williams & Wilkins; 2007.
15. Bankart A. The pathology and treatment of recurrent dislocation of the shoulder joint. BMJ 1938;26:23.
16. Townley CO. The capsular mechanism in recurrent dislocation of the shoulder. J Bone Joint Surg Am 1950;32:370.
17. Speer KP, Deng X, Borrero S, et al. Biomechanical evaluation of a simulated Bankart lesion. J Bone Joint Surg Am 1994;76:1819.
18. Bach BR, Warren RF, Fronek J. Disruption of the lateral capsule of the shoulder. A cause

of recurrent dislocation. J Bone Joint Surg Br 1988;70:274.

19. Bigliani LU, Kelkar R, Flatow EL, et al. Glenohumeral stability. Biomechanical properties of passive and active stabilizers. Clin Orthop Relat Res 1996;330: 13–30.

20. Bigliani LU, Pollock RG, Soslowsky LJ, et al. Tensile properties of the inferior glenohumeral ligament. J Orthop Res 1992;10:187.

21. Cole BJ, Warner JJ. Arthroscopic versus open Bankart repair for traumatic anterior shoulder instability. Clin Sports Med 2000;19:19.

22. Levine WN, Flatow EL. The pathophysiology of shoulder instability. Am J Sports Med 2000;28: 910.

23. Araghi A, Prasarn M, St Clair S, et al. Revision anterior shoulder repair for recurrent anterior glenohumeral instability. Bull Hosp Jt Dis 2005;62:102.

24. Rowe CR, Zarins B, Ciullo JV. Recurrent anterior dislocation of the shoulder after surgical repair. Apparent causes of failure and treatment. J Bone Joint Surg Am 1984;66:159.

25. Tauber M, Resch H, Forstner R, et al. Reasons for failure after surgical repair of anterior shoulder instability. J Shoulder Elbow Surg 2004;13:279.

26. Young DC, Rockwood CA Jr. Complications of a failed Bristow procedure and their management. J Bone Joint Surg Am 1991;73:969.

27. Bahu MJ, Covey AS, Bigliani LU, et al. Open instability repair: the anterior-inferior capsular shift. Operat Tech Orthop 2008;18:62.

28. Green MR, Christensen KP. Arthroscopic versus open Bankart procedures: a comparison of early morbidity and complications. Arthroscopy 1993;9: 371.

29. Angelo RL. Arthroscopic Bankart repair for unidirectional shoulder instability. Instr Course Lect 2009;58: 305.

30. Hubbell JD, Ahmad S, Bezenoff LS, et al. Comparison of shoulder stabilization using arthroscopic transglenoid sutures versus open capsulolabral repairs: a 5-year minimum follow-up. Am J Sports Med 2004;32:650.

31. Rhee YG, Lim CT, Cho NS. Muscle strength after anterior shoulder stabilization: arthroscopic versus open Bankart repair. Am J Sports Med 2007;35: 1859.

32. Altchek DW, Warren RF, Skyhar MJ, et al. T-plasty modification of the Bankart procedure for multidirectional instability of the anterior and inferior types. J Bone Joint Surg Am 1991;73:105.

33. Yamaguchi K, Flatow EL. Management of multidirectional instability. Clin Sports Med 1995;14:885.

34. Balg F, Boileau P. The instability severity index score. A simple pre-operative score to select patients for arthroscopic or open shoulder stabilisation. J Bone Joint Surg Br 2007;89:1470.

35. Levine WN, Arroyo JS, Pollock RG, et al. Open revision stabilization surgery for recurrent anterior glenohumeral instability. Am J Sports Med 2000;28:156.

36. Cho NS, Hwang JC, Rhee YG. Arthroscopic stabilization in anterior shoulder instability: collision athletes versus noncollision athletes. Arthroscopy 2006;22:947.

37. Pagnani MJ, Dome DC. Surgical treatment of traumatic anterior shoulder instability in American football players. J Bone Joint Surg Am 2002;84:711.

38. Burkhart SS, De Beer JF. Traumatic glenohumeral bone defects and their relationship to failure of arthroscopic Bankart repairs: significance of the inverted-pear glenoid and the humeral engaging Hill-Sachs lesion. Arthroscopy 2000;16:677.

39. Larrain MV, Montenegro HJ, Mauas DM, et al. Arthroscopic management of traumatic anterior shoulder instability in collision athletes: analysis of 204 cases with a 4- to 9-year follow-up and results with the suture anchor technique. Arthroscopy 2006;22:1283.

40. Mazzocca AD, Brown FM Jr, Carreira DS, et al. Arthroscopic anterior shoulder stabilization of collision and contact athletes. Am J Sports Med 2005; 33:52.

41. Rhee YG, Ha JH, Cho NS. Anterior shoulder stabilization in collision athletes: arthroscopic versus open Bankart repair. Am J Sports Med 2006;34: 979.

42. Gerber C, Werner CM, Macy JC, et al. Effect of selective capsulorrhaphy on the passive range of motion of the glenohumeral joint. J Bone Joint Surg Am 2003;85:48.

43. Yamamoto N, Itoi E, Tuoheti Y, et al. The effect of the inferior capsular shift on shoulder intra-articular pressure: a cadaveric study. Am J Sports Med 2006;34:939.

44. Jaeger A, Braune C, Welsch F, et al. Postoperative functional outcome and stability in recurrent traumatic anteroinferior glenohumeral instability: comparison of two different surgical capsular reconstruction techniques. Arch Orthop Trauma Surg 2004;124:226.

45. Wang VM, Sugalski MT, Levine WN, et al. Comparison of glenohumeral mechanics following a capsular shift and anterior tightening. J Bone Joint Surg Am 2005;87:1312.

46. Sugalski MT, Wiater JM, Levine WN, et al. An anatomic study of the humeral insertion of the inferior glenohumeral capsule. J Shoulder Elbow Surg 2005;14:91.

47. Deutsch A, Barber JE, Davy DT, et al. Anterior-inferior capsular shift of the shoulder: a biomechanical comparison of glenoid-based versus humeral-based shift strategies. J Shoulder Elbow Surg 2001;10:340.

48. Ahmad CS, Freehill MQ, Blaine TA, et al. Antero-medial capsular redundancy and labral deficiency in shoulder instability. Am J Sports Med 2003;31:247.

49. Marquardt B, Potzl W, Witt KA, et al. A modified capsular shift for atraumatic anterior-inferior shoulder instability. Am J Sports Med 2005;33:1011.

50. Freedman KB, Smith AP, Romeo AA, et al. Open Bankart repair versus arthroscopic repair with transglenoid sutures or bioabsorbable tacks for Recurrent Anterior instability of the shoulder: a meta-analysis. Am J Sports Med 2004;32:1520.

51. Guanche CA, Quick DC, Sodergren KM, et al. Arthroscopic versus open reconstruction of the shoulder in patients with isolated Bankart lesions. Am J Sports Med 1996;24:144.

52. Lenters TR, Franta AK, Wolf FM, et al. Arthroscopic compared with open repairs for recurrent anterior shoulder instability. A systematic review and meta-analysis of the literature. J Bone Joint Surg Am 2007;89:244.

53. Steinbeck J, Jerosch J. Arthroscopic transglenoid stabilization versus open anchor suturing in traumatic anterior instability of the shoulder. Am J Sports Med 1998;26:373.

54. Brophy RH, Marx RG. The treatment of traumatic anterior instability of the shoulder: nonoperative and surgical treatment. Arthroscopy 2009;25:298.

55. Karlsson J, Magnusson L, Ejerhed L, et al. Comparison of open and arthroscopic stabilization for recurrent shoulder dislocation in patients with a Bankart lesion. Am J Sports Med 2001;29:538.

56. Hiemstra LA, Sasyniuk TM, Mohtadi NG, et al. Shoulder strength after open versus arthroscopic stabilization. Am J Sports Med 2008;36:861.

57. Mohtadi NG, Bitar IJ, Sasyniuk TM, et al. Arthroscopic versus open repair for traumatic anterior shoulder instability: a meta-analysis. Arthroscopy 2005;21:652.

58. Pulavarti RS, Symes TH, Rangan A. Surgical interventions for anterior shoulder instability in adults. Cochrane Database Syst Rev 2009;4:CD005077.

Index

Note: Page numbers of article titles are in **boldface** type.

A

Allograft reconstruction, in humeral head bone defect management, 421

Anterior and posterior load and shift test, in glenohumeral instability evaluation, 291–292

Anterior drawer test, in glenohumeral instability evaluation, 289–290

Anterior labroligamentous periosteal sleeve avulsion, 301–303

Anterior release and surprise test, in glenohumeral instability evaluation, 294

Anterior shoulder instability
anatomy of, 325–326
arthroscopic management of, **325–337**
anchors in, 334–335
capsular plication in, 335
guidelines in, 332–335
indications for, 332
labrum preparation in, 334
patient setup in, 333
portals in, 333–334
rehabilitation after, 335
evaluation of
glenoid and humeral head bone loss assessment in, 328–331
patient history in, 327
physical examination in, 327–328
radiographic examination in, 328
nonoperative management of, 331
pathology associated with, 331

Apprehension test, in glenohumeral instability evaluation, 293

Apprehension-relocation test, in glenohumeral instability evaluation, 294

Arthroscopic Latarjet procedure, **393–405**
clinical results of, 402–403
coracoid fixation in, 401–402
coracoid graft harvesting in, 399
coracoid soft tissue preparation in, 398–399
coracoid transfer in, 400–401
described, 393
exposure creation in, 398–399
for bony defects, 394–395
for complex soft tissue injuries, 394
free bone graft vs., 396–397
H portal defining in, 399–400
indications for, 394–396
introduction into surgical practice, 397–402
joint evaluation in, 398–399
modified Bristow procedure vs., 396
need for, 393–394
open procedure vs., 397
patient activity and, 396
postoperative management, 402
rotator interval opening in, 398
stability restored by, methods of, 396
subscapularis exposure in, 398
subscapularis split in, 399

Arthroscopy
in anterior shoulder instability management, **325–337**. See also Anterior shoulder instability, arthroscopic management of.
in posterior shoulder instability management, **339–356**. See also Posterior shoulder instability, arthroscopic management of.
in throwing shoulder evaluation, 314–315

B

Bankart lesion, 301
bony, glenoid bone loss and, 303

Bankart revision
arthroscopic, in recurrent shoulder instability management, 373–374
open, in recurrent shoulder instability management, 374

Bankart-Bristow-Latarjet 2B3 procedure, 388–391
bone block harvest in, 389
bone block positioning and fixation in, 389–391
described, 388
discussion of, 388–391
patient positioning for, 388
portal placement in, 388–389
subscapularis split in, 389

Biceps tendon, normal anatomy of, 300

Bone defects, of humeral head, **417–425**. See also Humeral head bone defects.

Bone graft, free, arthroscopic Latarjet procedure vs., 396–397

Bone loss
glenoid
arthroscopic Latarjet procedure for, 394–395
bony Bankart and, 303
humeral, arthroscopic Latarjet procedure for, 395

Bony defects, arthroscopic Latarjet procedure for, 394–395

Bristow-Latarjet coracoid transfer, **381–388**

Orthop Clin N Am 41 (2010) 437–440
doi:10.1016/S0030-5898(10)00039-8

orthopedic.theclinics.com

Bristow-Latarjet (*continued*)
  background of, 381–382
  described, 381
  postoperative care, 386–388
  surgical technique, 382–386
    axillary nerve identification and subscapularis splitting, 385
    capsulolabral repair, 386
    coracoid harvesting, 383–385
    coracoid transfer and fixation, 385–386
    glenoid preparation and drilling, 382–383
Buford complex, anatomic variants of, 300–301

C

Capsular plication, in arthroscopic management of MDI, 360
Capsulorrhaphy, thermal, in arthroscopic management of MDI, 360
Complete resurfacing/hemiarthroplasty, in humeral head bone defect management, 423
Complete tears, throwing shoulder–related, management of, 319–320
Coracohumeral ligament, normal anatomy of, 298–299

F

Free bone graft, arthroscopic Latarjet procedure vs., 396–397

G

Gagey hyperabduction test, in glenohumeral instability evaluation, 292
GLAD lesions. See *Glenolabral articular disruption (GLAD) lesions.*
Glenohumeral instability
  classification of, 287
  evaluation of, **287–295**
    anterior release and surprise test in, 294
    apprehension test in, 293
    apprehension-relocation test in, 294
    imaging in, 288–289
    instability tests in, 293–294
    laxity testing in, 289–293
      anterior and posterior load and shift test, 291–292
      anterior drawer test, 289–290
      Gagey hyperabduction test, 292
      humeral translation grading, 293
      posterior drawer test, 290
      sulcus sign, 292–293
    patient history in, 288
    physical examination in, 289
  normal glenohumeral laxity vs., 287–288
Glenohumeral joint
  described, 287
  stability of, pathoanatomy of, 367–368

Glenohumeral ligaments, humeral avulsion of, 303–304
Glenoid, bony reconstruction of, 407–408. See also *Glenoid bone defects, open Latarjet with congruent arc modification for.*
Glenoid bone defects, open Latarjet with congruent arc modification for, **407–415**
  complications of, 414–415
  described, 407–408
  patient selection for, 408
  postoperative rehabilitation, 413
  results of, 413–414
  salvage surgery, 415
  technique, 408–413
Glenoid bone loss
  arthroscopic Latarjet procedure for, 394–395
  bony Bankart and, 303
Glenolabral articular disruption (GLAD) lesions, 305

H

Hill-Sachs lesion, humeral bone loss and, 303
Humeral bone loss
  arthroscopic Latarjet procedure for, 395
  Hill-Sachs lesion and, 303
Humeral head bone defects, **417–425**
  anatomy related to, 418
  classification of, 419
  described, 417
  epidemiology of, 417–418
  imaging of, 418
  surgical treatment of
    allograft reconstruction in, 421
    complete resurfacing/hemiarthroplasty in, 423
    humeralplasty/disimpaction in, 419–420
    indications for, 419
    options in, 419–423
    partial resurfacing in, 422–423
    remplissage in, 420–421
    rotational osteotomy in, 421–422
Humeral translation grading, in glenohumeral instability evaluation, 293
Humeralplasty/disimpaction, in humeral head bone defect management, 419–420

I

Inferior glenohumeral ligament complex, normal anatomy of, 299
Instability. See also specific types.
  multidirectional. See *Multidirectional instability (MDI).*
Internal impingement theory, in throwing shoulder injury, 311
Intratendinous tear, management of, 319

L

Labrum
    normal anatomy of, 297–298
    superior, anterior and posterior lesions of, 304
        management of, 315–318
Latarjet procedure, arthroscopic, **393–405.** See also
    Arthroscopic Latarjet procedure.
Lesion(s), pathologic, of shoulder, 301–305. See also
    specific lesions and *Shoulder(s), pathologic
    lesions of.*

M

MDI. See *Multidirectional instability (MDI).*
Middle glenohumeral ligament
    anatomic variants of, 301
    normal anatomy of, 299
Modified Bristow procedure, arthroscopic Latarjet
    procedure vs., 396
Multidirectional instability (MDI), of shoulder
    anatomic considerations in, 357–358
    arthroscopic management of, **357–365**
        author's preferred technique in, 360–363
        capsular plication in, 360
        thermal capsulorrhaphy in, 360
        transglenoid technique in, 359–360
    described, 357
    diagnosis of, 358–359
    nonoperative management of, 359
    open inferior shift for, 359

N

Near complete tears, throwing shoulder–related,
    management of, 319–320
Normal glenohumeral laxity, 287
    pathologic instability vs., 287–288

O

Open capsular shift, **427–436**
    described, 429–430
    indications for, 428–429
    rationale for, 427
    rehabilitation after, 431–432
    results of, 432–434
    technique, 430–431
Open Latarjet with congruent arc modification, for
    glenoid bone defects, **407–415.** See also *Glenoid
    bone defects, open Latarjet with congruent arc
    modification for.*
Open shoulder stabilization, **427–436.** See also *Open
    capsular shift.*
Osteotomy, rotational, in humeral head bone defect
    management, 421–422
Overhead athlete. See also *Throwing shoulder.*
    evaluation of, 312–313

        imaging studies in, 313
        patient history in, 312
        physical examination in, 312–313

P

Partial articular-sided supraspinatus tendon avulsion
    lesions, management of, 318–319
Partial resurfacing, in humeral head bone defect
    management, 422–423
Posterior capsular contracture, operative
    management of, 315
Posterior capsular contracture theory, in throwing
    shoulder injury, 311
Posterior drawer test, in glenohumeral instability
    evaluation, 290
Posterior shoulder instability
    arthroscopic management of, **339–356**
        capsular plication in, 350–351
            isolated, 351
        clinical results of, 352–353
        diagnostic, 347–348
        examination under anesthesia in, 347
        labral repair in, 348–350
            capsular plication with, 350–351
            posterior capsular release with, 351
            preparation of, 348
        portal creation in, 347–348
        postoperative rehabilitation, 352
        rotator interval closure in, 351–352
        setup for, 347
    described, 339–340
    evaluation of
        imaging studies in, 344–346
        patient history in, 342–344
        physical examination of, 342–344
    nonoperative management of, 346
    pathoanatomy of, 340–342
    surgical management of, 346–347

R

Radiography, in anterior shoulder instability
    evaluation, 328
Rehabilitation
    after arthroscopic management of anterior
        shoulder instability, 335
    after arthroscopic management of posterior
        shoulder instability, 352
    after open capsular shift, 431–432
    after open Latarjet with congruent arc
        modification for glenoid bone defects, 413
    in throwing shoulder injury management, 318
    postoperative, after throwing shoulder injury
        management, 320
Remplissage, in humeral head bone defect
    management, 420–421

Rotational osteotomy, in humeral head bone defect management, 421–422
Rotator cuff
    injuries to, repair of, 319
    normal anatomy of, 299–300
Rotator interval, normal anatomy of, 298–299

S

Scapulothoracic function theory, in throwing shoulder injury, 311–312
Shoulder(s), **297–308**
    anterior instability of, arthroscopic management of, **325–337.** See also *Anterior shoulder instability, arthroscopic management of.*
    conditions in athletes, management of, 313–320. See also *Throwing shoulder, management of.*
    MDI of, arthroscopic management of, **357–365.** See also *Multidirectional instability (MDI), of shoulder, arthroscopic management of.*
    normal anatomy of, 297–300
        biceps tendon, 300
        coracohumeral ligament, 298–299
        inferior glenohumeral ligament complex, 299
        labrum, 297–298
        middle glenohumeral ligament, 299
        rotator cuff, 299–300
        rotator interval, 298–299
        superior glenohumeral ligament, 298–299
        variants of, 300–301
    pathologic lesions of, 301–305
        anterior labroligamentous periosteal sleeve avulsion, 301–303
        Bankart lesion, 301
            bony, glenoid bone loss and, 303
        GLAD lesions, 305
        Hill-Sachs lesion, humeral bone loss and, 303
        humeral avulsion of glenohumeral ligaments, 303–304
        of superior labrum, anterior and posterior lesions, 304
    posterior instability of, arthroscopic management of, **339–356.** See also *Posterior shoulder instability, arthroscopic management of.*
    throwing. See *Throwing shoulder.*
Shoulder instability. See also specific types and *Shoulder(s).*

osteoarticular pathology and, 374–376
recurrent, management of, 371–373
    arthroscopic Bankart revision in, 373–374
    arthroscopic Latarjet procedure in, 396
    open Bankart revision in, 374
    surgical, 373
surgical management of, failed
    clinical evaluation of, 368–371
        imaging studies in, 369–371
        patient history in, 369
        physical examination in, 369
    management of, **367–379**
Soft tissue injuries, complex, arthroscopic Latarjet procedure for, 394
Sublabral foramen, anatomic variants of, 300–301
Sulcus sign, in glenohumeral instability evaluation, 292–293
Superior glenohumeral ligament, normal anatomy of, 298–299
Superior labrum
    anatomic variants of, 301
    anterior and posterior lesions of, 304
        management of, 315–318

T

Thermal capsulorrhaphy, in arthroscopic management of MDI, 360
Throwing shoulder. See also *Overhead athlete.*
    asymptomatic adaptation, 310–312
    described, 309–310
    injuries to
        management of, **309–323.** See also specific injuries.
            arthroscopic evaluation in, 314–315
            examination under anesthesia in, 314–315
            nonoperative, 313–314
            operative, 315–320
            postoperative rehabilitation, 320
            rehabilitation in, 318
    overall motion of, 310
    patient evaluation, 312–313
        under anesthesia, 314–315
    patterns, 310–312
        internal impingement theory, 311
        posterior capsular contracture theory, 311
        scapulothoracic function theory, 311–312

.

Printed and bound by CPI Group (UK) Ltd, Croydon, CR0 4YY

12/10/2024

01773394-0001